Cancer Biomarkers in Body Fluids

Gabriel D. Dakubo

Cancer Biomarkers in Body Fluids

Biomarkers in Proximal Fluids

Springer

Gabriel D. Dakubo
Medical Sciences Division
Northern Ontario School of Medicine
Thunder Bay, ON, Canada

ISBN 978-3-030-24723-2 ISBN 978-3-030-24725-6 (eBook)
https://doi.org/10.1007/978-3-030-24725-6

This Springer imprint is published by the registered company Springer Nature Switzerland AG.
The registered company address is: Gewerbestrasse 11, 6330 Cham, Switzerland

To all who have survived or living with this disease
In memory of those passed from this disease

Blurb

The ability to measure and monitor cancer biomarkers in "body fluid biopsy" should greatly impact oncologic practice. *Biomarkers in Proximal Fluids*, the third of the Cancer Biomarkers in Body Fluids series, details cancer signatures in none or minimally circulating body fluids including saliva, sputum, bronchoalveolar lavage fluid, exhaled breath condensate, nipple aspirate fluid, gastric and pancreatic juice, stool, urine, and prostatic, peritoneal, and cerebrospinal fluid. These fluids are enriched with biomarkers, especially those emanating from cells of the proximal tissue.

Chapter 1 examines the global burden of cancer and the need for regional efforts at primary prevention, early detection, and patient care. Chapters 2, 3, 4, 5, 6, 7, 8, 9, 10, 11 and 12 address tissue-specific biomarkers in associated body fluids. The tumor interstitial fluid as a microenvironment rich in cancer biomarkers is detailed in Chap. 13, while Chap. 14 looks at the human body fluid microbiome and its evolving role in cancer. Commercially available assays using proximal fluids are examined at the end of the respective chapters. This book complements its predecessors and is equally useful to oncologists, cancer researchers, clinicians, medical students, nurses, diagnostic laboratory, and pharmaceutical industry personnel.

Preface

The future of cancer research and practice of oncology yearns for, and is currently reaping, the benefits of noninvasive or minimally invasive technologies of "body fluid biopsy" for cancer biomarker applications. While this feat is being realized, the discipline is still being vehemently pursued to discover the best biomarkers and applicable technologies that will offer the best care for the patient. Cancer biomarkers in body fluids, the adage of "body fluid biopsy," are convenient and acceptable not only for cancer screening, but also for management of patients, especially those unsuitable for serial invasive tissue biopsy sampling. A major limitation of tissue biopsy is not just the level of discomfort, but also its lack of complete representation of tumor heterogeneity. Thus, biomarkers in body fluids provide holistic evaluation of cancer and yet fit into routine clinical practice of oncology.

Cancer "Biomarkers in Proximal Fluids" examines two main categories of body fluids used in biomarker discovery and clinical applications. Both categories of proximal fluids are not only enriched with biomarkers from the cancer of the proximal tissues but also obviate the dilution effect and complexity of fluids, such as blood, in biomarker discovery. The first category of proximal fluids includes fluids such as saliva (for oral cancer), sputum and exhaled breath condensate (for lung cancer), nipple aspirate fluid (for breast cancer), stool (for colorectal cancer), and urine (for urinary bladder cancer) that offer biomarker targets for screening and risk assessment. The second proximal fluids, such as cerebrospinal fluid (for brain cancer), gastric and pancreatic juices (for gastric and pancreatic cancers, respectively), bile (for hepatobiliary tract cancer), pleural fluid (for lung cancer), and ovarian ascites (for ovarian cancer), are acquired in a more invasive fashion and hence serve as media for easy biomarker discovery and subsequent leveraging in noninvasively acquired proximal fluids such as in category one. The research relevance of exploring for biomarkers in tumor interstitial fluids and the emerging importance of human body fluid microbiome deserve special attention that has been fully addressed.

The fact is "science is a stationary truth that requires constant refinements." As technologies improve and new biomarkers are discovered, the landscape of proximal fluid cancer biomarkers will change for the better. Patience is what is needed as the science and commercialization processes are being advanced.

I am grateful to my project managers and coordinators, Ursula Gramm, Martina Himberger, Karthik Periyasamy, and Balaji Padmanaban for their patience and understanding throughout the publication process. To my family, I thank you once again for the lost time.

Thunder Bay, ON, Canada
April 2019

Gabriel D. Dakubo

Contents

About the Author

Gabriel D. Dakubo is an expert in Molecular Medicine and faculty in the Division of Medical Sciences at the Northern Ontario School of Medicine. He received his BSc and MBChB degrees from the University of Ghana, followed by a Postdoctoral Research Fellowship in Molecular Medicine at the Ottawa Hospital Research Institute, Canada. His passion is in noninvasive deployment of biomarkers for cancer management. While an expert in mitochondrial genetic alterations in cancer, he also has a keen interest in the inter-genomic communications that occur in the cancer cell, as well as the Slaughter's concept of field cancerization. He is well published and is a reviewer of a number of esteemed journals.

Chapter 1
Global Burden of Cancer and the Call to Action

1.1 Introduction

The 2018 GLOBOCAN figures indicate a rise in the global cancer statistics to 18.1 million new cases or 17.0 (excluding non-melanoma skin cancer – NMSC) and 9.6 million deaths or 9.5 million (excluding NMSC), while 43,841,302 people were living with the disease. The global regional distributions of new cases were Asia (8,751,000 or age-standardized ratio (ASR) of 164.5), Europe (4,230,000 or ASR of 281.5), North America (2,379,000 or ASR of 350.2), Latin America and the Caribbean (1,413,000 or ASR of 189.6), Africa (1,055,000 or ASR of 129.7), and Oceania (252,000 or ASR of 418.8). The corresponding mortalities were Asia (5,477,000 or ASR of 101.3), Europe (1,944,000 or ASR of 111.3), North America (698,000 or ASR of 91.2), Latin America and the Caribbean (673,000 or ASR of 86.5), Africa (694,000 or ASR of 89.5), and Oceania (69,974 or ASR of 99.3) (Figs. 1.1 and 1.2). The top five most commonly diagnosed cancer types were lung cancer (2.094 million or 11.6% of all cases), breast cancer (2.089 million or 11.6%), colorectal cancer (1.8 million or 6.1%), prostate cancer (1.3 million or 7.1%), and gastric cancer (1.0 million or 5.7%). The top five cancers that caused the most deaths were lung cancer (1.8 million or 18.4% of all deaths), colorectal cancer (881,000 or 9.2%), gastric cancer (783,000 or 8.2%), liver cancer (482,000 or 8.2%), and breast cancer (627,000 or 6.6%).

With both sexes combined, the cumulative risk for developing cancer was 20.2% and for dying from it was 10.6% by age 75 years. Approximately one in five men and one in six women will develop cancer, and one in eight men and one in ten women will die from the disease [1]. These ominous statistical estimates need to be curtailed, and regional variations and attributable risk factors are ought to be fully identified and understood by regional or sectorial authorities. Due to the obviously high population size and possibly multiple risk factors, including infectious causes of cancer, nearly half (48.4 million) of all new cases and over half (57.3 million) of cancer mortality will occur in the Asian continent alone. Though it represents

G. D. Dakubo, *Cancer Biomarkers in Body Fluids*,
https://doi.org/10.1007/978-3-030-24725-6_1

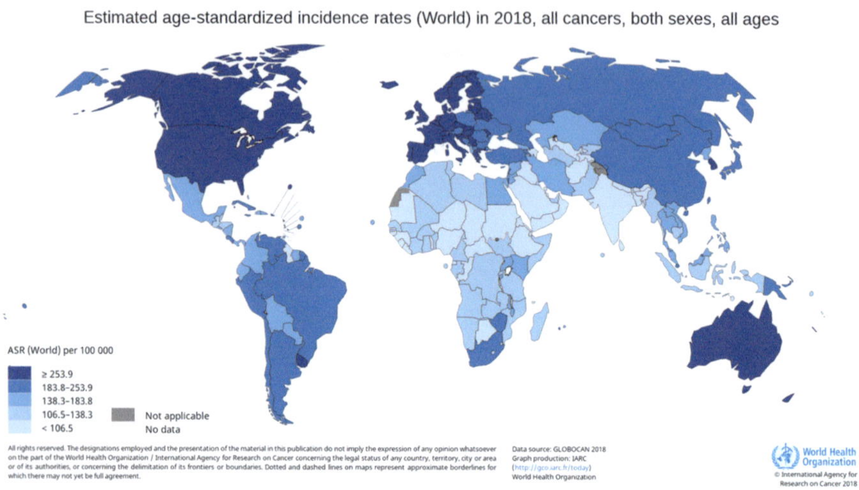

Fig. 1.1 Global age-standardized incident rates for all cancers

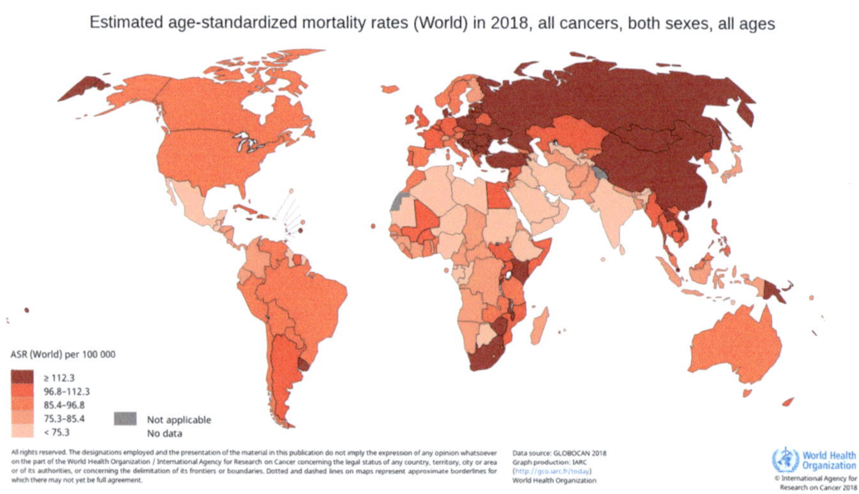

Fig. 1.2 Global age-standardized mortality rates for all cancers

only 9% of the global population, Europe is second according to the dismal statistics of cancer with an estimated incidence of 23.5% and mortality of 20.3%. Third come the Americas with incidence and mortality of 21.0% and 14.4%, respectively. This disturbing trend and the factors responsible will be discussed later. A critical look at these GLOBOCAN statistics reveals a disturbing pattern for Asia and Africa whereby mortality rates outstrip the incident rates. For instance, in China, the incident rate was 48.6% compared to a mortality figure of 57.3%. Similarly in Africa, an incident rate of 5.8% was a little lower than the mortality rate of 7.3%. The disparity may reflect levels of regional socioeconomic development, which may be due to technological differences in cancer detection and management. The involved authorities must identify factors related to the types of cancers, as well as regional and sex distribution patterns among others so that appropriate preventive measures can be implemented. For both sexes, common cancers that increased morbidity included lung, breast, colorectal, prostate, stomach, and liver cancer. Lung cancer, with incidence and mortality of 11.6% and 18.4%, respectively (note the mortality is greater that the incidence), has been the worse. This incident rate is identical to breast cancer (11.6%) followed by colorectal cancer (10.2%). For mortality data, lung cancer remains number one, while colorectal cancer comes second with 9.25%, followed by stomach with 8.2% and liver with 8.2% of all cancers. The sex distribution pattern is similar. For example, lung cancer remains the most diagnosed cancer and the leading cause of mortality in men. Prostate and colorectal cancers lead in incidence, while liver and stomach cancer lead in mortality among this sex. Unlike males, female breast cancer remains the most diagnosed and the leading cause of cancer-related death. For incidence, colorectal cancer is second, lung cancer is third, and cervical cancer comes fourth in women. The geographic and sex distribution patterns reflect causative factors that are identifiable for prevention, early detection, and targeted care.

1.2 Global Distribution Patterns of the Leading Cancers

The most commonly diagnosed cancer and leading cause of cancer-related deaths have been described above. As expected, there will be global diversity consistent with their distribution in incidence, mortality, and quality of care from resource availability and leadership. Ten and nine leading cancers mediate most of the incidence and mortality in men, respectively, while six types of cancer are mostly responsible for cancer-related mortality in women. In many geographical regions, prostate cancer is the most commonly detected cancer followed by lung cancer in 37 countries and liver cancer in 13 countries. There are also cancer clusters, some of which may be due to environmental exposures and/or genetic predisposition (e.g., Kaposi sarcoma in Eastern Africa, Burkitt lymphoma in West Africa, and lip and oral cancer in Southern Asia). For most part, the distribution pattern is heterogeneous. Globally, lung cancer (93 countries), prostate cancer (46 countries), and liver cancer (20 countries) are the most common causes of cancer morbidity. In the female population, breast cancer ranked as number one in 154 countries, while cervical cancer was most commonly diagnosed in 28 of the remaining 32 countries. Breast cancer (103 countries), cervical cancer (28 countries), and surprisingly lung cancer (28 countries) were the leading cause of cancer-related deaths worldwide in women.

1.3 Global Cancer Incidence and Distribution According to the Four-Tier Human Development Index

Based on the importance of national policies besides economic growth, the United Nations Development Program (UNDP) has divided the world into four-tier human development indices, namely, low, medium, high, and very high Human Development Index (HDI) (UNDP-HDI; Box 1.1). Cancer incidences and mortality patterns have also been illustrated according to the UNDP-HDI regional definition. Expectedly, due to the myriads of negative factors, cancer incident rates for 2018 were estimated at two- to three-fold higher in the low-to-medium- than the high-to-very high-HDI countries. Mortality patterns were also similar with higher case fatalities in the lower than higher-HDI countries. This calls for immediate action to equalize global health, which in turn will help solve many of the issues facing the world including emigration/immigration. Neglect is not an option or a solution. Despite enormous disparities in incidence between low-to-medium- and high-to-very high-HDI countries, lung cancer ranked first, while prostate cancer ranked second in mortality in both HDI countries. Second in mortality was colorectal cancer for the high-to-very high-HDI countries and lip and oral cavity cancers in the low-to-medium-HDI countries, mostly in India, which accounted for the majority of the population of low-to-medium-HDI countries. Incidence of breast cancer in women was high in both dichotomized HDI countries, while colorectal cancer was higher in high-to-very high- than low-to-medium-HDI countries, and the reverse was true for cervical cancer. Once again actions need to be taken to bridge the gap between these cancer incident disparities in the world.

Box 1.1 UNDP-HDI

- The UNDP developed a statistical composite index as a measure of life expectancy, education, and per capita income as indicators for how countries are fairing. This index is referred to as the HDI.
- Countries are grouped into four tiers based on their ranking as low-, medium-, high-, and very high-HDI countries.
- A high score indicates high life expectancy, high educational levels, high per capita GDP, and thus the potential for human growth and development.
- The 2018 top five HDI countries were Norway (HDI of 0.953), Switzerland (HDI of 0.944), Australia (HDI of 0.939), Iceland (HDI of 0.938), and Germany (HDI of 0.936). Canada ranked 12th (HDI of 0.926), the USA ranked 13th (HDI of 0.924), and the UK ranked 14th (HDI of 0.922).

1.4 Incidence and Mortality Rates of the Different Types of Cancer According to Global Locations

Cancer disparities exist across the world. Age-standardized rate (ASR) of cancer incidences in 2018 at 218 per 100,000 in men was much higher than the 182 per 100,000 in women. The variability across regions was eminent with a sixfold variance in men with 571.2/100,000 in Australia/New Zealand to 95.6/100,000 in West Africa. The variation in incidence among females was much less at fourfold, with the highest incidence again in Australia/New Zealand at 362/100,000 to 96.2/100,000 in South Central Asia. More males (about 50%) were estimated to die from cancer than women in 2018. Again, among males, there were regional variations with rates ranging from 171.0/100,000 in Eastern Europe to 67.4/100,000 in Central America. Another notable disparity was the 120.7/100,000 estimated deaths in Melanesia compared to 67.4/100,000 in Central American and Eastern Asia (except China). In women, the rates varied from 11.4% in East Africa to the estimated risk of 9.1% in Northern Europe, 8.6% in North America, and 8.1% in Australia/New Zealand. For the next sections, the global burden for a select number of cancers will be described.

1.4.1 Non-melanoma Skin Cancer

One of the frequently diagnosed cancers in North America and Australia/New Zealand is non-melanoma skin cancer (NMSC). With an estimated over a million cases to be diagnosed in 2018, and 65,000 deaths in the same year, NMSC deserves some attention. Incident rates are two times higher in men than women. Precautionary measures including the use of effective sunscreens and clothing should help reduce the incident rates, especially in endemic areas such as Australia/New Zealand.

1.4.2 Lung Cancer

Lung cancer remains the commonest and deadliest cancer globally. For 2018, 2.1 million new cases and 1.8 million deaths were expected, which represents 18.4% of all diagnosed cancers. The incidence of lung cancer was highest among men in Micronesia/Polynesia and Eastern Asia where rates were as high as 40/100,000. China, Japan, and the Republic of Korea, as well as much of Europe, especially Eastern Europe, also harbored high incidences with rates as high as 77.4/100,000. The lowest incidence remains in Africa, though there is no need for complacency because rates are cropping up to as high as 28.2/100,000 to 31.9/100,000 in Morocco among men in 2018. Analysis of incident trend in recent years uncovered a decreasing rate among men aged 35–64 years in Eastern Europe but was still on the rise in Bulgaria [2]. A disturbing trend also exists in some parts of the developing world. For example, in several African countries, lung cancer rates are increasing for the next decades. In India, lung cancer risk from cigarette smoke was similar to bidi smoke. In China and Indonesia, smoking among women has either peaked or continues to climb [3].

Lung cancer in women is still of a lesser concern than in men, though regional variations exist that require some attention. Despite this positive observation, many countries continue to observe an increasing trend in the female population [2, 4]. However, women in the USA and UK of a certain cohort have shown signs of a peak and decline, which is encouraging. In US whites, lung cancer incidence among young women are now much higher than men, and this trend is evidenced in non-Hispanic whites and Hispanics [4]. Among 28 countries, lung cancer was the leading cause of death among women, with the highest rates observed in North America, Northern and Western Europe (especially Denmark and the Netherlands), as well as Australia/New Zealand. At the pinnacle of these lung cancer deaths among women was Hungary.

1.4.3 *Breast Cancer*

In many countries (154 of 185 countries), breast cancer is the most commonly diagnosed female cancer. Globally, an estimated 2.1 million cases were diagnosed in 2018. It is also the primary cause of death among women in over 100 countries, except Australia/New Zealand, Northern Europe, North America, and many sub-Saharan African countries. Incident rates vary considerably, and the highest are in countries such as Australia/New Zealand, the UK, Sweden, Finland, Denmark, the Netherlands, France, and Italy and countries in North America. Belgium has the highest global rate. Mortality though is less variable across countries, but the highest death rates were in Melanesia, where Fiji topped the list globally. Incident rates for breast cancer have been rising for many low-to-medium-HDI countries over the past decades. Such regions include Africa, Asia, and South America [5]. A fall in incidence was observed in the USA, Canada, the UK, France, and Australia partly due to the decline in the use of postmenopausal hormone replacement therapy that has been linked to increased breast cancer risk [6, 7].

1.4.4 *Esophageal Cancer*

There were an estimated 472,000 new and 509,000 deaths from esophageal cancer in 2018. Note the incidence closely matches the mortality figure. Esophageal cancer was responsible for 1 in every 20 cancer-related deaths in 2018. It is more common in men who account for about 70% of all cases. It is twofold higher in high-HDI countries among men. The incidence of esophageal cancer is seventh globally (in both sexes), but mortality decreases to fifth in high-HDI countries.

The commonest cases of esophageal cancer were found in many Eastern and Southern African countries. It was the leading cause of cancer mortality in Kenyan men, and Malawi harbored the highest incidence globally in both men and women. Men in Eastern African region ranked 5th globally in incidence. Some of the highest rates were observed in Eastern Asian men, with Mongolia and China being among the top five globally.

There are two types of esophageal cancer with different risk factors, geographic distribution, and pathologies: esophageal squamous cell carcinoma (ESCC) and esophageal adenocarcinoma (EAC). In general, ESCC is common in low-to-medium-HDI countries, while EAC occurs more commonly in high-to-very high-HDI countries. Smoking and heavy alcohol drinking are established risk factors for ESCC in the Western world. However, in sub-Saharan Africa and Asia, where over 90% of all cases occur, the risk factors are not well understood. Betel quid chewing in India and very hot mate drinking in South America are other postulated risk factors for ESCC. Gastroesophageal reflux disease (GERD) and obesity that predisposes to GERD are identified risk factors for EAC. Noteworthy, the incidence of ESCC is declining, while EAC is on the rise, partly due to increased obesity epidemic, GERD, and decreasing *Helicobacter pylori* (*H. pylori*) infections [8].

1.4.5 Gastric Cancer

Globally, gastric cancer is of a significant impact on society. In 2018, over 1 million new cases and 783,000 deaths were estimated to occur, reflecting a 1 in every 12 deaths from the disease. It is the fifth most diagnosed and third leading cause of cancer-related deaths. The prevalence is twofold more in men than women and among men is the most commonly diagnosed cancer and the leading cause of cancer-related deaths in Western Asian countries such as Kyrgyzstan, Iran, and Turkmenistan. The incident rates are also markedly increased in Eastern Asian countries such as Japan, Mongolia, and the Republic of Korea that has the highest global incident rates in both sexes. The rates in Africa, North America, and Northern Europe are low. Multiple environmental factors are implicated as risk factors of gastric cancer. Food preserved in salt, alcohol abuse, and tobacco smoking, as well as low fruit intake, are known risk factors for developing gastric cancer. A bacterium strongly implicated in about 90% of non-cardia gastric cancer is *H. pylori* infection. Cancers from the cardia and pyloric regions of the stomach are quite different from cancers from the body of the stomach. Incidence of distal non-cardia gastric cancers (near the pylorus) has been decreasing, being attributable to decreasing *H. pylori* infection and improved food preservation. Cancers of the gastric cardia are similar to EAC in etiology and pathology.

1.4.6 Colorectal Cancer

Colorectal cancer remains a disease of importance despite considerable improvements in uncovering its molecular genetics. For instance, over 1.8 million new cases and 881,000 deaths were estimated for 2018, which accounted for 1 in 10 cancer cases and deaths. While third in incidence, colorectal cancer is the second cause of cancer-related deaths. The rates are higher (threefold) in high-to-very high- than low-to-medium-HDI countries. For global distribution, the highest colorectal cancer incidences were found in Hungary, Slovakia, the Netherlands, Norway, Australia/New Zealand, North America, Japan, the Republic of Korea, and Singapore. Hungary and Norway ranked first among males and females, respectively. Uruguay also harbored high rates in both sexes. Rectal cancer incidences were highest in the Republic of Korean males and in female Macedonians. In Africa and Southern Asia, colorectal cancer incidences were low compared to other regions of the world.

Colorectal cancer distribution varies six to eightfold across the world, which may reflect socioeconomic advancements because the levels tend to rise with increasing HDI. Indeed, Arnold et al. uncovered three regional variations in colorectal cancer associated with socioeconomic development: (i) the Baltic countries, China, Russia, and Brazil with increasing colorectal cancer incidence and mortality; (ii) Denmark, Canada, the UK, and Singapore with increasing incidence but reduced mortality; and (iii) the USA, France, and Japan that have both decreasing incidence and mortality [9]. Efforts of these latter countries need to be emulated by all. While mortality remains high in low-to-medium-HDI countries, it is declining in the high-to-very high-HDI countries partly due to adoption of best practices in cancer detection and management such as practiced by the "Cancer Treatment Centers of America" that uses state-of-the-art team and personalized approach to cancer care.

Risk factors for colorectal cancer include dietary factors, obesity, genetics, and other lifestyle factors. There are established evidence that processed meat, alcoholic drinks, and increased body fat all elevate the risk for developing colorectal cancer. On the contrary, physical activity protects against this cancer.

1.4.7 Liver Cancer

Cancer of the liver has been a problem in some regions of the world and, despite its deleterious effects in the past, could be curtailed in the future due to effective public health measures. Liver cancer that comprises 75–85% hepatocellular carcinoma (HCC) and 10–15% cholangiocarcinoma and other very rare subtypes was predicted to be the sixth most commonly diagnosed cancer and the fourth cause of cancer-related death globally in 2018. The incident rates are more common (two to three times) in men than women globally. It ranked fifth in case incidences and second in mortality among men. Similar to other cancers, the incident rate was high (twofold) in low-to-medium-HDI countries, with the highest rates being among the lowest

HDI countries. Countries most affected included Egypt, the Gambia, Guinea, Mongolia, Cambodia, and Vietnam. The rates in Cambodia astonishingly far exceeded any other country. The estimated 2018 Mongolian cases were four times higher than among men in China and the Republic of Korea.

The primary risk factors for HCC are chronic hepatitis B virus (HBV) or hepatitis C virus (HCV) infections or coinfections, consumption of aflatoxin-containing food, heavy alcohol intake, smoking, obesity, and type II diabetes. There are regional variations in these risk factors. For example, in the high-risk zones, namely, East Africa and China, chronic HBV infections and aflatoxin consumption are the main key risk factors, whereas in countries such as Egypt and Japan, HCV infections are the predominant causes. HBV and HCV infections as well as coinfections of HBV carriers with hepatitis delta agent, as well as alcohol abuse, are major contributors to HCC in Mongolia [10]. In low-risk areas, the rising obesity crises are being blamed for the increasing rise in HCC [11]. The introduction of HBV vaccine in the early 1980s should help curtail the incidence of HCC in the future. It has been recommended by the WHO to be included in routine infant vaccination, and by 2016, 186 countries had adopted this practice, with greater than 80% coverage for complete doses. It has helped decrease the incidence of HCC especially in the high-risk countries. There is no vaccine for HCV, but the use of safe transfusion practices and clean needles should help reduce the rate of transmission.

1.4.8 *Pancreatic Cancer*

Pancreatic cancer is the seventh leading cause of cancer deaths in both males and females. Rates are three- to fourfold higher in high-HDI countries. Incident rates are highest in Europe, North America, and Australia/New Zealand. Pancreatic cancer is a disease that requires identification of authentic and validated early detection biomarkers to enable detection when it is curable, because of its poor prognosis. The number of new cases in 2018 (459,000) matches the mortality rate (432,000), and this is associated with low disease prevalence. A disease with such poor prognosis requires due attention and efforts to discover noninvasive biomarkers for its early detection and timely curtailment.

1.4.9 *Urothelial Bladder Cancer*

With an estimated incidence and mortality of 549,000 and 200,000, respectively, urothelial bladder cancer ranked tenth among cancers globally in incidence. In general, it is more common in men than women probably due to occupational exposures. Among the male population, it was the sixth most common and the ninth leading cause of cancer-related death. The incident and mortality rates were 9.6 and 3.2 per 100,000 in men, respectively. Incident rates are highest in men globally, with

Spain, Greece, Italy, Belgium, the Netherlands, and North America being among the high incident countries; however, estimates put the highest rate among Lebanese women. Cigarette smoking is the primary risk factor for bladder cancer. Additionally, exposures to various chemicals, water contaminants, and infections (e.g., schistosomiasis infection of the bladder) are risk factors. With increasing cigarette smoking among women, especially in the USA, the attributable risk for urothelial bladder cancer will approximate those of men.

1.4.10 Prostate Cancer

Prostate cancer is the most commonly diagnosed cancer in men globally (i.e., in 105 of 185 countries). In 2018, an estimated 1.3 million new cases and 359,000 deaths were expected, making it rank as the second most diagnosed and fifth leading cause of cancer-related death. It is commonly diagnosed in North America, Northern and Western Europe, Australia/New Zealand, and several sub-Saharan African countries. Asia is the least region of prostate cancer diagnosis. It is a major cause of cancer death in sub-Saharan Africa and the Caribbean, with the highest incidence and mortality in Guadeloupe and Barbados, respectively. Prostate cancer is quite prevalent in Australia/New Zealand, Northern and Western Europe, Norway, Sweden, Ireland, and North America, especially the USA where the incidence is also high, but mortality rates are low. Elevated mortality rates of prostate cancer are found in sub-Saharan African countries of Benin, South Africa, Zambia, and Zimbabwe, as well as in the Caribbean.

Surprisingly, despite its high frequency, the etiology of prostate cancer is enshrined in mystery, making control measures difficult. Because it is very common in African-American and Caribbean men, a proposed ethnic and genetic predisposing factor has been entertained, and expectedly several linkage genes have been identified and characterized; yet none explains all the causes of the disease. Body adiposity, for example, has also been linked to advanced-stage prostate cancer.

With the advent of the prostate-specific antigen (PSA) testing in the middle of the 1980s, latent prostate cancers have been diagnosed, which otherwise will not have harmed or caused death to the individual, leading to the concept of overdiagnosis and overtreatment. The PSA test increased the incident rate of prostate cancer in several countries including the USA, Europe, several Nordic countries, Australia, and Canada. The US Preventive Services Task Force recommended against the routine use of the PSA test in 2012 but later revised this to be based on an individual decision. This action caused prostate cancer rates to decline in countries such as Finland, Denmark, and Sweden in the 2000s and stable in Norway. However, the UK, Japan, Brazil, Costa Rica, and Thailand where PSA testing continued to be widely used have seen rates on the rise. Cases also continue to rise in some sub-Saharan African countries such as Uganda and Zimbabwe. However, prostate cancer mortality has been on the decline especially in countries such as North America, Oceania, Northern and Western Europe, developed part of Asia, and the USA. These achievements have been attributed to screening for early detection of curable cancers, as well as effective treatment technologies. Unfortunately, in low-to-medium-HDI countries such as Central and Eastern Europe, Cuba, Brazil, the Philippines, Singapore, Bulgaria, and Russia, mortality has been on the rise, which may be due to late diagnosis and ineffective management.

1.4.11 Cervical Cancer

Cervical cancer is the fourth most frequently diagnosed cancer (with an estimated 570,000 new cases expected in 2018) and also the fourth leading cause of cancer-related mortality (at least 311,000 deaths were expected in 2018). In lower-HDI countries, it ranked second in incidence and mortality behind breast cancer. The vast majority of countries where it is commonly diagnosed (28 countries) and where most mortality occurs (42 countries) are in sub-Saharan Africa and Southeastern Asia. Swaziland had the highest incident rate, while Malawi and Zimbabwe harbored the highest mortality.

Twelve human papilloma viruses (HPVs) classified as group 1 carcinogen in the International Agency for Research on Cancer (IARC) monograph are necessary but not sufficient to cause cervical cancer. Other causative cofactors identified include smoking, immunosuppression, multiparity (high number of full-term pregnancies), and use of oral contraceptives.

In general, cervical cancer incidence and mortality have been declining globally over the past few decades. This is attributable in part to avoidance or reversal of some of the known risk factors. These factors include screening for early detection of curable cancers, improved socioeconomic factors, reduced HPV infection or virulent factors, improved genital hygiene, reduced parity, and reduced incidence of sexually transmitted infections, among other yet to be identified factors. Unfortunately, with all these gains, there are pockets of geographic regions where these are not being realized. For example, in areas of ineffective screening such as Eastern Europe and Central Asia (including Republic of the former Soviet Union), an increase in premature cervical cancer deaths have been reported in recent generations [12]. Similarly, in sub-Saharan Africa, a rise in cervical cancer has been reported in Zimbabwe and Uganda.

The available HPV vaccine should make a tremendous impact on cervical cancer eradication or reduced burden. Indeed, screening and vaccination should be intensified in those high-risk countries. The World Health Organization (WHO) currently recommends two doses of the vaccine to girls aged 9–13 years. In Australia/New Zealand and North America, there is a generation of women born between the 1930s and 1950s who are at elevated risk for cervical cancer because of changes to their sexual behaviors [13, 14]. Another recommendation by the WHO is the screening of women aged 30–49 years through visual inspection with acetic acid in low-resource setting, Papanicolaou cervical cytology every 3–5 years, or HPV testing every 5 years. This should enable identification of early lesions for timely intervention. In a randomized trial in India, HPV testing for the detection of precursor lesions offered greater protection against invasive cervical cancers than visual inspection with acetic acid or Papanicolaou cytology [15]. With effective implementation of the available technologies by the various health authorities, the burden of cervical cancer can be markedly reduced.

1.4.12 Thyroid Cancer

Thyroid cancer is more common in women than men. The 2018 estimated incidence of 567,000 cases worldwide placed it in the ninth position of all cancers. The global incident rate in women (10.2 per 100,000 people) was three times higher than in men. Despite these statistics, the mortality rates are low (estimated at 41,000 deaths in 2018), with ASR per 100,000 being as low as 0.4 and 0.5 for men and women, respectively. The incident rate varies little between low-to-medium- and high-to-very high-HDI countries, although mortality rates do not differ. The Republic of Korea harbors the highest rate in the world in both males and females. In high incident regions such as North America (Canada), Australia/New Zealand, and Eastern Asia, the Pacific including New Caledonia and French Polynesia, incident rates remain higher in women than men. Overdiagnosis accounts in part for the increasing incident rates of thyroid cancer due to introduction of new diagnostic techniques and technologies. For example, overdiagnosis was estimated to account for 90% of newly diagnosed women in South Korea. Similarly, 70–80% of newly diagnosed cases in the USA, Italy, France, and Australia/New Zealand were due to overdiagnosis [16].

1.5 Global Burden of Cancer in Adolescents and Young Adults

Cancers among children and adolescents and young adults aged 20–39 years deserved attention. The global incidence and mortality of cancer reported for adolescents and young adults in 2012 were 975,396 and 358,392 cases, respectively. But this cancer burden was disproportionately more common among women than men. The top ten new cases and causes of mortality are shown in Tables 1.1 and 1.2. The reported male to female ratio for incidence and mortality were 0.5 and 0.8, respectively, and the incidence and mortality ASR were 43.3 and 15.0 cases per 100,000 people per year, respectively. Also of importance was the annual burden being more common among young adults than children aged 0–19 years, which was about four times greater for new cases and about three times greater for cancer-related deaths. While disproportionately higher in young adults than children and adolescents, these figures were still lower than those among middle-aged (40–49 years) and older adults (60 years and above).

Table 1.1 The top ten new cases of cancer in adolescents and young adults in 2012

	Both sexes		Men		Women	
Cancer site	New cases	%	New cases	%	New cases	%
All cases except NMSC	358,397	100	163,954	100	194,438	100
Breast	48,774	13.6	–	–	48,774	25.1
Leukemia	36,253	10.1	20,874	12.7	15,379	7.9
Liver	36,228	10.1	28,864	17.6	7364	3.8
Cervical	27,887	7.8	–	–	27,887	14.3
Brain	20,783	5.8	12,262	7.5	8521	4.4
Colorectal	20,659	5.8	10,536	6.4	10,123	5.2
Gastric	18,365	5.1	9521	5.8	8844	4.5
NHL	17,281	4.8	10,145	6.2	7136	3.7
Lung	15,544	4.3	9388	5.7	6156	3.2
Lip and oral cavity	10,121	2.8	7686	4.7	2435	1.3

NMSC non-melanoma skin cancer, *NHL* non-Hodgkin lymphoma

Table 1.2 The top ten causes of cancer mortality in adolescents and young adults in 2012

	Both sexes		Men		Women	
Cancer site	New cases	%	New cases	%	New cases	%
All cases except NMSC	975,396	100	342,721	100	632,675	100
Breast	191,105	19.6	–	–	191,105	30.3
Cervical	110,749	11.4	–	–	110,749	17.5
Thyroid	78,568	8.1	15,681	4.6	62,887	9.9
Leukemia	49,293	5.1	28,020	8.2	21,373	3.4
Colorectal	41,117	4.2	21,055	6.1	20,062	3.2
Liver	40,720	4.2	31,767	9.3	8953	1.4
Brain	40,363	4.1	22,822	6.7	17,541	2.8
NHL	40,212	2.1	23,746	6.9	16,466	2.6
Testis	30,580	3.1	30,580	8.9	–	–
Ovary	29,262	3.0	–	–	–	–

NMSC non-melanoma skin cancer, *NHL* non-Hodgkin lymphoma

In regard to global incidence and mortality according to types of cancer, the commonest in this young adult population in several countries were brain and cervical cancers. Together their contribution to cancer incidence and mortality were 301,854 (30.9%) and 76,661 (21.4%), respectively. The ASR for incidence and mortality for breast cancer was 17.0 cases per 100,000 people per year and 4.41 cases per 100,000 people per year, respectively. The corresponding figures for cervical cancer were 9.9 cases per 100,000 people per year and 2.5 cases per 100,000 people per year, respectively. Other relevant cancers contributing to the cancer burden in this age group include thyroid cancer with an incidence and ASR of 78,568 new cases and 3.5 cases per 100,000 people per year, respectively; leukemia with 49,293 new cases and 2.3 cases per 100,000 people per year, respectively; and colorectal cancer with 41,117 new cases and 1.8 cases per 100,000 people per year. Thyroid cancer was four times more common in females than males. In terms of mortality, leukemia, liver cancer, and brain cancer were the major burdens. With global death rates of 36,253 (10.1%) cases for leukemia, 36,228 (10.1%) cases for liver and an ASR of 1.6 cases per 100,000 people per year for both leukemia and liver cancer, and 20,783 (5.8%) cases and an ASR of 0.9 cases per 100,000 people per year for brain cancer, these three cancers (leukemia, liver and brain cancer) contributed mostly to the mortality burden among this young group in 2012.

1.5.1 Geographic Distribution of Cancers of Adolescents and Young Adults

Obviously the global burden of cancer will differ between the defined four-tier levels of HDI countries and geographic regions based on numerous factors such as socioeconomic and health logistics. Interestingly, while the absolute numbers of cancers in young adults were much higher in high-HDI countries, the incident rates were the reverse, being highest in the very low-HDI countries with an ASR of 64.5 new cases per 100,000 people per year compared to the high-HDI countries with an ASR of 46.2 new cases per 100,000 people per year.

In all HDI countries, the top five cancers accounted for 50% of all estimated cancers. In low-, medium-, and high-HDI countries, brain and cervical cancers were the first and second most commonly diagnosed cancers, respectively. While breast cancer remained first in the very high-HDI countries, cervical cancer fell to fifth position. Also commonly diagnosed in the very high-HDI countries were thyroid cancer, melanoma, and testicular cancer. Probably because of the increased prevalence of infectious diseases in the low economic countries, infectious causes of cancer including HPV (cervical cancer), HBV and HCV (liver cancer), and *H. pylori* (gastric cancer) were more frequent in low-HDI than high-HDI countries. Indeed, in low-HDI countries, 1:3 (33.3%) cases of cancers were of infectious causes compared to 11.3% attributed to infections in high-HDI countries.

Findings from Fidler et al. also indicate that the incidence and causes of cancer in young adults differ geographically within the four-tier HDI regions [17]. For instance, in this study, the incidence of cancer was highest in Australia/New Zealand, as well as North American and European countries. On the contrary, Western and Southern Asia as well as parts of Africa registered the lowest incidences. The case profiles also differed geographically. With breast cancer, for instance, the ASR of 14.0 cases per 100,000 people per year in Australia/New Zealand contrasted sharply with that of 6.6 cases per 100,000 people per year in the lowest incident regions. Similarly, cervical cancer was the highest and lowest cause of cancer burden in this group in South and North Africa, respectively. Other cancers including Kaposi's sarcoma, testicular cancer, melanoma, and thyroid cancer also demonstrated such marked geographic variations. For instance, melanoma and testicular cancers were clustered in North America, Europe, and Australia/New Zealand, while Kaposi's sarcoma was more prevalent in East and South Africa that harbored 84.5% of all estimated new cases, which might be explained by the then human immunodeficiency virus (HIV) epidemic. Thyroid cancer was more common in North Africa where the incidence was 45 times higher than in Middle Africa. Equally worrisome was the substantial number of thyroid cancer cases in Australia/New Zealand, Europe, and Western Asia.

Despite the incidence of cancer being higher in the high-HDI than low-HDI countries, the mortality trend was the reverse. Cancer mortality burden and disparities will first be described for the HDI regions before examining their burden in specific geographic regions of the world. The overall case fatalities for cancer in this group were 55.0%, 49.1%, and 14.3% for the low-HDI, medium-HDI, and very high-HDI countries, respectively. Regarding the types of cancers, breast cancer, cervical cancer, and leukemia were the highest causes of cancer deaths in all these HDI countries. Gastric and colorectal cancers were the most fatal cancers in medium-HDI countries, while Kaposi's sarcoma and liver cancer were the most contributors to cancer mortality burden in low-HDI countries. Surprisingly, liver cancer was the leading cause of death among high-HDI countries. For the very high-HDI countries, brain and colorectal cancers were the primary cause of cancer-related deaths in young adults. There was an observed huge disparity in cancer mortality, whereby melanoma, Hodgkin lymphoma, prostate cancer, testicular cancer, thyroid cancer, kidney cancer, and breast cancer case fatalities were at least five times higher in low-HDI than high-HDI countries [17].

Cancer mortality burden among this demographic group was highest in parts of Africa and Asia. The highest was in Africa, which accounted for 64.3% of cases. Cancer mortality proportions over 50% were also observed in Middle Africa and Southern Asia. All these figures were importantly higher than those of Australia/New Zealand (11.3%), Western Europe (12.5%), and Northern Africa (12.5%). Variations were also uncovered in high-income countries (HICs), with the highest being breast cancer mortality in West, Middle, and East Africa. Cervical cancer mortality varied 31-fold with the highest mortality (ASR of 5.1 per 100,000 people per year) found in Melanesia, Polynesia, and Micronesia and the lowest with an ASR of 0.2 per 100,000 people per year in North Africa and Western Asia.

1.5.2 Probable Causes of Cancer in Adolescents and Young Adults

For every problem to be solved, the underlying factors to the problem must be identified so that appropriate solutions can be offered. Although cancer is the most common cause of death among this age group, the issue has been neglected until quite recently. For the diverse geographic distribution of young adult cancers, disparate causes must be accountable for them, and these have been explored for curtailment. Before examining possible causes and solutions, a number of issues need to be considered:

- The problem needs to be recognized and acknowledged.
- The global burden of cancer in this age group must be determined.
- The distribution patterns of the common causes should be identified.
- Availability and judicious use of screening strategies must be in place.
- The complex genetics of the cancers must be known.
- How do we limit the case fatalities, especially in low-to-medium-income countries (LMICs)?
- What preventive measures do we have for these cancers, and are we effectively using them?
- What are the barriers to early diagnosis?
- Is this age group aware of harmless and cost-effective screening procedures?
- Are these young adults aware of the burden of these cancers?
- Are there available high-caliber care team and technologies for dealing with these cancers?
- Are plans in place to acquiring the needed investments for young adult oncology?

Now let us address these points in a little more detail. The global incidence and mortality among young adults are quite high at 43.3 cases per 100,000 people per year and 15.9 cases per 100,000 people per year, respectively. These high figures urge us to identify the necessary awareness needed and resources required to help reduce this cancer burden among this subpopulation of our globe. Two important points that stood out in the Fidler et al. study were as follows: (i) though geographically variable, the burden of breast and cervical cancer was observed globally among this age group, and (ii) there was a disproportionate number of infectious causes of cancer in this age group residing in low-HDI countries [17]. While several other findings from this study were also important and will be addressed, these two need some immediate attention.

Breast cancer is a disease that is more often diagnosed after the age of 40 years; hence cases diagnosed before 40 need interrogation for possible underlying genetic causes. The increased diagnosis of such early-age cancers especially in high-HDI countries such as North America, Australia/New Zealand, and Europe where the incidence of BRCA1 and BRCA2 mutations is common deserves to be interrogated further. Indeed, studies need to be conducted to uncover what proportion of these mutations actually cause cancer in young adult women. Although frowned upon by some oncologist as inaccurate, simple self-breast examination, possibly followed by clinical breast examination, is harmless and yet could detect some early-stage cancers for curable measures. Proximal fluid biomarkers such as those in nipple aspirate fluids should augment such early detection efforts. A conundrum is the fact that the incidence of breast cancer in West Africa is similar to those in Western countries. For instance, it has been shown that the mean age for breast cancer diagnosis in West African women is 35–45 years, similar to those in high-HDI countries [18].

Many of these cancers carry poor prognosis, and yet the etiologic factors are enigmatic. A putative explanation is that it could be a mixed combination of genetic and environmental factors. This is an area that requires intense study. The internal carcinogenic environment should always be taken into account during such studies.

Another cancer of interest in this subpopulation is colorectal cancer. Early-age diagnosis of colorectal cancer should also prompt consideration of genetic factors such as mutations in *APC*, *AXIN2*, *MLH1*, *MSH2*, *MSH6*, *PMS2*, *GTBP*, *LKB1*, *STK11*, *MYH*, *PTEN*, *BMPR1a*, and *DPC4*.

Similarly, cervical cancer could be detected early or even completely prevented from developing through screening and vaccination. Periodic clinical examination, possibly by visual inspection with ascetic acid screening, especially in LMIC, could detect some early-stage cancers amenable to curative interventions. Additionally, in the advent of HPV, a virus known to contribute to the development of cervical and other cancers, the recommendation by the WHO for the vaccine to be given to girls aged 9–13 years should quickly help curtail HPV-associated cancers. Again effective coverage, especially in girls in LICs where resources are limited and accessibility is poor, deserves special attention.

Another issue of the burden of cancer in this subpopulation is overdiagnosis and overtreatment, which simply means finding and treating otherwise harmless "cancers." For example, thyroid cancer incidence is high in very high-HDI countries, and a study by Vaccarella et al. suggested the increased epidemic of thyroid cancer in these very high-HDI countries such as the USA, Canada, Australia/New Zealand, Europe, and other HICs in Asia may be due to overdiagnosis from the availability of sensitive diagnostic equipment [16].

The human microbiome and its dysbiosis are possible etiologic factors of several cancers (this concept is addressed in Chap. 14). For now we will restrict our discussion on infectious causes of cancer to those that directly cause the disease within the organ they infect such as HPV that causes cervical cancer, HBV that causes hepatocellular cancer, HIV that causes Kaposi's sarcoma, HHV8 that also causes Kaposi's sarcoma, and rarely primary effusion lymphoma. Vaccination with HPV and HBV has reduced the incidence of cervical cancer and hepatocellular carcinoma, respectively. Similarly, with the curtailment of the HIV epidemic, there has been a reduction in the number of Kaposi's sarcoma.

Fatal cancers tend to occur more commonly in LMICs. Fidler et al. noted that even within the same cancer type such as breast, kidney, and testicular cancers, as well as leukemia and lymphoma, mortality was still higher in LMICs, suggesting that other factors needed to be identified and dealt with [17]. Multiple explanations were offered to explain this disparity in cancer mortalities between HIC and LMIC: (i) a fractured health infrastructure that fails to detect cancer early in LMICs, (ii) ineffective screening tests or no early detection procedures in LMICs, and (iii) poor access to available treatment protocols in LMICs. Added to this problem are psychological and social factors, cultural norms that may hinder seeking Western medicine early, and difficult geographic accessibility, which all could be obstacles to early detection of curable diseases. Finally, once diagnosed, high-quality care is needed for this "neglected" subpopulation, and this is often unavailable in LMICs.

1.5.3 Cancer Survival in Adolescents and Young Adults

While the hitherto discussed situation may look dismal, the incidence of some adolescent and young adult cancers is decreasing, but others are increasing. On the brighter side, application of modern technologies is improving the survival of this population with diverse cancers. A few illustrations will suffice.

Some adolescent and young adult cancers such as those of the uterine cervix, lung, larynx, bladder, and ovary have been decreasing in incidence since 1975. Decreasing cervical cancer incidence reflects the development of the Papanicolaou smear. Also with education and reduced smoking among this population, lung, laryngeal, and bladder cancer incidences have decreased. The observed decrease in ovarian cancer among this population is as yet inexplicable.

On the gloomy side, some cancers are increasing in incidence, but with intense education, others are beginning to show a decrease. For example, (i) anorectal cancer that has been linked to HPV infection has been increasing faster than colorectal cancer among this population; (ii) the increase in testicular cancer linked to recreational marijuana use may have geographic variation in incidence, but self-examination of the testicles should help early detection of some of these cancers; (iii) increase in acute lymphoblastic leukemia is also linked to HPV infections, which should hopefully decrease with vaccination; (iv) increased multiple myeloma detection is associated with overdiagnosis due to sensitive immunoassays; and (v) the increase in other cancers, such as Ewing sarcoma and female non-Hodgkin lymphoma, is unexplained.

Kaposi's sarcoma had been a worrisome diagnosis because it carries a poor prognosis. The epidemic peaked during the HIV pandemic. With the decrease and settlement of HIV infections due to effective treatment, the incidence of Kaposi's sarcoma has decreased. The observed survival of thyroid cancers is not due to any efficient intervention, but to overdiagnosis. The cancers that received the most dramatic improvements in the USA among this population are (i) chronic myeloid leukemia with the discovery of *BCR-ABL* (Philadelphia chromosome) tyrosine kinase inhibitor, imatinib mesylate (Gleevec), and (ii) multiple myeloma due to improved hematopoietic stem cell transplantation in conjunction with successful treatment using combination chemotherapy with histone deacetylase and proteasomal inhibitors. Putatively, lung, pancreatic, and liver cancers in young adults have the worse prognosis, but immense progress is being made in their treatment due to modern advancements. These advancements include proper disease staging, which is critical to effective management, as well as use of multimodal therapy that includes efficient surgery, chemotherapy, radiotherapy, and recent molecularly targeted therapies. Finally, while sarcomas have relatively good prognosis with 5-year survival rates of 60–90%, the overall progress is dismal. For example, young adults with sarcomas have decreased cancer-specific survival, of which chondrosarcoma, osteosarcoma, rhabdomyosarcoma, and soft tissue sarcomas are noteworthy.

1.6 Summary

- Despite geographic and regional variations due to HDI, the incidence of cancer is on the rise globally.
- Lung cancer was the highest in incidence and mortality in both sexes, and in some countries, this was even higher than breast cancer among women.
- The vast majority of the causative factors of cancer are environmental and occupational exposures, as well as lifestyle choices such as tobacco and alcohol use, and habits that lead to increased body mass index. Thus, primary prevention should curb the rising trend in cancer incidence.
- The reported 2012 cancer incidence and mortality among adolescents and young adults are substantial, especially among females.
- In children and young adults, leukemia, hepatoma, and brain cancer were the leading causes of cancer mortality.
- While the burden of young adult cancers in most countries were from brain and cervical cancers, the top three cancers according to incidence were breast, cervical, and thyroid cancers.

References

1. Bray F, Ferlay J, Soerjomataram I, Siegel RL, Torre LA, Jemal A. Global cancer statistics 2018: GLOBOCAN estimates of incidence and mortality worldwide for 36 cancers in 185 countries. CA Cancer J Clin. 2018;68(6):394–424. https://doi.org/10.3322/caac.21492. PubMed PMID: 30207593
2. Lortet-Tieulent J, Renteria E, Sharp L, Weiderpass E, Comber H, Baas P, et al. Convergence of decreasing male and increasing female incidence rates in major tobacco-related cancers in Europe in 1988–2010. Eur J Cancer. 2015;51(9):1144–63. https://doi.org/10.1016/j.ejca.2013.10.014. PubMed PMID: 24269041
3. Jha P. Avoidable global cancer deaths and total deaths from smoking. Nat Rev Cancer. 2009;9(9):655–64. https://doi.org/10.1038/nrc2703. PubMed PMID: 19693096
4. Jemal A, Miller KD, Ma J, Siegel RL, Fedewa SA, Islami F, et al. Higher lung cancer incidence in young women than young men in the United States. N Engl J Med. 2018;378(21):1999–2009. https://doi.org/10.1056/NEJMoa1715907. PubMed PMID: 29791813
5. Bray F, McCarron P, Parkin DM. The changing global patterns of female breast cancer incidence and mortality. Breast Cancer Res. 2004;6(6):229–39. https://doi.org/10.1186/bcr932. PubMed PMID: 15535852; PubMed Central PMCID: PMCPMC1064079
6. Rossouw JE, Anderson GL, Prentice RL, LaCroix AZ, Kooperberg C, Stefanick ML, et al. Risks and benefits of estrogen plus progestin in healthy postmenopausal women: principal results from the Women's Health Initiative randomized controlled trial. JAMA. 2002;288(3):321–33. PubMed PMID: 12117397
7. Ravdin PM, Cronin KA, Howlader N, Berg CD, Chlebowski RT, Feuer EJ, et al. The decrease in breast-cancer incidence in 2003 in the United States. N Engl J Med. 2007;356(16):1670–4. https://doi.org/10.1056/NEJMsr070105. PubMed PMID: 17442911
8. Arnold M, Laversanne M, Brown LM, Devesa SS, Bray F. Predicting the future burden of esophageal cancer by histological subtype: international trends in incidence up to 2030. Am J Gastroenterol. 2017;112(8):1247–55. https://doi.org/10.1038/ajg.2017.155. PubMed PMID: 28585555

9. Arnold M, Sierra MS, Laversanne M, Soerjomataram I, Jemal A, Bray F. Global patterns and trends in colorectal cancer incidence and mortality. Gut. 2017;66(4):683–91. https://doi.org/10.1136/gutjnl-2015-310912. PubMed PMID: 26818619
10. Chimed T, Sandagdorj T, Znaor A, Laversanne M, Tseveen B, Genden P, et al. Cancer incidence and cancer control in Mongolia: results from the National Cancer Registry 2008–12. Int J Cancer. 2017;140(2):302–9. https://doi.org/10.1002/ijc.30463. PubMed PMID: 27716912
11. Marengo A, Rosso C, Bugianesi E. Liver cancer: connections with obesity, fatty liver, and cirrhosis. Annu Rev Med. 2016;67:103–17. https://doi.org/10.1146/annurev-med-090514-013832. PubMed PMID: 26473416
12. Bray F, Carstensen B, Moller H, Zappa M, Zakelj MP, Lawrence G, et al. Incidence trends of adenocarcinoma of the cervix in 13 European countries. Cancer Epidemiol Biomarkers Prev. 2005;14(9):2191–9. https://doi.org/10.1158/1055-9965.EPI-05-0231. PubMed PMID: 16172231
13. Bray F, Loos AH, McCarron P, Weiderpass E, Arbyn M, Moller H, et al. Trends in cervical squamous cell carcinoma incidence in 13 European countries: changing risk and the effects of screening. Cancer Epidemiol Biomarkers Prev. 2005;14(3):677–86. https://doi.org/10.1158/1055-9965.EPI-04-0569. PubMed PMID: 15767349
14. Bray F, Lortet-Tieulent J, Znaor A, Brotons M, Poljak M, Arbyn M. Patterns and trends in human papillomavirus-related diseases in Central and Eastern Europe and Central Asia. Vaccine. 2013;31(Suppl 7):H32–45. https://doi.org/10.1016/j.vaccine.2013.02.071. PubMed PMID: 24332296
15. Islami F, Goding Sauer A, Miller KD, Siegel RL, Fedewa SA, Jacobs EJ, et al. Proportion and number of cancer cases and deaths attributable to potentially modifiable risk factors in the United States. CA Cancer J Clin. 2018;68(1):31–54. https://doi.org/10.3322/caac.21440. PubMed PMID: 29160902
16. Vaccarella S, Franceschi S, Bray F, Wild CP, Plummer M, Dal ML. Worldwide thyroid-cancer epidemic? The increasing impact of overdiagnosis. N Engl J Med. 2016;375(7):614–7. https://doi.org/10.1056/NEJMp1604412. PubMed PMID: 27532827
17. Fidler MM, Gupta S, Soerjomataram I, Ferlay J, Steliarova-Foucher E, Bray F. Cancer incidence and mortality among young adults aged 20–39 years worldwide in 2012: a population-based study. Lancet Oncol. 2017;18(12):1579–89. https://doi.org/10.1016/S1470-2045(17)30677-0. PubMed PMID: 29111259
18. Vanderpuye V, Olopade OI, Huo D. Pilot survey of breast cancer management in Sub-Saharan Africa. J Glob Oncol. 2017;3(3):194–200. https://doi.org/10.1200/JGO.2016.004945. PubMed PMID: 28717760; PubMed Central PMCID: PMCPMC5493219 manuscript. All relationships are considered compensated. Relationships are self-held unless noted. I = Immediate Family Member, Inst = My Institution. Relationships may not relate to the subject matter of this manuscript. For more information about ASCO's conflict of interest policy, please refer to http://www.asco.org/rwc or ascopubs.org/jco/site/ifc. Verna D.N.K. VanderpuyeNo relationship to discloseOlufunmilayo I. OlopadeOther Relationship: Co Founder, CancerIQDezheng HuoNo relationship to disclose

Chapter 2
Breast Cancer Biomarkers in Proximal Fluids

2.1 Introduction

Breast cancer (BrCa) is one disease that recent molecular and genetic research efforts have contributed tremendously to the understanding of its molecular pathology and hence has led to effective disease management. This feat has translated into improved patient survival outcomes. For example, the 5-year survival rate has improved from about 63% in the 1960s to about 90% in recent times. However, BrCa remains a disease of importance, being the second most common cancer in the world (after lung), and the first and second most common cause of cancer-related deaths in the less and more developed parts of the world, respectively. Globally, 2,088,849 new cases were diagnosed, and 626,679 people died from the disease in 2018 (GLOBOCAN 2018). The 5-year global prevalence was 6,875,099, and this was the highest among all cancer types. This survival effect is partly attributed to early detection and effective management such that many women are now living longer with the disease.

Early cancer detection offers the best opportunity for cure. Indeed, patients with early BrCa confined to the breast have a 5-year survival rate of about 99%, compared to a woeful 26% rate for those diagnosed with advanced-stage disease. Late-stage BrCa patients are treated with hormonal, chemotherapeutic, and biologically targeted agents, yet metastatic relapse occurs in a vast majority of cases, and this accounts for the poor prognosis. Established in cancer is the concept of field cancerization, which should enable the discovery of early detection biomarkers for BrCa.

Screening strategies, including mammography, have proven useful in early detection and improved survival of BrCa patients. Current screening efforts detect about 63% of BrCa at an early stage. This is probably because mammography has limited utility in premenopausal women with dense breast tissue, and yet they contribute to about 12% of all BrCa. Cautioned by the Director of the International Agency for Research on Cancer (IARC), Dr. Christopher P. Wild, "Mammography is really only applicable in places with–developed health service"…"One of the major challenges globally is to find an alternative to mammography that can be

G. D. Dakubo, *Cancer Biomarkers in Body Fluids*,
https://doi.org/10.1007/978-3-030-24725-6_2

applied to screening and early detection of breast cancer in low- to middle-income countries." Measurement of serum cancer antigen 14-3 (CA15-3) has also been helpful in the management of some women with metastatic BrCa. The need for novel accurate and validated biomarkers for early BrCa detection and management is hence acute, and there has been a plethora of confirmatory BrCa biomarkers. However, biomarkers in body fluids (circulation, nipple fluid, urine, or saliva) should enable acceptable screening of all women at risk, especially premenopausal women and women in resource-poor communities of the world. Body fluid biomarkers should also fit into the ease of serial longitudinal sampling necessary for making important clinical decisions required for personalized BrCa oncology. However, proximal fluids of the breast should be enriched for BrCa-specific biomarkers to enable accurate disease detection. Because some approaches such as ductal lavage (DL) and random periareolar fine needle aspiration (RPFNA) are minimally invasive, biomarkers discovered in these media could be applied only to women at high risk and leveraged in circulating body fluid or nipple aspirate fluid (NAF) for use in average risk women.

2.2 Anatomy and Histology of the Breast

The breast is a modified sweat gland (the mammary gland) embedded in the thoracic cutaneous connective tissue stroma and covered by the skin. The structure of the breast is very important in understanding BrCa histopathology, as well as why certain proximal body fluids may not be representative of the entire breast tissue. Each breast contains between 15 and 25 lobes that are embedded in adipose tissue and demarcated into individual units by collagenous connective tissue septa (Fig. 2.1). The lobes are variable in sizes, with each lobe being made up of tubuloacinar glands. Regarding BrCa assays based on breast proximal fluid analysis, it is noteworthy that only about 15–20 large lobes connect to the surface by lactiferous ducts that dilate into lactiferous sinuses just before opening onto the surface at the nipple. Ducts of smaller lobes end blindly in the breast connective tissue. Within a lobe, the main lactiferous duct subdivides into terminal ducts that connect to lobules forming a terminal duct or lobular unit. The ducts in a terminal duct or lobular unit are referred to as intralobular ducts. These are lined by cuboidal or low columnar epithelium, the base of which is lined by contractile myoepithelial cells and the basement membrane. The myoepithelial cells contract to help in expulsion of secretions. Large interlobular ducts surround the lobules and intralobular ducts. The nipple is surrounded by areola cutaneous tissue that is pigmented and contains sebaceous glands without hair.

2.3 The Sick Lobe Theory of Breast Cancer

The sick lobe hypothesis postulated for the evolution of BrCa posits that carcinoma in situ and invasive BrCa are lobar diseases. It asserts that most BrCa develops from a single "sick lobe" that is more susceptible to carcinogenic insults. Pioneered and

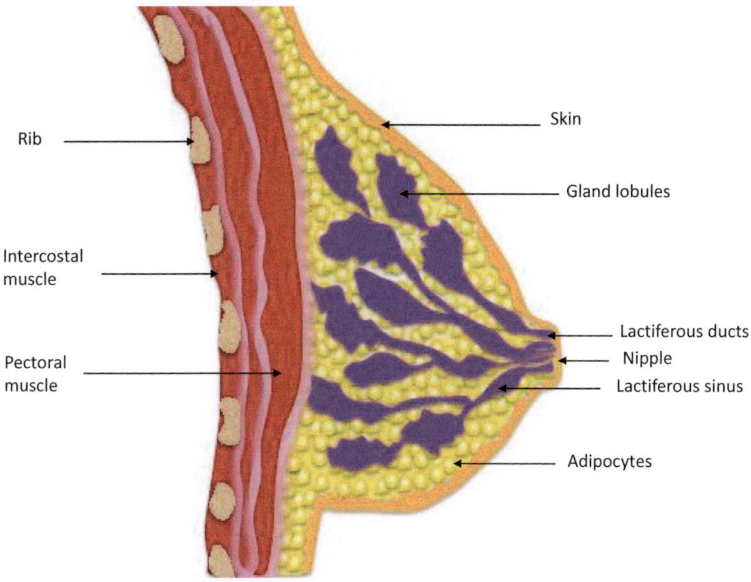

Fig. 2.1 Structure of the female breast

championed by Dr. Tibor Tot, Professor at the University of Uppsala, this theory is based on evidence from breast developmental biology, genetic analysis, and breast cytoarchitecture. Putatively, from early embryogenesis, cells in the sick lobe harbor genetic instabilities. These genetically altered progenitor cells that are confined to a specific lobe accumulate more mutations, epigenetic alterations, and chromosomal instabilities that drive them through progressive stages of cancer development. Even multifocal tumors are deemed to have evolved from many distinct lobules in the sick lobe. Thus, targeted destruction of the sick lobe should almost completely treat BrCa in an individual. This theory has numerous implications for early BrCa detection and prevention of invasive disease in high-risk women by the intraductal approach. However, synchronous and metachronous contralateral BrCas from carcinogen-exposed field cancerization are not readily explicable by this hypothesis.

2.4 Historic Overview of Proximal Fluids in Breast Cancer Risk Assessment

Interests in using breast proximal fluids for risk assessment have been entertained since the 1940s; however, Susan Love in the 1990s championed the sampling of ductal cells and fluid for analysis to detect abnormal cells. Before then, other surgeons and investigators had tried these methods for BrCa detection. In 1946, Raul Leborgne catheterized ducts, infused them with saline, and then washed to sample ductal fluid, which he referred to as "ductal rinse." George Papanicolaou in 1958 used a suction approach to sample nipple fluid for analysis, which he also referred to as "breast Pap smear." He was successful in this approach to even detect ductal carcinoma in situ (DCIS). In about a decade of dormancy, much enthusiasm rekindled in the 1970s, and many investigators began asking questions about the clinical importance of the intraductal approach. Works by Gertrude Buehring, Otto Sartorius, as well as Eileen King and Nicholas Petrakis are noteworthy. In general, these investigators were successful in obtaining nipple fluid from about 80% and 50% of premenopausal and postmenopausal women, respectively. Ed Sauter improved upon the nipple aspirate fluid (NAF) technique for sampling the breast and was able to obtain NAF from almost all women in his cohort. Studies with large samples from patients who were followed for long periods of time provide informative conclusions. Typically, all the works from these pioneers indicate that:

- Women unable to produce NAF (had dry breasts) had the lowest risk of developing BrCa, with an incidence of 4.7%.
- Women who produced NAF with cells had increased risk of developing BrCa.
- Women who produced NAF containing normal cells had mild risk, with BrCa incidence of 8.2%.
- Women who produced NAF containing hyperplastic cells had moderate risk, with BrCa incidence of 10.8%.
- Women who produced NAF containing atypical cells had the highest risk of cancer, with BrCa incidence of 13.8%.
- Women with atypical NAF cells and first-degree relative with BrCa had two times the risk of BrCa compared to women with atypical cells without a family history of BrCa.

Susan Love highly improved upon the ductoscopy and lavage procedure. She developed a double-lumen catheter technique whereby fluid was infused through one catheter to wash the ducts and collected via the other catheter. This method improved the cellular content of NAF. Ductal lavage (DL) was more sensitive at detection of abnormal cells (three times more frequently) than NAF.

2.5 Proximal Fluids of the Breast

Proximal fluids of the breast commonly used for biomarker mining include NAF, DL fluid (DLF), and random periareolar fine nipple aspiration fluid (RPFNAF). These fluids have their merits and demerits in regard to BrCa risk assessment (Table 2.1).

2.5.1 Nipple Aspirate Fluid

Secretions into the duct system of non-lactating women can be collected noninvasively by spontaneous discharge, means of pumps, and breast massage. This fluid and exfoliated cells in the ductal system can be aspirated, and this is referred to as

Table 2.1 Comparison of breast proximal fluids

Attributes	NAF	DLF	RPFNA
Mode of acquisition	Noninvasive	Invasive	Invasive
Level of discomfort	Mild to nothing	Severe	Moderate
Screening utility	Yes	No	No
Duration of procedure (minutes)	15	60	30
Cellularity (% of cells)	23–66	60	95
Ease of biomarker analysis	Not	Easy	Easy
Ability to localize lesion	No	Yes	No
Cost	Least expensive	Most expensive	Intermediate expensive

NAF nipple aspirate fluid, *DLF* ductal lavage fluid, *RPFNA* random periareolar fine needle aspiration

NAF. Physiologically, nipple fluid flows down the main ducts and ampullae via breast alveolar glands into the lymphatic and blood circulation, which could be a mechanism for BrCa biomarker release into the peripheral circulation and possibly other body fluids such as saliva and urine.

Nipple discharge is simply breast "body fluid" from the nipple. This could be NAF that is easily obtained using modified breast pumps, or spontaneous pathologic nipple discharge, which is fluid that emanates usually from only one breast that may harbor a benign or malignant lesion. Both types of nipple fluid can be collected in a noninvasive fashion and yet contain secreted biomolecules and cells from the ductal epithelium of the breast.

The successful production of NAF in healthy women is very variable, being obtained in about 48–94% of all women, depending on ethnicity and menopausal status. Caucasian and black women are good NAF yielders (about 75% produce NAF) compared to Asian women from whom NAF is obtained successfully in under 35% of them. Similarly, women aged 30–55 years most successfully produce NAF, with many postmenopausal women being unable to do so. The volume and ease of NAF production and the presence of cytological atypia are predictors of BrCa risk.

NAF composition is variable, being influenced by both endogenously produced biomolecules and exogenous bio-compounds such as macronutrients and micronutrients from dietary sources. The endogenously produced compounds are many, including lipids, proteins, hormones, antigens, growth factors, and several other biomolecules. In addition, NAF contains mammary epithelial cells, cell free nucleic acids, proteins, and metabolites of intermediary metabolism. Passive filtration of plasma and secretion by apocrine breast cells in association with selective accumulation determines the levels of exogenous compounds.

Depending on the technique used and the experience of the collector, sufficient NAF can be successfully obtained from up to 70% of all women. However, a novel method employing NAF extraction under oxytocin induction has been successful in about 94% of women. Vacuum aspiration, a method originally reported by Sartorius, is the primary mode of NAF collection. In this procedure, the nipple is first cleansed with a detergent, followed by removal of keratin with OmniPrep™ paste, and then cleaned and let dry with alcohol. A plastic cup that is connected to a 10 ml syringe is attached to the nipple. The participant is then instructed to compress or massage the breast from the base to the nipple, while the attendant or operator simultaneously retracts the plunger of the syringe to about the 5 ml position. NAF may or may not flow out depending on patient yield. If there is no NAF, further retraction of the plunger can be applied to about the 10 ml position and held for about 15 s. The procedure can be repeated two more times if required. But, if NAF still fails to be extracted after such repeats, the individual can be considered a nonproducer. NAF at the nipple is collected either with a capillary tube or a micropipette and stored or processed for the specific indicated analysis. In producers, up to 200 ul of NAF can be collected, but a majority of women will yield between 20 and 40 ul. A major contraindication to NAF collection is any procedure that causes nipple distortion, e.g., from surgery or retracted nipples.

Oxytocin can be used to induce NAF production. This procedure is preceded by single spray of oxytocin (4 IU) into each nostril. This medication works in about 5 min after spray with a half-life of 3–17 min, which is a sufficient time for NAF collection. Oxytocin causes contraction of the myoepithelial cells of the breast acinar to squeeze out NAF. This procedure is very tolerable by many women, and because the drug is clinically safe (as it is used to promote nursing), the procedure can be adopted, especially in women with poor NAF yield.

NAF is processed for cytologic, genomic, transcriptomic, proteomic, or metabolomic analysis. For cytologic evaluation, NAF is rinsed with 3% polyethylene glycol in denatured alcohol, cyto-centrifuged onto a glass slide, and stained and examined under a microscope. A number of issues might be encountered with only cytological evaluation of NAF for BrCa risk assessment. These include acellularity or limited cellularity of NAF that may limit efficient cytologic evaluation, atypia that may be from benign lesions, requirement for a specialist cytopathologist, subjectivity as with all histopathologic evaluations, and normal cytology that does not necessarily preclude molecular and genetic changes possibly from precancer fields.

NAF can be stored in the refrigerator (4 °C) or freezer (−20 °C) and DNA extracted later for analysis. For RNA preservation, it is recommended to quickly freeze NAF in liquid nitrogen and stored at −80 °C for subsequent use. Alternatively, NAF can be collected in RNA protective reagents. For proteomic analysis, NAF is rinsed into centrifuge tubes containing about 500 ul sterile phosphate-buffered saline (PBS) and protease inhibitors. Centrifugation is performed at 1500 rpm for 10 min to pellet cells and other insoluble materials. The supernatant is collected for proteomic analysis or, if not used immediately, stored at −80 °C.

2.5.2 *Ductal Lavage Fluid*

"Lavage" is a French word for "rinse or wash." Ductal lavage is a procedure developed initially by D. Susan Love (Pro-Duct Health, acquired by Cytyc Corporation) for the collection of ductal fluid and cells for examination as a complement to breast examination and mammography for BrCa risk assessment. Evidently, this sample is suitable for cancer genetic signature analysis as well, as has been conducted by several groups. The intraductal approach, which includes nipple aspiration, DL, and mammary ductoscopy (MD), enables direct visualization, biopsy, and washes (lavage) of the breast ducts. This minimally invasive procedure, often performed on high-risk women such as those with abnormal nipple discharge without noticeable masses, contributes to the diagnosis of intraductal lesions.

The procedure involves invasive cannulation and washing of NAF-producing breast ducts via a dustoscope. DL increases the cellularity of nipple fluid for cytological examination and BrCa risk assessment. DL can produce a median epithelial cell count of 13,500 compared to NAF counts of 120 [1]. Biomarker exploration therefore appears facile as a complement in determining accurately the risk of a woman for developing BrCa and hence the possible recommendation for prophylactic surgery, tamoxifen chemoprevention, or oophorectomy in premenopausal women. Accurate risk assessment is critical because each of these interventions is associated with possible serious psychological and physical side effects. However, DL is minimally invasive, can be painful or uncomfortable, and increases psychosomatic adverse effects in women leading to poor compliance and acceptance for screening purposes.

There are some issues with NAF as risk-associated breast proximal fluid that can be overcome by DL. First, in some instances, target molecules are insufficient in NAF for analysis. With the development of sensitive technologies, this problem is being resolved with successful analysis of many biomolecules. Second, not all women produce NAF. However, women who fail to produce NAF may be considered low risk for developing BrCa; hence this may not be an important factor. Finally, if not performed properly, NAF could be obtained only from the periareolar region, thus missing deep-seated breast tissues. Hence, some tumors will be missed using such NAF as a screening material. Ductal lavage provides a solution to these problems. However, not all these procedures can detect lesions in lobules and ducts that fail to open at the nipple.

During the DL procedure, NAF-producing ducts are cannulated by means of microcatheter. Just as the tip of the microcatheter enters the duct orifice, 2–3 ml of 1% lidocaine can be infused to anesthetize the ductal tree prior to saline lavage. Local anesthesia can first be provided via periareolar infiltration of about 5 ml of 1% lidocaine. Saline or other physiologic solutions are infused, the breast is massaged, and the lavage effluent is aspirated and placed in a tube containing a fixative. Repeat infusions of 2 ml solutions up to a total volume of about 10 ml are acceptable.

The procedure is well tolerated but less so than NAF collection with median pain of 24 mm compared to 8 mm for NAF on a 0–100 mm visual analogue scale. Cytologically evaluable samples are obtainable in up to 60% of women undergoing risk assessment [1, 2]. But successful DL has been performed in >80% of high-risk women [3]. Failure to obtain sufficient epithelial cells for analysis is attributed to a number of factors including skill of the operator, lack of NAF production, inability to cannulate ducts, and inadequate cells in the effluent. Difficulty of catheter passage through the nipple sphincter is an obstacle that can be overcome with use of nitroglycerin paste to relax the sphincter. Lack of NAF-producing ducts to guide catheter insertion is also an obstacle to successful DL. However, investigators skilled at the procedure have been able to perform DL on non-NAF-producing ducts. Epithelial cell yield is up to 5000 cells per duct when performed by experienced investigators.

Of the various BrCa screening procedures (breast exam, mammographic evaluation, magnetic resonance imaging (MRI), NAF and DL specimen analysis), both perceived and experienced distress and discomfort appear worse with DL. Expectedly, preexisting psychological distress augments the experienced pain, and this contributes to the high rates of attrition among women needing subsequent procedures. A major source of procedural pain is forced dilatation of the sphincter at the nipple by the catheter. Local anesthesia works well just at the surface of the nipple in some cases, and smooth muscle relaxants (e.g., topical nitro-paste) may not be adequate. Thus, general anesthesia is employed in some cases for ductoscopy and lavage. Psychological, educational, and procedural improvements are needed for even the high-risk patient including women already diagnosed with BrCa. Though useful for BrCa surveillance, DL cannot be recommended for screening.

2.5.3 Random Periareolar Fine Nipple Aspiration

Random periareolar fine nipple aspiration (RPFNA) is a minimally invasive method of sampling "normal" breast tissue for risk assessment. The procedure differs from fine needle aspiration (FNA), which involves sampling of suspicious nodular lesions for evaluation. RPFNA is based on the thesis that women at risk for developing BrCa often harbor multifocal and multicentric proliferative lesions (from "field cancerized" breast) as evidenced in autopsy series and prophylactic mastectomy samples from high-risk women. Apart from histopathologic appearance, there is ample evidence of molecular field cancerization of the breast in disease state.

RPFNA is generally an outpatient procedure performed by a trained expert. It is often conducted as part of some research protocol to evaluate BrCa risk or response to treatment in an interventional trial. Following breast physical examination, ice is used to numb the breast, which also serves to reduce bleeding during the procedure. After about 20 min, the ice is removed, and the skin cleansed with antiseptic swabs. First the skin, followed by the deeper tissues, is anesthetized with 1% lidocaine. About 12–16 21G needles attached to 10 ml syringes containing sterile saline are used to aspirate 0.5–1 ml of samples from the four breast quadrants. While referred to as "random," preferential sampling occurs in areas where resistance is felt, which is suggestive of possibly harboring proliferative or neoplastic lesions. Usually three to four syringes are used per quadrant. The samples, made up of cells (epithelial and immune) and tissues (adipose and stroma), are rinsed in 10 ml CytoLyt® and transferred to PreservCyt® solutions. The samples are pooled into two separate tubes, one for each breast, or into a single tube, depending on experimental protocol, for cytomorphologic and biomarker analyses. Precautions taken to prevent post-procedural bleeding or hematoma formation include instructing women to discontinue nonsteroidal anti-inflammatory drugs (NSAIDs), vitamin E, and fish oil products for 3 weeks and administration of 10 mg vitamin K for 3 days prior to the procedure. Additional safety measures include application of ice on sampled areas for 20 min and instructing clients to wear tight-fitting sports bra for several days and to avoid activities that will cause significant breast movements.

2.6 Breast Cancer Biomarkers Amenable to Proximal Fluid Evaluation

Alterations in the epigenome, especially CpG island hypermethylation, are prevalent in BrCa samples. Although these tumor markers are yet to be clinically validated and translated, the promise to use these biomarkers in early detection and prognostication is not far from reality. Of even more clinically important is the sensitive detection of these cancer-specific epigenome changes in minimally invasive samples including blood, NAF, DL, and FNA of patients. Several methylated genes detected in body fluids are potential biomarkers of early BrCa detection. Whereas these genes demonstrate variable sensitivities, they appear very specific (up to 100%) for BrCa even in body fluid samples. Commonly methylated in BrCa include *RASSF1A, APC, CDKN2A, CCND2*, Stratifin (*SFN*), *RAR-β*, and *TWIST*. *CDKN2A* methylation is detected in up to 23% of cancer tissues and 8–14% of plasma samples. *CDH1* methylation can be detected in 20% of plasma samples. Methylations of *APC* and *RASSF1A* in serum are biomarkers of survival, and methylations of *CCND2*, *RARβ*, and *TWIST* are detectable in ductal fluid samples.

BrCa is a disease of chromosomal instability including loss of heterozygosity (LOH), aneuploidy, as well as epigenetic alterations and mutations of specific genes. Together, these lesions interfere with normal functioning of pathways important in cellular maintenance such as apoptosis, DNA repair, senescence, cell cycle, and cellular proliferation and differentiation. Several chromosomal regions are amplified, simply deleted, or rearranged in BrCa. Affected chromosomal regions include 1, 3, 4, 6, 7, 8, 9, 10, 11, 12, 13, 15, 16, 17, 18, 19, 20, and 22. That these instabilities are causative and/or drivers of BrCa progression is the fact that benign breast pathologies such as fibroadenoma rarely harbor these genetic alterations, with premalignant cells containing intermediate proportions of chromosomal instabilities, but levels become markedly increased in aneuploid BrCa. DNA sequence anomalies have been detected in many genes including *BRAC*, *TP53*, *EGFR*, *VEGF*, and *ERBB2 (HER2/neu)*, among several others.

There are over 30 endogenous BrCa metabolites identified in tissue biopsy studies. The BrCa metabolome includes increased glycerophosphocholine, phosphocholine, and free choline. Spectroscopic resonances of these metabolites show a broad single peak referred to as "total choline-containing compounds." However, in vitro studies identify elevated phosphocholine as the major metabolite responsible for the peak. Levels of phosphocholine also parallel disease stage as disease progression correlates with increases. Other BrCa metabolite changes include increased taurine, myoinositol, and phosphoethanolamine and low glucose levels. In vivo magnetic resonance spectroscopy imaging (MRSI) analysis of choline levels can yield a sensitivity of 100% in BrCa detection.

2.7 Breast Cancer Risk Assessment Using Breast Proximal Fluids

There are a number of biomarkers for assessing the risk of a woman developing BrCa. These include germline mutations in *BRCA1* and *BRCA2* and single nucleotide polymorphisms in genes controlling DNA repair and metabolism of carcinogens and hormones. However, the low prevalence of BRAC mutations in the general population (about 1%) and women with BrCa (5–10%) precludes their use as screening biomarkers for the average risk woman. In postmenopausal women, elevated levels of estradiol (>2.7 pg/ml) or testosterone are associated with relative BrCa risk of about 4. Moreover, levels of serum IGF and IGFBP3 confer BrCa risk in premenopausal women. Because of their subjectivity to modulation by disease progression, mammographic breast density and intraepithelial neoplasia (IEN) have been attractive screening and monitoring biomarkers for BrCa. The relative BrCa risk associated with IEN are 1.4–2 for hyperplasia, 4–5 for atypical hyperplasia, and 10–20 for carcinoma in situ. Thus, in high-risk women, screening for BrCa risk in proximal fluids has relied on detecting degrees of IEN.

Among high-risk women for BrCa, ~16% will have cellular atypia detected in DL fluid. However, the majority of these women with atypical cells in their breast tissue do not subsequently develop BrCa. Therefore, the use of only histology in analysis of breast proximal fluid (i.e., NAF or DL cytology) is unlikely to be useful in early BrCa detection in the general population. Complementary molecular approaches are more likely to be useful, because cancer begins with epigenomic and genomic changes prior to evident cellular morphologic features of cancer. Genomic approaches could potentially identify molecular subtypes of hyperplasia such that those with increased risk of progression provided with active surveillance to enable early detection.

2.7.1 *Proliferative Breast Lesions*

The prior commonly diagnosed fibrocystic breast disease represents a spectrum from minimal insignificant changes to worrisome proliferative lesions including carcinoma in situ. Because fibrocystic breast disease is associated with elevated BrCa risk, Page and colleagues categorized these changes into relevant prognostic groups. These categories include nonproliferative breast disease that carries no risk for BrCa, proliferative breast disease without atypia that is associated with 1.5–2.0 times risk for BrCa, and proliferative breast disease with atypia, which confers 4–5 times BrCa risk. Carcinoma in situ was associated with 8–10 times risk for BrCa [4, 5].

The cytomorphological features of the Page and colleague's prognostic categories were not well defined in FNA samples. In view of this, Masood et al. performed a prospective study with cytologic-histologic correlation using mammographically guided FNA biopsy (FNAB) and follow-up needle localization excision biopsy to define cytomorphology of high-risk proliferative breast disease [6]. A semiquantitative cytologic grading system was developed and used to evaluate the needle aspirate samples on the basis of cellular arrangement, degree of cellular pleomorphism and anisonucleosis, the presence or absence of myoepithelial cells and nucleoli, and chromatin pattern. They assigned values from 1 to 4 to each of these criteria and calculated a score based on the sum of the individual values for each case (the Masood cytologic index). This index ranges from a minimum score of 6 to a maximum of 24. This cytologic index is used to categorize fibrocystic changes into nonproliferative breast disease (score of 6–10), proliferative breast disease without atypia (score of 11–14), proliferative breast disease with atypia (score of 15–18), and BrCa (score of 19–24). This categorization was validated by the high degree of concordance between their cytologic evaluation and histologic diagnosis from needle-localized excision biopsy.

2.7.2 Breast Cancer Risk Assessment Models

The Gail and its improved Tyrer-Cuzick models are used for BrCa risk assessment (Table 2.2). The Gail risk model was developed using data from the BrCa Detection Project and relies on five elements, namely, current age, age at menarche (younger age is associated with elevated risk), age at first live birth (older age is associated with elevated risk), number of breast biopsies (more biopsies is associated with elevated risk), and number of first-degree relatives who developed BrCa (elevated risk with increasing number of involved relatives). Additionally, this model considers whether a biopsy contained atypical ductal hyperplasia (ADH), which elevates the risk as well. This model has been validated in a population of women undergoing BrCa screening. The initial model considered a 5-year risk of >1.67% as being relevant for concern. Modified 5-year, 10-year, 20-year, and 30-year risk models based on race are available on the National Cancer Institute (NCI) website. While useful, this model has only modest discriminatory ability to inform decision-making that is associated with potential adverse effects. For example, the benefit from tamoxifen chemoprevention therapy in Caucasian women aged 35–70 years based on the Gail risk model is <25% in the at risk population. Tyrer et al. included more risk variables in an attempt to improve the Gail model of risk assessment. The variables, which were obtained from the International BrCa Prevention Study I, included weight, height, family history of ovarian cancer, BrCa in second-degree relatives,

Table 2.2 Gail risk model for predicting BrCa development

Risk factor	Modifier	Risk		
Age at menarche (years)	≥14	1.00		
	12–13	1.10		
	≤12	1.21		
Number of repeat biopsy procedures		Age <50 years		Age ≥50 years
	0	1		1
	1	1.7		1.27
	≥2	2.88		1.62
ADH on biopsy	Absent	0.93		
	Present	1.83		
Age at first live birth (years)		# of first-degree relatives with BrCa		
		0	1	2
	<20	1	2.61	6.80
	20–24	1.24	2.68	5.78
	25–29	1.55	2.76	4.91
	≥30	1.93	2.83	4.17

ADH atypical ductal hyperplasia

age, and unilaterality or bilaterality of BrCa [7]. With addition of these parameters, this model offers a much better cancer prediction for women at average risk because the model used data from BrCa prevention study.

2.7.3 Nipple Aspirate Fluid Cytomorphology for Risk Assessment

The ability to produce NAF is influenced by a number of factors. Cohort selection, increasing number of attempts, spontaneous nipple discharge, contralateral BrCa, young age, prior lactation, and non-Asian descent are all factors associated with increased NAF production. For example, about 80% of women were able to produce NAF after five or more attempts [8]. While 39–66% of women could produce NAF independent of BrCa risk, this percentage increased to 50–95% [9, 10] in women at elevated BrCa risk [1, 8, 11, 12]. Oxytocin nasal spray also increases the volume of NAF [13]. About 53–83% of women are able to produce at least 100 epithelial cells for cytomorphologic analysis, and the median number of epithelial cells in NAF is reported to be 120 [1, 10].

NAF production and epithelial cell analysis has been extensively evaluated for detection of proliferative lesions including atypia. Ample evidence implicates NAF cytomorphological analysis as useful adjunct to BrCa risk assessment. Additionally, incorporating NAF cytology helps stratify risks based on the Gail model. Not only does NAF yield increase with the number of attempts, but the frequency of atypia detection also increases. For example, in women where NAF was collected every

6 months for 2 years, atypia was detected in 6.7% in the initial NAF but increased to 18.2% by the fifth attempt [14]. There is a stepwise increase in relative risk from non-NAF producers to NAF producers without proliferative lesions, with proliferative lesions, and with proliferative lesion and atypia [9]. The presence of atypia was associated with a relative risk five times that of non-NAF-producing women. In a median follow-up of 21 years, the relative risk of BrCa in women producing NAF-containing proliferative lesions with or without atypia was 2.4–2.8-fold than that of non-NAF producers [10]. In a cohort of 6904 women with 100,000 patient years of follow-up, incorporating NAF cytomorphology to the Gail risk model improved model fit [15]. The relative BrCa incidence comparing the highest to the lowest quintile was 3.2 for only the Gail model, but increased to 5.3 when NAF cytology was incorporated in model prediction.

2.7.4 Ductal Lavage Fluid Cytomorphology for Breast Cancer Risk Assessment

DL is usually performed on NAF-producing ducts to obtain epithelial cells for cytomorphologic analysis. In the multicenter study by Dooley and colleagues, 83% of the 500 women at high risk for developing BrCa could produce NAF, of which DL was successfully performed on 92%, with 78% producing enough epithelial cells (>10 cell) for cytomorphologic analysis [1]. This percentage of women producing sufficient cells in DL fluid was superior to that obtained from NAF (27%). The median number of epithelial cells in DL fluid was 4,000 or 13,500 (depending on type of microcatheter used) versus 120 in NAF samples. Cytomorphologic assessment uncovered mostly mild atypia in 8% of NAF and 18% of DL samples; however, concordance was poor between the two sample types. Fifty percent of the women with NAF atypia were sored as benign in their DL samples. Moreover, other investigators have failed to reproduce the high epithelial cell yield by the multicenter study, requiring standardization to DL procedure.

Use of DL atypia in risk assessment had inferior sensitivity to mammography (61–81%) in a population of young screening women [16, 17] or MRI (79%) in a high-risk population [18]. But in young high-risk women, the sensitivity of DL atypia was similar to mammography at 33% [18]. For example, in the study of 44 breasts from 39 women with BrCa, 87% of cancerous breasts produced NAF. However, mild or marked atypia and marked atypia or presence of cancerous cells were observed in 42% and 13%, respectively, of the cases [19]. The sensitivity was 13–42% depending on the definition of threshold of mild or marked atypia used. A number of factors, including duct anatomy and cancer location within the breast, accounted for this low sensitivity of DL. Many ducts are inaccessible by DL, because they either do not communicate with the skin surface or taper to a minute orifice. Only a minority (22%) of ductal carcinoma in situ (DCIS) or invasive BrCa (IBC) involves the nipple or central duct [20]. Moreover, minority of ducts drains the majority of the breast tissue volume [21]. However, it is suggested that standard risk reduction options such as tamoxifen chemoprevention be offered to women with DL-detected atypia [22], while ductoscopy may be offered to women presenting with moderate to marked atypia.

2.7.5 Random Periareolar Fine Needle Aspiration Cytomorphology for Breast Cancer Risk Assessment

The rationale for using RPFNA in BrCa risk assessment is based on the "field effect" concept of breast carcinogenesis, whereby women at elevated risk for developing BrCa will present with multifocal premalignant lesions in both breasts. Multifocal proliferative lesions have been demonstrated in autopsy samples [23, 24] and prophylactic mastectomy tissues from high-risk women [25]. These findings also suggest that women at elevated risk for developing BrCa will harbor high density of these proliferative lesions, which should increase the chances of detecting these lesions using RPFNA.

Studies have affirmed the value of RPFNA cytology and biomarker analysis in BrCa risk assessment. Four-quadrant FNA was performed on first-degree relatives of cancer patients in comparison to age-matched controls with relatives without cancer [26]. This initial study detected proliferative lesions with or without atypia in 35% of the high-risk women who had cancer relatives compared to 13% of the controls. Fabian et al. refined the technique to increase the probability of premalignant lesion detection [27, 28]. Their sampling was based on the frequent anatomic location of BrCa, being highest in the upper-outer followed by the upper-inner quadrants. Thus, two sites at approximately 1 cm from the areolar in both the upper-inner and upper-outer quadrants of both breasts were aspirated. Epithelial cells obtained were pooled, preserved, and used to make up to four slides for cytomorphologic and biomarker analysis. As expected, the number of epithelial cell yield was directly related to the cytomorphology, being highest in the breast with atypia, followed by hyperplasia and nonproliferative lesions. Findings of proliferative breast lesions including hyperplasia and atypia in RPFNA aspirates are also associated with elevated BrCa risk. RPFNA was performed on a cohort of 480 women (60% premenopausal) with median 10-year Gail risk of 4%. A follow-up procedure was performed in 82% of them 6–12 months after the initial, and the results from both combined as baseline dataset. Subjects were then followed and monitored for cancer development. With 94% of subjects producing adequate cells for cytomorphologic analysis, the combined baseline dataset uncovered 30% nonproliferative cytology, 49% hyperplasia, and 21% hyperplasia with atypia. The 21% atypia frequency contrasts with the 12% uncovered in only the initial samples [28]. Thus, multiple sampling increases atypia detection. Women (both premenopausal and postmenopausal) on hormone replacement therapy (HRT) had significantly higher frequency of atypia than postmenopausal women not on HRT ($p = 0.001$) [28]. At 45-month median follow-up, both 10-year Gail risk of >4% and RPFNA atypia could predict the risk of cancer development. Baseline hyperplasia with atypia was predictive of subsequent development of DCIS and/or IBC. Similarly, women with both 10-year Gail risk above 4% and atypia had a 15% incidence of DCIS and/or IBC compared to 4% in those with 10-year Gail risk of less than 4%. Thus, RPFNA cytology could predict subsequent BrCa development as well as stratify women with 10-year Gail risk index of 4% into very high and moderately high-risk groups [28].

2.7.6 Features of Nipple Aspirate Fluid as Breast Cancer Risk Factors

Various characteristics of NAF have been associated with an elevated risk for developing BrCa. The ability to produce NAF, and features of NAF including volume, appearance, cellularity, micronutrients, and microbiome, have all been predictive of BrCa development. The ability to produce NAF depends on a number of factors including age, ethnicity, prior lactation history, early menarche, consumption of high-fat diet, and dietary intake of lactose. Premenopausal women aged 30–50 years who had early menarche and lactated tended to produce more NAF than nulliparous women of comparable age [29]. Moreover, premenopausal nulliparous women of Asian descent are less likely to produce NAF compared to their white American counterparts. NAF micronutrients and estrogen levels have also been associated with BrCa risk. In premenopausal women aged 34–44 years, high dietary fat is positively associated with ease of NAF production. On the contrary, diets high in fruits and vegetables were associated with reduced NAF production and hormone levels [30]. The levels of estrone, estradiol, cholesterol, cholesterol epoxides, and perioxidated lipids, as well as breast surgery or biopsy procedures prior to NAF collection, influence the color of NAF. Thus, the color of NAF varies considerably, from being clear to pale yellow, brown, dark yellow, bloody, black, white, or even green. A study found that the risk for developing BrCa was higher in women who produced bloody (nonsurgery related) or brown nipple discharge than those with creamy, white, or green NAF. Additionally, the frequency of red or brown NAF increased with progression from breast precancer to cancer [31].

Evidence has implicated gut microbial dysbiosis as risk factor of BrCa. Indeed, NAF microbiome may also be associated with elevated BrCa risk. One study found ductal microbiome to be distinctly different from the microbiome of nipple and areolar [32], and there may be differences in the incidence of particular microbial genus between BrCa patients and healthy control women.

2.8 Breast Cancer Biomarkers in Nipple Aspirate Fluid

Cytologic and ploidy image analysis of both NAF and DL fluid samples complement each other to enhance sensitivity of cancer detection. Except in high-risk population, cytologic analysis of breast proximal fluids is prohibitive for screening purposes. Atypical cells from benign breast lesions such as papilloma can confound diagnosis by creating false-positive calls. Thus, molecular signature biomarkers should complement these procedures even in the above-average-risk woman.

Proteins from ductal epithelial cells are the major constituents of NAF. Thus, proteins are more abundant in NAF than plasma, with NAF protein concentration being as high as 170 mg/ml [33]. BrCa protein biomarkers identified in NAF include testosterone, prostate-specific antigen (PSA), superoxide dismutase 1 (SOD1), protein deglycase DJ-1 or Parkinson disease protein 7 (PARK7), cytokines, Thomsen-Friedenreich (TFr) and Tn antigens, urokinase-type plasminogen activator (uPA), plasminogen activator inhibitor-1 (PAI-1), ferritin (FTN), serotransferrin (TF), and C-reactive protein (CRP). In addition to these proteins, proteomic approaches have been applied to identify candidate protein profiles in NAF. Testosterone levels in NAF could predict BrCa risk in postmenopausal women [34]. Additionally, non-albumin-bound or free testosterone in NAF was much higher in premenopausal women with BrCa and may therefore be a predictive biomarker in this population [35]. TFr proteins and Tn antigens are O-linked monosaccharide or disaccharide associated with cell surface glycoproteins. These proteins have been linked to progression of skin, breast, colorectal, and prostate cancers. Analysis of NAF from women with BrCa and non-cancerous controls found that over 90% of cancer patients had high levels of both proteins compared to healthy control women [36]. Even in women with atypia, the levels of TFr and Tn antigens were much higher than healthy control women, and TFr was found to be more predictive of atypical hyperplasia and BrCa than Tn antigens [37]. The levels of the prostate cancer biomarker, PSA or KLK3, in NAF may also be a BrCa biomarker. While elevated in men with prostate cancer, PSA levels are lower in NAF from women with precancerous lesions and invasive BrCa than healthy controls [8], and the levels are inversely proportional to tumor stage, size, nodal status, and distant metastasis [38]. It is established that levels of cellular reactive oxygen species (ROS) can mediate cancer initiation and progression and levels of redox antioxidant enzymes in NAF are suggested to be predictive of BrCa risk. Thus, the levels of the antioxidant enzyme, SOD1, were low in NAF from women with compared to those without BrCa [39]. In contrast, the levels of the antioxidant oncoprotein, DJ-1, were high in NAF from BrCa patients compared to women with benign papillomas [40].

Inflammatory and immune mediators in NAF have been explored as BrCa biomarkers. While levels of cytokines and chemokines in NAF from cancerous and non-cancerous women do not significantly differ, it appears that levels of aluminum in NAF might influence cytokine levels. Thus, NAF from BrCa women with high levels of aluminum as component of breast micronutrient demonstrated higher levels of IL-1β, IL-6, IL-8, IL-12, p70, TNF-α, MCP1, and MIP-1α than cancer patients with low aluminum levels [41]. Iron metabolism might be important in BrCa progression, because BrCa cells expressed higher levels of transferrin receptors and also contained higher levels of transferrin (TF) and ferritin (FTN) than normal breast epithelial cells [42]. Thus, TF and FTN have been explored in NAF as BrCa biomarkers. A preliminary study found high levels of both proteins in NAF from postmenopausal BrCa patients compared to normal controls [43]. PAI-1 may promote BrCa invasion, and significantly higher levels of both PAI-1 and uPA have been detected in NAF from BrCa women [44, 45]. Elevated CRP in NAF has been positively correlated with Gail model of BrCa risk [46].

Application of proteomics technologies using NAF has enabled discovery of potential BrCa biomarkers. Because initial experiments failed to uncover differences in NAF proteome between BrCa patients and healthy controls, improvements were made to protocols and instrumentation that subsequently enabled identification of discriminatory biomarkers. Differential protein profiles were observed in NAF from women with and without BrCa [47]. Additionally, differences in protein patterns were demonstrated in NAF from healthy controls and women with early-stage BrCa. However, in the disease cohort, no differences were observed between the involved and contralateral uninvolved breast [48], probably due to field cancerization. Five differentially expressed protein profiles were demonstrable in NAF from over 75% of women with IBC compared to <10% of NAF from healthy controls [49]. Using ion trap mass spectrometry (MS) to analyze immune-depleted NAF samples enabled identification of 64 candidate BrCa protein biomarkers. Of interest, 15 of these proteins including osteopontin and cathepsin D had previously been demonstrated to have altered expression in primary BrCa tissues and sera from patients [50]. Alexander et al. used 2D PAGE separation of proteins followed by in-gel trypsinization and MALDI-TOF MS to uncover 41 altered components in NAF from BrCa women. Prolactin-inducible protein, apolipoprotein D, and α1-acidic glycoprotein were among the proteins that were demonstrated to correlate with cancer stage and menopausal status [51]. With optimized protocols, the number of proteins/peptides identified in NAF has increased considerably. Isotope-coded affinity tag (ICAT) tandem MS analysis of NAF identified 353 peptides from 39 proteins in NAF from BrCa patients. Specifically altered in NAF from BrCa women were increased lipophilin B, β-globin, hemopexin, and vitamin D binding protein, as well as decreased α-2-HS-glycoprotein [52]. Another pilot study of NAF using LTQ-Orbitrap XL MS was successful in identifying 854 unique proteins. Similarly, this signature also included established BrCa biomarkers such as cathepsin D, tissue plasminogen activator (tPA), and uPA [53]. Brunoro et al. uncovered 557 differential levels of proteins in NAF from BrCa patients [54]. Shaheed and colleagues also uncovered over 1,900 unique NAF protein profiles involved in multiple cell biologic processes [55]. These include established BrCa biomarkers, growth factors, and cell adhesion molecules. Additionally, 46 candidate BrCa biomarkers were uncovered and evaluated by the National Cancer Institute-Early Detection Research Network (NCI-EDRN) program. Another preliminary investigation that compared NAF samples from healthy women and those with benign lesions, DCIS, or IBC uncovered more than 1,200 proteins per sample [55]. Matched NAF samples were similar in profile, but significant variations were found between individuals. This finding was consistent with another study of NAF using SDS-PAGE and 2D-DIGE [56].

2.9 Breast Cancer Biomarkers in Ductal Lavage Fluid

Ductal lavage proteomics have been unfavorable due to protein dilution by the lavage fluid. However, an improved ductal aspiration with multiple collections increased the recovery rate in up to 90% of women [57]. Additionally, this approach yielded over 1000 cells with 50% of the women producing >20,000 cells at 80–100% epithelial cell purity, suitable for biomarker exploration.

Biomarkers of epigenetic and metabolic alterations in BrCa have been successfully explored in DL fluid samples. Gene promoter methylation was assessed in DL fluid from women with known *BRCA1* and *BRCA2* mutations. Methylation of *CDKN2A* was associated with known *BRCA1* mutation status and in women with history of contralateral BrCa [58]. *RASSF1A* methylation in DL fluid was also associated with development of BrCa. Another epigenetic biomarker in DL fluid is miRNA alterations. Profiling of 742 miRNAs in DL fluid identified differential levels of 17 between cancer and paired normal samples [59]. Systems biology analysis implicated these altered miRNAs in MAPK, ERB, PI3K-AKT, p53, mTOR, TFGβ, and WNT signaling pathways involved in breast carcinogenesis. Moreover, some of these DL fluid miRNAs have been detected in other body fluids including plasma (miR-200a), breast milk (miR-181a), and serum (miR-23b, miR-133b, miR-181a, miR-338-3p, and miR-625) samples from BrCa patients.

Untargeted metabolomic analysis of DL fluid identified endogenous BrCa metabolites to include amino acid derivatives such as N-acetyl-DL-tryptophan and products of lipid metabolism including N-linoleoyl taurine, trans-2-dodecenoylcarnitine, lysophosphatidylcholine, glycerophospholipids, and phosphatidylserine [60]. Controlling for race, menopausal status, smoking, tumor grade, and TNM stage, 21 metabolites were selected for predictive conditional logistic regression model, which provided diagnostic performance at a sensitivity, specificity, and area under the receiver operating characteristic curve (AUROCC) of 90.7%, 88.4%, and 0.959%, respectively, for BrCa detection.

In a study using DL fluid to measure biomarkers of tamoxifen action (ERα, Ki-67, and cyclooxygenase-2), greater reductions in Ki-67 and ERα in the tamoxifen compared to control observation group were uncovered [61]. However, the authors concluded that DL fluid was unsuitable for longitudinal patient monitoring because of poor reproducibility of biomarkers in the observation group, the high (53%) attrition rate from recruitment to biomarker analysis, and the cost implications of the procedure.

2.10 Breast Cancer Biomarkers in Random Periareolar Fine Needle Aspiration Fluid

Developed by Carol J. Fabian in 1998, RPFNA is used to sample cells from the breast of asymptomatic women at an elevated risk for developing BrCa [27, 28]. While this procedure may be useful in this population of women, it is unlikely to be a screening procedure for women at an average risk of developing BrCa, due to the discomfort associated with the procedure.

The RPFNA procedure requires anesthetization of the breast with 1% lidocaine followed by five needle aspirations on the lateral breast and four from the medial aspect of each breast. The advantage of this procedure is that the cell yield is higher than in DL fluid, and the procedure can be performed in almost all women. However, the aspirate contains heterogeneous cells, including epithelial, stromal, adipose, and immune cells that may introduce high background noise in molecular analysis [28]. Zalles et al. performed a clinical trial of RPFNA on 480 women at elevated risk for BrCa (10 year Gail risk of 4%) and concluded that the procedure increased detection of cytological atypia [64]. Indeed, 20 women from this cohort subsequently developed DCIS or invasive BrCa after 45 months of follow-up. In 119 high-risk women on chemoprevention trial with α-difluoromethylornithine (DFMO), RPFNA cytology and molecular markers, including TP53, PCNA, and EGFR failed to demonstrate any change [65]. Proteomic studies have also been performed on RPFNA samples with identification of up to 60 phosphoproteins [66]. Apart from identifying women at elevated risk for BrCa, profiling of RPFNA fluid from precancerous lesions should enable discovery of early BrCa biomarkers.

2.11 Breast Cancer Biomarkers in Other Breast Proximal Fluids

Although less common, BrCa biomarkers have also been assayed in breast cystic fluids, milk, and colostrum. Two types of breast cysts are recognized based on morphological and cellular features: type I or apocrine and type II cysts. Apocrine cysts have higher $K+/Na +$ ratio than type II cysts. Ample evidence suggests apocrine cysts are related to BrCa risk. Over 81 proteins have been identified in cystic breast fluids, with prolactin-inducible protein, albumin, apolipoprotein, and zinc-α2-glycoprotein being the most abundant. However, only 3-hydroxymethylglutaryl-CoA reductase and 15-hydroxy-prostaglandin dehydrogenase in cystic fluid have been associated with primary BrCa [62]. These metabolites were specifically expressed by apocrine type I cysts, as well as apocrine metaplastic cells in type II microcysts, terminal ducts, and intraductal papillary lesions. More studies are required to identify cystic fluid proteins that carry risk for BrCa development. Proteomic studies have identified over 1000 proteins in milk and over 100 in colostrum for non-oncologic applications. Because BrCa is rare in lactating mothers, cancer biomarker discovery using these fluids is uncommon. However, profiling of milk proteins in a small cohort of lactating women with BrCa identified unique proteins [63].

2.12 Clinical Translation of Commercial Products

As a result of the extensive exploration and validation works on breast proximal fluids, a number of these efforts have been translated into patient care. Among these are HALO® Breast Pap test and the Mammary Aspirate Specimen Cytology Test (MASCT) systems.

2.12.1 *HALO® Breast Pap Test*

Neomatrix developed the HALO® Breast Pap test for quick noninvasive collection of NAF for cytologic examination and BrCa risk assessment. The HALO® nipple aspiration fluid system is an FDA-approved device that is easy to use in any family practice office. It requires no specialization for an attendant to operate, and it is a mobile device such that it can be moved from room to room. The device has three components: (i) a console that is controlled by microprocessor to monitor the aspiration event and maintain specific requirements for delivery of temperature and compression, (ii) a patient interface cassette that has adjustable breast cups to fit any breast, and a fluid reservoir, and (iii) disposable sample collection cups, swabs, and pads for preparing the breasts. The fluid reservoir is connected to the console via connection tubes that enable the delivery of warmth, suction, and massage. The cups are replaced every 2–3 months. Operating the HALO® NAF collecting system is easy such that many attendants at the primary practice office can operate it. To operrate the system, disposable sample collection cups are inserted into the adjustable breast cups. The nipples are then cleansed with alcohol swaps. The adjustable cups are comfortably placed on the patient's breast. The HALO® console is then operated. It automatically generates gentle suction on both breasts and simultaneously warms and massages the breasts to aspirate NAF. At the end of each of the 5-minute cycle, the cups are removed and the aspirated NAF is collected using a swab. The collected samples are placed in a fluid-containing cytology vial, labeled, and shipped for analysis.

2.12.2 *Mammary Aspirate Specimen Cytology Test System*

Atossa Genetics Inc. has patented technologies for the collection of NAF samples for cytologic and "omic" analyses as risk assessment tools for BrCa detection. The name "Atossa" signifies the first woman to be diagnosed with BrCa (~470 BC). She was the daughter of Cyrus the Great and wife of King Darius I. The company has developed an FDA-cleared device and system for NAF collection and analysis named Mammary Aspirate Specimen Cytology Test (MASCT) system. As with all NAF aspiration, the device uses cycles of negative pressure (similar to breast suckling by a baby) to extract NAF from the ducts by capillary action. The MASCT device augments NAF yield by employing a hydrophilic membrane that comes into contact with the nipple. The device enables NAF collection at the point-of-care in just 10 min (5 min per breast). It is easy to use, requiring no special training. Because of the ease and rapidity of NAF collection, the procedure fits well within a woman's clinic visit for regular mammography, Pap smear, or just annual physical examination. The device is able to collect between 1 and 37 ul of NAF (average 7 ul) in over 90% of women.

2.12.3 BCtect Test

While not based on breast proximal fluids, the BCtect test is another noninvasive commercial system for BrCa risk assessment. With the concept that diseases react, and the body responds by producing unique imprints that circulate, DiaGenic has developed tests based on proprietary circulating markers of various diseases. One such test is the BCtect for breast cancer that is based on expression profiling of unique circulating BrCa markers. In a multicenter (five sites) validation study based on qPCR targeting 96 genes (includes control genes), the CE-marked test detected early stage cancer (stage 0 and 1) and lobar carcinoma in women (premenopausal and postmenopausal) with an accuracy of 75–85%. Turnaround time is 7 days from sample shipment to core laboratory. Results are reported as normal (negative) or abnormal (positive) and interpreted in conjunction with other tests and patient clinical information.

2.13 Summary

- Malignant transformation of breast epithelial cells remains the number one cause of cancer in women.
- Improved management has led to increased prevalence of BrCa, despite its associated morbidity and socioeconomic and psychological impacts.
- Biomarkers that enable detection of curable premalignant lesions are currently needed.
- Biomarkers enriched in breast proximal fluids are available for risk assessment in the above-average-risk woman.
- Because of its noninvasive mode of acquisition, NAF biomarkers should be acceptable for BrCa screening, especially in premenopausal NAF-producing women with dense breast tissue that hampers mammographic sensitivity in cancer detection.
- In expert centers, proximal fluid biomarkers augment cytomorphology in BrCa risk management.

- The global burden of BrCa will benefit from leveraging technologies that enable screening of all women at risk, especially those in low-to-medium human development index countries and other remote areas.
- Technologies such as HALO®Breast Pap test (Neomatrix) and MASCT (Atossa Genetics) are useful BrCa risk assessment tools using NAF.
- Making the above technologies available to women in low-to-medium HDI countries where BrCa incidence is equally on the rise but with limited resources is strongly recommended.

References

1. Dooley WC, Ljung BM, Veronesi U, et al. Ductal lavage for detection of cellular atypia in women at high risk for breast cancer. J Natl Cancer Inst. 2001;93:1624–32.
2. Francescatti DS, Kluskens L, Shah L. Ductal lavage using medically aseptic technique in women at high risk for breast cancer. Clin Breast Cancer. 2004;5:299–302.
3. Bhandare D, Nayar R, Bryk M, et al. Endocrine biomarkers in ductal lavage samples from women at high risk for breast cancer. Cancer Epidemiol Biomark Prev. 2005;14:2620–7.
4. Page DL. Cancer risk assessment in benign breast biopsies. Hum Pathol. 1986;17:871–4.
5. Dupont WD, Parl FF, Hartmann WH, et al. Breast cancer risk associated with proliferative breast disease and atypical hyperplasia. Cancer. 1993;71:1258–65.
6. Masood S, Frykberg ER, McLellan GL, et al. Prospective evaluation of radiologically directed fine-needle aspiration biopsy of nonpalpable breast lesions. Cancer. 1990;66:1480–7.
7. Tyrer J, Duffy SW, Cuzick J. A breast cancer prediction model incorporating familial and personal risk factors. Stat Med. 2004;23:1111–30.
8. Sauter ER, Daly M, Linahan K, et al. Prostate-specific antigen levels in nipple aspirate fluid correlate with breast cancer risk. Cancer Epidemiol Biomark Prev. 1996;5:967–70.
9. Wrensch MR, Petrakis NL, King EB, et al. Breast cancer incidence in women with abnormal cytology in nipple aspirates of breast fluid. Am J Epidemiol. 1992;135:130–41.
10. Wrensch MR, Petrakis NL, Miike R, et al. Breast cancer risk in women with abnormal cytology in nipple aspirates of breast fluid. J Natl Cancer Inst. 2001;93:1791–8.
11. Kurian AW, Mills MA, Jaffee M, et al. Ductal lavage of fluid-yielding and non-fluid-yielding ducts in BRCA1 and BRCA2 mutation carriers and other women at high inherited breast cancer risk. Cancer Epidemiol Biomark Prev. 2005;14:1082–9.
12. Sharma P, Klemp JR, Simonsen M, et al. Failure of high risk women to produce nipple aspirate fluid does not exclude detection of cytologic atypia in random periareolar fine needle aspiration specimens. Breast Cancer Res Treat. 2004;87:59–64.
13. Zhang L, Shao ZM, Beatty P, et al. The use of oxytocin in nipple fluid aspiration. Breast J. 2003;9:266–8.
14. King EB, Chew KL, Hom JD, et al. Multiple sampling for increasing the diagnostic sensitivity of nipple aspirate fluid for atypical cytology. Acta Cytol. 2004;48:813–7.
15. Tice JA, Miike R, Adduci K, et al. Nipple aspirate fluid cytology and the Gail model for breast cancer risk assessment in a screening population. Cancer Epidemiol Biomark Prev. 2005;14:324–8.
16. Humphrey LL, Helfand M, Chan BK, Woolf SH. Breast cancer screening: a summary of the evidence for the U.S. preventive services task force. Ann Intern Med. 2002;137:347–60.
17. Carney WP, Neumann R, Lipton A, et al. Potential clinical utility of serum HER-2/neu oncoprotein concentrations in patients with breast cancer. Clin Chem. 2003;49:1579–98.

18. Kriege M, Brekelmans CT, Boetes C, et al. Efficacy of MRI and mammography for breast-cancer screening in women with a familial or genetic predisposition. N Engl J Med. 2004;351:427–37.
19. Khan SA, Wiley EL, Rodriguez N, et al. Ductal lavage findings in women with known breast cancer undergoing mastectomy. J Natl Cancer Inst. 2004;96:1510–7.
20. Badve S, Wiley E, Rodriguez N. Assessment of utility of ductal lavage and ductoscopy in breast cancer-a retrospective analysis of mastectomy specimens. Mod Pathol. 2003;16:206–9.
21. Going JJ, Moffat DF. Escaping from Flatland: clinical and biological aspects of human mammary duct anatomy in three dimensions. J Pathol. 2004;203:538–44.
22. O'Shaughnessy JA, Ljung BM, Dooley WC, et al. Ductal lavage and the clinical management of women at high risk for breast carcinoma: a commentary. Cancer. 2002;94:292–8.
23. Bhathal PS, Brown RW, Lesueur GC, Russell IS. Frequency of benign and malignant breast lesions in 207 consecutive autopsies in Australian women. Br J Cancer. 1985;51:271–8.
24. Nielsen M, Thomsen JL, Primdahl S, et al. Breast cancer and atypia among young and middle-aged women: a study of 110 medicolegal autopsies. Br J Cancer. 1987;56:814–9.
25. Hoogerbrugge N, Bult P, de Widt-Levert LM, et al. High prevalence of premalignant lesions in prophylactically removed breasts from women at hereditary risk for breast cancer. J Clin Oncol. 2003;21:41–5.
26. Skolnick MH, Cannon-Albright LA, Goldgar DE, et al. Inheritance of proliferative breast disease in breast cancer kindreds. Science. 1990;250:1715–20.
27. Fabian CJ, Zalles C, Kamel S, et al. Prevalence of aneuploidy, overexpressed ER, and overexpressed EGFR in random breast aspirates of women at high and low risk for breast cancer. Breast Cancer Res Treat. 1994;30:263–74.
28. Fabian CJ, Kimler BF, Zalles CM, et al. Short-term breast cancer prediction by random periareolar fine-needle aspiration cytology and the Gail risk model. J Natl Cancer Inst. 2000;92:1217–27.
29. Zhao YS, Pang D, Wang F, et al. Nipple aspirate fluid collection, related factors and relationship between carcinoembryonic antigen in nipple aspirate fluid and breast diseases in women in Harbin, PRC. Cancer Epidemiol Biomark Prev. 2009;18:732–8.
30. Djuric Z, Chen G, Ren J, et al. Effects of high fruit-vegetable and/or low-fat intervention on breast nipple aspirate fluid micronutrient levels. Cancer Epidemiol Biomark Prev. 2007;16:1393–9.
31. Sauter ER, Winn JN, Dale PS, Wagner-Mann C. Nipple aspirate fluid color is associated with breast cancer. Cancer Detect Prev. 2006;30:322–8.
32. Chan AA, Bashir M, Rivas MN, et al. Characterization of the microbiome of nipple aspirate fluid of breast cancer survivors. Sci Rep. 2016;6:28061.
33. Djuric Z, Visscher DW, Heilbrun LK, et al. Influence of lactation history on breast nipple aspirate fluid yields and fluid composition. Breast J. 2005;11:92–9.
34. Sauter ER, Babb J, Daly M, et al. Prostate-specific antigen production in the female breast: association with progesterone. Cancer Epidemiol Biomark Prev. 1998;7:315–20.
35. Sauter ER, Tichansky DS, Chervoneva I, Diamandis EP. Circulating testosterone and prostate-specific antigen in nipple aspirate fluid and tissue are associated with breast cancer. Environ Health Perspect. 2002;110:241–6.
36. Kumar SR, Sauter ER, Quinn TP, Deutscher SL. Thomsen-Friedenreich and Tn antigens in nipple fluid: carbohydrate biomarkers for breast cancer detection. Clin Cancer Res. 2005;11:6868–71.
37. Deutscher SL, Dickerson M, Gui G, et al. Carbohydrate antigens in nipple aspirate fluid predict the presence of atypia and cancer in women requiring diagnostic breast biopsy. BMC Cancer. 2010;10:519.
38. Sauter ER, Klein G, Wagner-Mann C, Diamandis EP. Prostate-specific antigen expression in nipple aspirate fluid is associated with advanced breast cancer. Cancer Detect Prev. 2004;28:27–31.

39. Mannello F, Tonti GA, Pederzoli A, et al. Detection of superoxide dismutase-1 in nipple aspirate fluids: a reactive oxygen species-regulating enzyme in the breast cancer microenvironment. Clin Breast Cancer. 2010;10:238–45.
40. Oda M, Makita M, Iwaya K, et al. High levels of DJ-1 protein in nipple fluid of patients with breast cancer. Cancer Sci. 2012;103:1172–6.
41. Mannello F, Ligi D, Canale M. Aluminium, carbonyls and cytokines in human nipple aspirate fluids: possible relationship between inflammation, oxidative stress and breast cancer microenvironment. J Inorg Biochem. 2013;128:250–6.
42. Kabat GC, Miller AB, Jain M, Rohan TE. Dietary iron and heme iron intake and risk of breast cancer: a prospective cohort study. Cancer Epidemiol Biomark Prev. 2007;16:1306–8.
43. Mannello F, Tonti GA, Medda V, et al. Analysis of aluminium content and iron homeostasis in nipple aspirate fluids from healthy women and breast cancer-affected patients. J Appl Toxicol. 2011;31:262–9.
44. Duffy MJ. Urokinase plasminogen activator and its inhibitor, PAI-1, as prognostic markers in breast cancer: from pilot to level 1 evidence studies. Clin Chem. 2002;48:1194–7.
45. Qin W, Gui G, Zhang K, et al. Proteins and carbohydrates in nipple aspirate fluid predict the presence of atypia and cancer in women requiring diagnostic breast biopsy. BMC Cancer. 2012;12:52.
46. Lithgow D, Nyamathi A, Elashoff D, et al. C-reactive protein in nipple aspirate fluid associated with Gail model factors. Biol Res Nurs. 2007;9:108–16.
47. Paweletz CP, Trock B, Pennanen M, et al. Proteomic patterns of nipple aspirate fluids obtained by SELDI-TOF: potential for new biomarkers to aid in the diagnosis of breast cancer. Dis Markers. 2001;17:301–7.
48. Pawlik TM, Fritsche H, Coombes KR, et al. Significant differences in nipple aspirate fluid protein expression between healthy women and those with breast cancer demonstrated by time-of-flight mass spectrometry. Breast Cancer Res Treat. 2005;89:149–57.
49. Sauter ER, Zhu W, Fan XJ, et al. Proteomic analysis of nipple aspirate fluid to detect biologic markers of breast cancer. Br J Cancer. 2002;86:1440–3.
50. Varnum SM, Covington CC, Woodbury RL, et al. Proteomic characterization of nipple aspirate fluid: identification of potential biomarkers of breast cancer. Breast Cancer Res Treat. 2003;80:87–97.
51. Alexander H, Stegner AL, Wagner-Mann C, et al. Proteomic analysis to identify breast cancer biomarkers in nipple aspirate fluid. Clin Cancer Res. 2004;10:7500–10.
52. Pawlik TM, Hawke DH, Liu Y, et al. Proteomic analysis of nipple aspirate fluid from women with early-stage breast cancer using isotope-coded affinity tags and tandem mass spectrometry reveals differential expression of vitamin D binding protein. BMC Cancer. 2006;6:68.
53. Pavlou MP, Kulasingam V, Sauter ER, et al. Nipple aspirate fluid proteome of healthy females and patients with breast cancer. Clin Chem. 2010;56:848–55.
54. Brunoro GV, Carvalho PC, Ferreira AT, et al. Proteomic profiling of nipple aspirate fluid (NAF): exploring the complementarity of different peptide fractionation strategies. J Proteome. 2015;117:86–94.
55. Shaheed SU, Tait C, Kyriacou K et al. Nipple aspirate fluid-A liquid biopsy for diagnosing breast health. Proteomics Clin Appl 2017;11:9–10.
56. Brunoro GV, Ferreira AT, Trugilho MR, et al. Potential correlation between tumor aggressiveness and protein expression patterns of nipple aspirate fluid (NAF) revealed by gel-based proteomic analysis. Curr Top Med Chem. 2014;14:359–68.
57. Danforth DN, Warner AC, Wangsa D, et al. An improved breast epithelial sampling method for molecular profiling and biomarker analysis in women at risk for breast cancer. Breast Cancer (Auckl). 2015;9:31–40.
58. Antill YC, Mitchell G, Johnson SA, et al. Gene methylation in breast ductal fluid from BRCA1 and BRCA2 mutation carriers. Cancer Epidemiol Biomark Prev. 2010;19:265–74.
59. Do Canto LM, Marian C, Willey S, et al. MicroRNA analysis of breast ductal fluid in breast cancer patients. Int J Oncol. 2016;48:2071–8.

60. Matos Do Canto L, Marian C, Varghese RS, et al. Metabolomic profiling of breast tumors using ductal fluid. Int J Oncol. 2016;49:2245–54.
61. Khan SA, Lankes HA, Patil DB, et al. Ductal lavage is an inefficient method of biomarker measurement in high-risk women. Cancer Prev Res (Phila). 2009;2:265–73.
62. Celis JE, Gromov P, Moreira JM, et al. Apocrine cysts of the breast: biomarkers, origin, enlargement, and relation with cancer phenotype. Mol Cell Proteomics. 2006;5:462–83.
63. Schneider SS, Aslebagh R, Ngounou Wetie AG, et al. Using breast milk to assess breast cancer risk: the role of mass spectrometry-based proteomics. Adv Exp Med Biol. 2014;806:399–408.
64. Zalles CM, Kimler BF, Simonsen M, et al. Comparison of cytomorphology in specimens obtained by random periareolar fine needle aspiration and ductal lavage from women at high risk for development of breast cancer. Breast Cancer Res Treat. 2006;97:191–7.
65. Fabian CJ, Kimler BF, Brady DA, et al. A phase II breast cancer chemoprevention trial of oral alpha-difluoromethylornithine: breast tissue, imaging, and serum and urine biomarkers. Clin Cancer Res. 2002;8:3105–17.
66. Ibarra-Drendall C, Troch MM, Barry WT, et al. Pilot and feasibility study: prospective proteomic profiling of mammary epithelial cells from high-risk women provides evidence of activation of pro-survival pathways. Breast Cancer Res Treat. 2012;132:487–98.

Chapter 3
Head and Neck Cancer Biomarkers in Proximal Fluids

3.1 Introduction

According to GLOBOCAN 2018, head and neck cancers (HNCs) were the sixth most common cancer globally, with reported incidence, mortality, and 5-year prevalence of 887,659, 453,307, and 2,287,731, respectively. The annual global incidence, mortality, and 5-year prevalence according to anatomic sites were, respectively, 354,864, 177,384, and 913,514 for lip and oral; 177,422, 94,771, and 488,900 for laryngeal; 129,079, 172,987, and 362,219 for nasopharyngeal; 92,887, 51,005, and 280,508 for oropharyngeal; 80,608, 34,984, and 119,130 for hypopharyngeal; and 52,799, 22,176, and 123,460 for salivary gland cancers. The prevalence of HNC is higher in males than females, with a male-to-female ratio of about 3:1, which may reflect sex differences in risk-factor associated habits. High incident rates of up to 20 per 100,000 are observed in Central and Eastern Europe, Germany, Denmark, Scotland, Italy, Spain, France, Brazil, Hong Kong, the Indian subcontinent, South Africa, and Australia.

HNCs arise in epithelial lining of the upper aerodigestive tract. However, the commonest anatomic sites of HNC are the oral cavity (with over 250,000 cases diagnosed each year), larynx, nasopharynx, and oropharynx. It should be noted, however, that the etiologic and molecular features differ considerably among these cancer types. For example, salivary gland tumors are biologically distinct. The majority of HNC (>90%) is of squamous cell histology, and hence they are referred to as head and neck squamous cell carcinoma (HNSCC).

Known risk factors for developing oral squamous cell carcinoma (OSCC) include environmental and lifestyle factors, as well as genetic predisposition from mutations in genes such as *PIK3CA*, *TP53*, *CDKN2A*, and *FAT1*. Tobacco use is associated with oral and laryngeal cancers, while excess alcohol consumption causes more pharyngeal and laryngeal tumors. Additionally, human papillomavirus (HPV) infection of the oropharynx is an etiologic agent for oropharyngeal squamous cell carcinoma (OPSCC), while nasopharyngeal Epstein-Barr virus (EBV) infections

G. D. Dakubo, *Cancer Biomarkers in Body Fluids*,
https://doi.org/10.1007/978-3-030-24725-6_3

account for the majority of nasopharyngeal carcinoma (NPC), especially in endemic areas. HNCs are heterogeneous; however, based on etiology and molecular pathology, two main groups are currently established: non-HPV and HPV-positive cancers. With increasing education and adherence to tobacco cessation, the incidence of non-HPV cancers is declining; however, that of HPV-mediated OPSCC is on the rise, especially in the Western world.

Modern salvage or organ-sparing surgeries coupled with chemoradiation are improving the quality of life for patients with HNC, although no change in the overall survival rate is accomplished due probably to the concept of "field cancerization," whereby a vast expanse of the oral epithelium is at an elevated risk for developing cancer due to carcinogen exposure. Thus, locoregional recurrences are common. Additionally, the 5-year survival rate is about 60%, and this declines with advanced tumor stage. Thus, biomarkers that can be used for early detection (when treatment, including administration of chemopreventive remedies, is optimal), prognosis, and therapy selection can improve patient management and hence survival. Noninvasive screening assays targeting biomarkers in saliva or blood among high-risk groups such as smokers, excessive alcohol users, and those involved in oral sex, as well as individuals in endemic areas of EBV infections, could lead to early detection, with possible curative interventions, given that only 33% of all cases are currently detected at an early stage.

Early detection and personalized or precision medicine will benefit from point-of-care diagnostic and monitoring tools. The use of portable devices to assess and monitor health status of an individual should enhance early detection and timely provision of individualized care based on disease characteristics. Salivary point-of-care tools based on technologies such as microfluidics, electrochemistry, photometric portable biosensors, and electronic noses are being developed. One such potential development is the electric field-induced release and measurement (EFIRM) technology. EFIRM is an electrochemical detection system developed at the University of California, Los Angeles, that uses immobilized probes and readout enzymes to detect biomarkers in body fluids.

Given the origins of saliva, this fluid may not only be amenable to detection and management of cancers of the oral cavity, salivary glands, and larynx but also cancers located elsewhere in the body. Thus, although this chapter is focused on HNC biomarkers in saliva, it also briefly examines biomarkers of other cancers in saliva.

3.2 Saliva

Saliva is a complex biological fluid primarily produced by the major and minor salivary glands as a filtrate of blood (Fig. 3.1). It, however, receives inputs from other sources, which reflect on its chemical, molecular, and cellular composition. In addition to salivary glandular secretions are those from gingival crevices and the nasopharynx, as well as oral mucosal transudates, erythrocytes and leukocytes, desquamated oral epithelial cells, bacteria, and transiently ingested substances such as food and drugs. The diverse source of whole saliva is also the basis for the

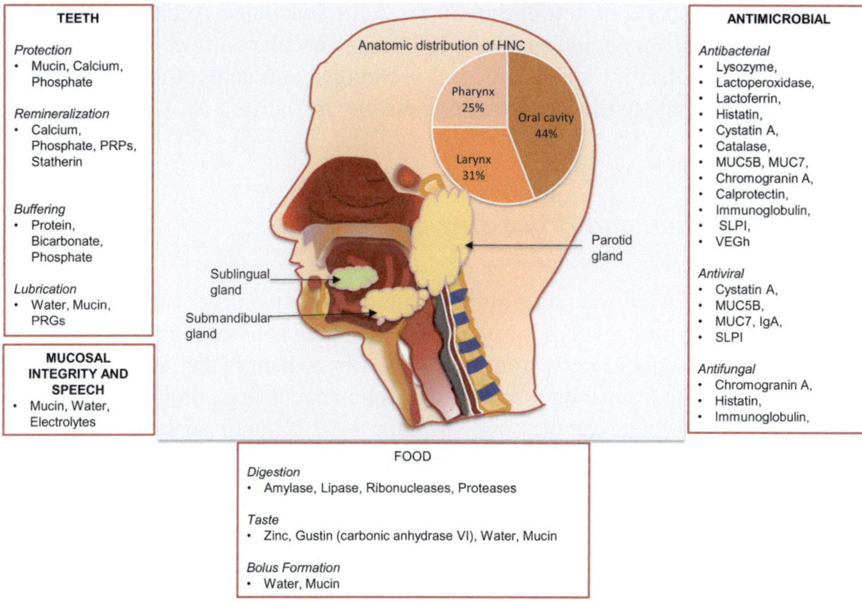

Fig. 3.1 Salivary glands and anatomic distribution of head and neck cancer. Illustrated are the major functions of saliva

discipline of "salivary diagnostics," whereby this medium is amenable not only for the detection of oral cancer but also the diagnosis of cancers located elsewhere in the body, as well as dental, infectious, metabolic, renal, cardiovascular, and several other diseases, and in drug and toxicology testing.

While primarily composed of water (98–99%) and electrolytes (1–2%), saliva also contains several compounds including mucus (mucopolysaccharides and glycoproteins), cytokines, minerals, digestive enzymes, growth factors, nucleic acids, as well as antibacterial agents (IgA and H_2O_2) and enzymes (lysozyme, thiocyanate, lactoferrin, and lactoperoxidases) that serve numerous functions. This oral fluid serves the important functions of oral lubrication, food digestion, and protection against microbial invasion. While its main function is to lubricate the mouth, saliva also plays an important role of beginning food digestion (carbohydrates by amylases and fat by lipases). About a liter of saliva is produced each day, with most (about 75%) produced by the submandibular gland and the rest by the parotid, sublingual, and other minor salivary glands. Each millimeter of saliva contains about 8 million human and 500 bacterial cells. The composition of saliva varies with age, gender, diet, circadian rhythm, and physiological state. Also stimulated and non-stimulated saliva may vary in composition.

There are diverse sources of biomarkers in saliva. The different origins of whole saliva suggest biomarkers in this medium are equally from different sources reflective of the local head and neck environment as well as the systemic circulation. Filtration of blood in salivary glands produces a significant portion of salivary biomarkers. These circulating biomarkers in saliva could be produced by passive diffusion, active transport, or ultrafiltration via tight junctions. Adding to this are secretions from salivary gland epithelial cells and crevicular outflow. Within the oral cavity, local cell death, trauma, mucosal secretions, and active transport mechanisms also contribute to the biomarker composition of saliva.

3.2.1 Collection and Processing of Saliva

Saliva can be collected with or without induction. Sample processing ought to be performed within minutes to hours of collection. This is usually accomplished by centrifugation to separate cells from fluid. The supernatant is then gently removed and transferred into a separate tube. A stabilization agent (e.g., protease inhibitors) could be added to both samples and stored at −80 °C until analysis. While not encouraged, freeze-thaw for up to five cycles may not affect proteome and metabolome biomarkers; however, nucleic acid biomarkers may lose integrity.

3.2.2 Salivary Diagnostics

Saliva is similar to the skin that is reflective of several general systemic diseases. Salivary diagnostics is the use of salivary biomarkers for the noninvasive detection of multiple systemic diseases and not just HNC. Given that saliva is in part a filtrate of the circulating blood, other systemic biomarkers are reflective in saliva as well, and these have been explored.

Nicotine and cotinine levels for example have been measured in smokers using saliva [1, 2]. Saliva is an easy noninvasive medium for monitoring pharmacodynamics of drug levels and response in the body, and this has been demonstrated in epileptic patients [3]. Steroids, hormones, and viral antibodies (e.g., HIV, hepatitis) can be detected in saliva. Excess alcohol use [4] and drug [5] have also been assessed using saliva. Another potential use of salivary biomarkers is in the early detection of periodontal disease and general oral hygiene. Saliva is beneficial to the oral cavity. It contains many antimicrobial agents such as lysozyme, lactoferrin, lactoperoxidases, thiocyanate, H_2O_2, and IgA that can kill bacteria or prevent their invasion. It also contains useful bacteria called normal microbiota (or oral microbiome) that prevents colonization of the mouth by harmful bacteria. Poor oral hygiene can lead to an imbalance between the good and bad bacteria leading to oral diseases such as dental caries and periodontitis, which is chronic inflammation of the periodontium that supports the teeth. Diagnostics of periodontitis can be delayed due a number of factors such as late presentation from lack of defined symptoms. Lectin staining of saliva to identify oral pathogens is an assessment for risk for developing dental caries. Several systemic diseases including diabetes mellitus [6], cystic fibrosis [7, 8], Sjogren's syndrome [9], myocardial infarction [10–14], and Parkinson's disease

[15–17] are associated with altered salivary transcriptome. Salivary troponin, for example, may be a biomarker for myocardial infarction [13, 14]. Matrix metalloproteinase levels are elevated in patients with vesiculo-erosive diseases [18]. Finally, several other cancer biomarkers are measurable in saliva.

3.3 Salivary Head and Neck Cancer Biomarkers

A number of salivary biomarkers demonstrate clinical potential for the management of HNSCC (Table 3.1).

3.3.1 Salivary Head and Neck Cancer Mitochondrial Genome Biomarkers

As an established risk factor for a number of cancers including head and neck, esophageal, lung, and bladder cancers, the toxins in tobacco smoke and other genotoxins can damage mitochondrial DNA (mtDNA) and possibly contribute to the development of these cancers. Mitochondrial DNA content changes were measured in saliva of smokers and nonsmokers. Saliva from smokers, including those who had stopped smoking, contained significantly high levels of mtDNA compared to those from people who never smoked [19].

Table 3.1 HNSCC biomarkers in saliva

Target	Biomarkers
Epigenome	*DAPK, DCC, MINT-31, TIMP-3, MGMT, CDKN2A, CCNA1, KIF1A, EDNRB, NID2, HOXA9, IL-11, INSR, GABRB3PXN, NTRK3, NOTCH3, PTCH2, ERBB4, ADCYAP1, CEBPA, EPHA5, HLF, FGF3, TWIST, TNFSF10, TMEFF1*
Genome	*Nuclear:* chromosome 9p loss, *CCND1* amplification, MSI (markers D3S1234, D9S156, D17S799), *TP53* mutations (in codon 63)
	Mitochondrial: mutations and content variations
	Viral: HPV, EBV DNA
Transcriptome	*Coding: IL-8, IL-1β, S100P, OAZ1, H3F3A, DUSP1, Spermine N1-acetyltransferase (SAT)*
	Noncoding: miR-31, miR-125a, miR-200a, HOTAIR
Proteome	IL-8, IL-1β, M2BP, S100A9/MRP14, CD59, catalase, profilin
Metabolome	Taurine, cadaverine, alpha-aminobutyric acid, alanine, C5H14N5, piperidine, piperideine, pipercolic acid, C4H9N, C8H9N, pyrroline hydroxycarboxylic acid, betaine, C6H6N2O2, leucine, isoleucine, tyrosine, histidine, tryptophan, beta-alanine, glutamic acid, threonine, serine, glutamine, choline, carnitine, C4H5N2O11P, phenylalanine, valine, lactic acid
Redox species	Peroxidase, GSTP1, SOD, 8-OHdG, reactive nitrous species (NO, NO2, and NO3), glutathione, malondialdehyde

Mitochondrial DNA copy number or content alterations have been measured in HNCs and matched saliva using quantitative polymerase chain reaction (qPCR). In an initial study of head and neck tumor tissues of various clinical grades reminiscence of disease progression, it was found that increased mtDNA content positively correlated with histopathologic grade [20]. In a follow-up study, oral rinse samples were collected from patients with HNSCC as well as individuals without cancer for mtDNA content analysis [21]. Mitochondrial DNA levels were significantly higher in saliva from cancer patients than controls. Importantly, primary tumors also had higher levels of mtDNA than pretreatment saliva, suggesting the elevated levels of mtDNA in saliva of cancer patients were tumor-derived. In another study, the effect of treatment on mtDNA levels was examined in patients with HNSCC [22]. Analysis of pretreatment and posttreatment saliva revealed a significant decrease in mtDNA content in posttreatment samples. In addition, saliva from patients who had radiation treatment and those who never smoked contained lower levels of mitochondrial genomes than in saliva from non-irradiated and smoking counterparts. Thus, the harmful effects of smoking on mtDNA appear to be chronic and irreversible.

Mutations in the mitochondrial genome are present in early-stage HNCs. Microarray-based resequencing of the entire mitochondrial genome was conducted on a panel of HNSCC samples, and mutations were found in nearly half of the tumors [23]. Sequencing of dysplastic adjacent tissues of one tumor identified the same mutation in both tumor and margin samples, suggesting mtDNA mutations occurred early in this particular tumor and could be involved in disease progression. To demonstrate the possible utility of mtDNA mutations as a tool for early cancer detection in clinical samples, Fliss et al. used manual sequencing to study mtDNA mutations in primary HNCs and matched available saliva [24]. Six of the 13 solid tumors had mutations that were also detected in 6 of 9 saliva samples. MitoChip resequencing of salivary rinses from patients with known tumor mtDNA mutations was studied by Mithani et al., for possible presence of same mutations in noninvasively collected body fluids [25]. Using a proprietary algorithm, heteroplasmic mutations could be detected at even a dilution of 1:200. This sensitive methodology enabled these investigators to uncover tumor mutations in saliva from 77% of the patients. Thus, mtDNA content changes and mutations can be measured in saliva for diagnosis and management of HNSCC.

3.3.2 Salivary Head and Neck Cancer Epigenetic Biomarkers

The robustness of detecting gene promoter methylation in body fluids has been tested in salivary samples for HNSCC detection. Following the feasibility study whereby methylation in at least one of *CDNK2A*, *MGMT*, and, *DAPK* was detected in 65% of matched saliva, several groups have confirmed the clinical relevance of methylation of cancer-related genes in saliva from HNSCC patients [26]. Another proof of concept study used methylation array to generate gene classifiers from 34 methylated genes in preoperative saliva. Using panels consisting of four to ten genes from this list, a sensitivity of 62–77% and a specificity of 83–100% were achieved for OSCC detection [27].

Methylation of *EDNRB* and *DCC* in saliva could potentially classify people at risk of developing oral premalignant and malignant disease. In a prospective study of high-risk population, methylation of *EDNRB*, *DCC,* and *HOXA9* in salivary rinses was significantly associated with premalignant and malignant diseases, but only *EDNRB* and *DCC* achieved significant associations with histologic diagnosis in multivariate modeling [28]. The combination of methylated *DCC*, *EDNRB,* and clinical risk classification based on lesion examination by an expert pathologist achieved an optimal area under the receiver operating characteristic curve (AUROCC) of 0.67 in detection of premalignant and malignant lesions. Additionally, methylation of *HOXA9* and *NID2* in saliva achieved AUROCC of 0.75 and 0.73, respectively, for early detection of OSCC [29].

Saliva methylated gene panels have also been examined for HNSCC detection. In oral rinse samples, a methylation panel consisting of *CDH1*, *TMEFF2*, *RARβ*, and *MGMT* achieved a sensitivity and specificity of 100% and 87.5%, respectively, for OSCC detection [30]. However, methylation of three of these genes (*CDH1*, *TMEFF2*, and *MGMT*) as a panel sufficed accurate detection of OSCC at a sensitivity of 97.1% and specificity of 91.7%. Another panel consisting of methylated *RASSF1A*, *DAPK1*, and *CDKN2A* in saliva achieved a sensitivity of 94% and specificity of 87% in detecting early-stage HNSCC [31]. In a validation study of methylated genes in saliva, *CCNA1*, *DAPK*, *DCC*, and *TIMP3* were highly specific for OSCC [32]. Thus, a panel consisting of *CCNA1*, *DCC*, and *TIMP3* reached optimal sensitivity and specificity each of 92.5% for OSCC detection. Of interest, methylation of *DAPK*, *DCC*, and *TIMP3* was found in about 90% of early-stage (T1/T2) disease. Development of local recurrence is prevalent in HNSCC patients, and this is often associated with poor prognosis. Patients with *TIMP3* methylation in post-treatment salivary rinses had lower local recurrence-free survival ($p = 0.008$), and this was an independent prognostic factor for local recurrence in multivariate analysis [33]. The various consistent findings confirm and validate the clinical relevance of using panels of methylated genes in saliva for the noninvasive management of HNSCC patients.

3.3.3 Salivary Head and Neck Cancer Genomic Biomarkers

Genetic biomarkers in saliva for oral cancer detection have been investigated with promising findings. Genome alterations including mutations, amplifications, and microsatellite instability (MSI) in saliva are associated with HNSCC. Huang et al. demonstrated a 66% and 50% loss of heterozygosity (LOH) in *TP53* exon 4 and intron 6, respectively, in exfoliated cytologic samples from OSCC patients [34]. Subsequently, this group demonstrated the exon 4 codon 63 mutation in salivary samples from 62.5% of OSCC patients and in 18.5% of healthy subjects [35]. Of interest, another study confirmed the presence in saliva of the C-deletion in codon 63 of exon 4 in as many as 93.3% of OSCC patients, but not in healthy controls [36], and this mutation was related to betel nut and tobacco lime quid chewing habits. Using a multiplex ligation-dependent probe amplification assay, genetic alterations (losses and gains) of 11 genes (*PMAIP1*, *PTPN1*, *ERBB2*, *ABCC4*, *UTY*, *DNMT1*, *CDKN2B*, *CDKN2D*, *NFKB1*, *TP53,* and *DCC*) in saliva could potentially identify HNSCC patients. However, based on classification and regression tree analysis, alterations in only *PMAIP1* and *PTPN1* sufficed discrimination between all patients and controls [37].

MSI has equally been demonstrated in salivary samples from HNSCC patients. Previously known allelic losses in primary tumor samples were detectable in 84% of mouthwashes and lesion brushings from these patients [38]. The findings were tumor stage independent, which suggests their potential as early detection biomarkers. In another study, the selection of 23 microsatellite markers from chromosomal loci known to have high probability of allelic loses in HNSCC enabled detection of MSI in 86% of primary tumor samples [39]. Matched salivary samples were positive in 76% of cases, including 92.3% of patients with small primaries. Microsatellite analysis of chromosomal regions frequently altered in HNSCC identified MSI in 86% of tumor samples and 49% of saliva in at least one of 25 microsatellite markers studied [40]. While markers D3S1234, D9S156, and D17S799 identified the majority (72.2%) of salivary MSI, those specific for primary tumors were D3S1234, D8S254, and D9S171, which were associated with 84.3% of tumors. The heterogeneity in these markers provides support for the genetic preconditioning of the head and neck mucosal epithelium. In another analysis, eight microsatellite markers detected alterations in 22% of primary HNSCC, but as high as 80% of these MSIs were detectable in salivary samples [41], an important feat that supports the use of saliva for diagnosis of these cancers.

3.3.4 Salivary Head and Neck Cancer Transcript Biomarkers

The stability of coding transcripts has been a problematic issue when questioning their ease and authentic measurements in many body fluids as clinical biomarkers. However, salivary transcriptomics for oral cancer detection and management has been successfully examined [42, 43]. The salivary transcriptome comprises over 3000 mRNAs. Li et al. found four genes from this transcriptome to be very accurate (ROC 0.95) in discriminating between cancer and non-cancer patients [42]. These genes included IL-8, ornithine decarboxylase, spermidine acetyltransferase, and IL-1β. The importance of tissue-derived fluids for respective tissue-associated cancer biomarkers evaluated by Wong's group compared saliva and blood biomarkers for oral cancer detection, which showed much worse performance for blood compared to saliva (AUROCC; saliva 0.95 vs. blood 0.88) [42, 44].

3.3.4.1 Coding Transcripts

While the mechanism of RNA release into saliva is not well understood, they appear very stable in this medium. Possible reasons for their stability include their inclusion in extracellular vesicles. Additionally, AU-rich elements (ARE) sequence structures in the 3′UTRs of mRNA could recruit ARE-binding proteins to help protect them from degradation. Thus, mRNA molecules are present as intact and fragmented forms in saliva and have been successfully assayed as biomarkers of various diseases (e.g., Sjogren's syndrome) and cancer (OSCC, breast, pancreatic, and ovarian cancers). Mostly, saliva transcriptomics has been achieved by global microarray profiling, followed by qPCR validation. However, low template amounts and the need to detect tumor-associated low-abundant targets have necessitated the initial universal transcript amplification for microarray discovery studies. This is often followed by a multiplex pre-amplification strategy for qPCR validation analysis.

The salivary transcriptome is of both human and microbial origins. Using next-generation sequencing, Spielmann et al. demonstrated that 25% and 30% of the sequences in cell-free saliva (CFS) were from human and oral microbial genomes, respectively [45]. In total, >4000 coding and noncoding sequences from both sources are represented in saliva. A number of transcripts have been discovered in saliva as OSCC biomarkers. The seminal work of Li et al. in 2004 uncovered increased levels of transcripts to *IL-8*, *IL-1β*, *DUSP1*, *S100P*, *OAZ1*, *H3FP3A*, and *SAT* in saliva from OSCC patients [42]. The sensitivity and specificity of a panel consisting of four of these mRNAs (*IL-8*, *IL-1β*, *SAT*, and *OAZ1*) were 91% each with AUROCC of 0.95 for OSCC detection. A number of other studies have validated these transcripts for OSCC. The robustness of these biomarkers was demonstrated in a Serbian population study [46]. The National Cancer Institute-Early Detection Research Network-Biomarker Research Laboratory (NCI-EDRN-BRL) provided another validation of these biomarkers. However, in this independent cohort, the top performers in terms of accuracy were *IL8* and *SAT* transcripts [47]. Their performance in detection of early-stage (T1/T2) disease has also been demonstrated [48]. In this setting, *IL-8*, *IL-1β*, *SAT*, and *OAZ1* achieved an AUROCC of 0.799 for OSCC detection (but not for leukoplakia with dysplasia). However, the combination of *IL-8* and *SAT* with AUROCC of 0.755 may suffice accurate cancer detection. The expression of *MMP1* and *MMP9* is associated with progression of dysplasia to OSCC. *MMP1* mRNA levels are much higher in saliva from OSCC patients than controls [49, 50]. However, although specificity was high (100%), sensitivity was at a dismal 20%, making the authors suggest the need for technical improvement in salivary *MMP1* detection.

3.3.4.2 Noncoding Transcripts

Noncoding RNAs (ncRNAs) have been characterized in salivary samples and demonstrate diagnostic potential for various diseases including HNSCC. The characterization of miRNA in 12 body fluids including saliva revealed higher number of miRNAs in saliva, breast milk, and seminal fluids than in cerebrospinal fluid, pleural fluids, and urine. A unique profile was uncovered for miRNA in blood that was suggestive of its representation of almost all tissues of the body [51]. In reference to saliva, there are variations in ncRNA between whole saliva and cell-free saliva (CFS). The ability to isolate high-quality RNA from whole saliva enabled the detection of several miRNAs inclusive of five known salivary miRNAs (miR-16, miR-24, miR-191, miR-203, and miR-223) [52]. Using massively parallel sequencing of whole saliva and CFS, it was however uncovered that there are more microbial RNAs in whole saliva than CFS, which tend to mask human RNA detection in whole saliva [45].

Given the unique role of exosomes in packaging miRNAs, attention has been focused on examining miRNAs in exosomes isolated from saliva. Due to cellular contamination and high viscosity, isolating exosomes from whole saliva has been technically challenging. However, in an experiment whereby RNA was extracted from exosomes in pellet and from exosome-depleted supernatant, it was demonstrated that salivary miRNAs are predominantly exosomal [53]. Moreover, using next-generation sequencing (NGS) of salivary exosomes and whole saliva, it was further concluded that many small RNAs (e.g., snoRNA, miRNA, and piRNA) are indeed carried in salivary exosomes [54]. Another in-depth characterization of salivary small ncRNAs involved the use of RNA-seq and bioinformatic analysis of CFS from healthy people [55]. While piRNAs were abundant in CFS compared to other body fluids, miRNA expression profiles were similar to those in serum and CFS. Additionally, this study uncovered over 400 circular RNAs in CFS.

A number of clinical studies have also uncovered the potential of salivary miRNAs in disease detection. In a pilot study by Park et al., 50 miRNAs were detected in both CFS and whole saliva [56]. Of interest, the levels of miR-125a and miR-200a were significantly lower in saliva from OSCC patients than healthy controls. Promoter methylation and silencing of miR-137 are associated with HNSCC, and this was uncovered in oral rinses from 21.2% of patients. Among cases, methylated miR-137 was associated with female gender (OR, 5.30) and inversely with body mass index (OR-0.88) [57]. Wiklund et al. confirmed the methylation of miR-137 in oral cancer [58]. Additionally, the levels of miR-137 and miR-200a, coupled with methylation of miR-200c-141 in oral rinse and saliva, could differentiate OSCC patients from healthy controls. Liu et al. uncovered elevated plasma miR-31 in OSCC patients with diagnostic AUROCC of 0.82. Similar increases were demonstrated in salivary samples from these patients [59]. Subsequent analysis of saliva confirmed the elevated levels in OSCC cases of all stages including patients with very small tumors. However, the elevated levels were not present in precursor lesions (verrucous leukoplakia). The levels in saliva were much higher than in circulation, but both decreased following surgery [60]. Salivary levels of miR-9, miR-134, and miR-191 were significantly different between HNSCC patients and controls [61]. As potential diagnostic biomarkers, the AUROCC were 0.85 (miR-9), 0.74 (mi-134), and 0.98 (miR-191). Saliva from different groups of patients and healthy controls were analyzed using NanoString nCounter miRNA expression array to identify differential OSCC miRNAs [62]. Of over 700 tested miRNAs, 13 were significantly dysregulated in saliva from patients. The levels of miR-24 and miR-27b were higher, while those of miR-136, miR-147, miR-148a, miR-220a, miR-323-5p, miR-503, miR-632, miR-646, miR-668, miR-877, and miR-1250 were reduced. Of interest, the reduced miR-136 could differentiate OSCC patients from both healthy controls and OSCC patients in remission, while elevated miR-27b was equally discriminatory (inclusive of patients with lichen planus). Thus, increased miR-27b appears as a useful salivary OSCC-associated miRNA. To identify risk biomarkers for lesion progression from low-grade to high-grade dysplasia and cancer, miRNA microarray was used to identify candidate-dysregulated miRNAs, which were then demonstrated in saliva using RT-qPCR [61]. Twenty-five (12 upregulated and 13 downregulated) miRNAs could predict lesion progression, and these were measurable in salivary samples. To enable deployment of salivary miRNA for OSCC detection at the point-of-care (POC), Wang et al. developed a magnetic-controllable electrochemical RNA biosensor device that has enhanced analytical sensitivity (can detect attomolar levels of target miRNAs) as well as miRNA selectivity for OSCC [63]. Putatively, this device is easy to fabricate and operate, with short analytical time and good stability and reusability, which are good attributes for its utility for early detection of OSCC at the point-of-care.

A meta-analysis was conducted to determine the diagnostic performance of miRNAs in serum, plasma, blood, saliva, and tissue samples for OSCC [64]. Of 23 studies from 10 articles composed of 598 cases and 320 controls, the pooled sensitivity, specificity, and AUROCC were 75.9%, 77.3%, and 0.832, which suggested some value in using these noninvasive biomarkers for OSCC detection. However, there was heterogeneity between studies in reference to types of samples and ethnicity of patients.

The potential of salivary lncRNA is uncovered in a pilot study. MALAT1 was detected in all nine, while HOTAIR was present in five out of nine whole salivary samples from OSCC patients [65]. Their clinical relevance awaits further investigation.

3.3.5 Salivary Head and Neck Cancer Proteomic Biomarkers

A number of proteins demonstrate dysregulated levels of expression in HNSCC. He et al. found HSP60, HSP27, α-β-crystalline, ATP synthase β, calgranulin β, myosin, tropomyosin, and galectin 1 to be significantly altered in cancers of the tongue [66]. Chen et al. uncovered buccal squamous cell carcinoma proteomic signature, which included heat shock proteins, tumor antigens, glycolytic enzymes, cytoskeletal proteins, antioxidant and detoxification enzymes, mitochondrial proteins, and intracellular signaling proteins [67]. The salivary proteome comprises over 300 targets of interest in oral cancer detection. IL-8, IL-1β, and ferritin mRNAs were significantly increased in oral cancer tissues and matched saliva from patients. Specifically, IL-8 expression was increased in oral cancer tissues. This highly elevated marker was increased at the protein level as well in saliva of patients using ELISA analysis [68]. Dual matched comparison of mRNA and protein revealed downregulation of calgranulins A and B and annexins 1 and 2 at both the message and protein levels in HNSCC [69].

The diagnostic potential of salivary proteins for OSCC has been extensively investigated. Differential salivary protein levels between HNSCC patients and healthy individuals have been uncovered, and their clinical relevance demonstrated. Various proteomic technologies including mass spectrometry (MS), Western blotting, ELISA, and bead-based (Luminex xMAP) assays have been applied for salivary protein biomarker discoveries. These efforts have yielded a plethora of potentially valuable HNSCC biomarkers, although just a handful has received extensive clinical scrutiny. Indeed, except for transferrin, statherin, and α-amylase, many of the potentially useful OSCC biomarkers are proteins, often in low abundance. Of the numerous salivary protein biomarkers, IL-8, IL-1b, M2BP, MRP14, CD59, catalase, and profilin appear to have diagnostic utility as single or panel biomarkers of HNSCC. As single biomarkers, only IL-8 has proven useful as accurate salivary protein for HNSCC detection [70]. Hu et al. used LC MALDI-MS to uncover diagnostic proteomic biomarkers in oral fluid samples from OSCC patients [71]. Tandem MS analysis enabled identification of thioredoxin as a useful biomarker that achieved a sensitivity, specificity, and AUROC of 70.8%, 70.8%, and 0.71, respectively. A panel protein biomarker composed of M2BP, S100A9/MRP14, CD59, catalase, and profilin achieved a diagnostic sensitivity of 90%, specificity of 83%, and AUROCC of 0.93 for OSCC detection. Salivary levels of myosin and actin enabled differentiation between patients with OSCC and premalignant dysplastic lesions in a pilot study. The diagnostic sensitivity and specificity were 100% and 75%, respectively, for actin and 67% and 83%, respectively, for myosin [72]. A study of 14 proteins known to be significantly elevated in saliva from OSCC patients was conducted in Hungarian population [73]. After an initial Luminex-based multiplex analysis of IL-1α, IL-1β, IL-6, IL-8, TNFα, and VEGF, as well as selected reaction monitoring (SRM)-based analysis of catalase, profilin-1, S100A9, CD59, galectin-3-bindig protein, CD44, thioredoxin, and KTR-19, validation of selected proteins was performed using ELISA. In this population, IL-6 and S100A9 were the best salivary biomarkers for OSCC detection. The authors noted the need for ethnic group-specific biomarker development, as this set was different for other populations. At a predictive probability cutoff value of 0.47, soluble CD44 in saliva could detect HNSCC at a sensitivity of 80.4% and specificity of 65.5%. Incorporating levels of total salivary protein could enhance this performance [74].

A number of salivary protein biomarkers are associated with stages of OSCC. Two-dimensional electrophoretic analysis of salivary samples from OSCC patients and healthy controls identified transferrin as OSCC biomarker [75]. The performance of this biomarker in OSCC detection was stage-dependent, achieving, respectively, sensitivity and AUROCC of 100% and 0.95 for stage T1, 86.6% and 0.94 for stage T2, and 100% and 0.91 for stage T3/T4 OSCC. In another study by this group, MS analysis of salivary peptidome uncovered three peaks that showed differential levels between OSCC patients and controls [76]. One of the peaks identified as a 24-mer peptide of zinc finger protein 510 (ZNF510) achieved an AUROCC of 0.95 for stage T1/T2 and 0.98 for stage T3/T4 OSCCC. The salivary transcript performance validation studies by Brinkmann et al. included measurement of three promising salivary proteins (IL8, IL1b, and M2BP) [43]. These proteins together with six transcripts were used to establish three panels for all, T1/T2, and T3/T4 OSCC. The panels achieved sensitivity, specificity, and AUROCC, respectively, of 89%, 78%, and 0.86 for all; 67%, 96%, and 0.85 for stage T1/T2; and 82%, 84%, and 0.88 for stage T3/T4 OSCC detection. Elashoff et al. performed a validation study of the seven mRNAs and three proteins elevated in saliva from OSCC patients in five independent cohorts from UCLA and NCI-EDRN-BRL. While IL-8 and subcutaneous adipose tissue (SAT) were the top performers as independent single biomarkers, including measurement of the three promising proteins (IL-8, IL-1β, and M2BP) enhanced the diagnostic accuracy of the transcripts for OSCC [47].

Protein peak biomarkers have also been demonstrated for OSCC. Four SELDI-MS peaks at m/z 2902, 3883, 4951, and 5797 as a panel biomarker achieved a sensitivity of 88.2% and specificity of 93.3% in OSCC detection [77].

3.3.6 Salivary Head and Neck Cancer Metabolomic Biomarkers

Alterations in the levels of salivary metabolites are potentially useful HNSCC biomarkers. Capillary electrophoresis TOF MS analysis of saliva coupled with multiple logistic regression models identified taurine, piperidine, and a peptide peak (m/z 120.081) as OSCC biomarkers [78]. As a panel, the diagnostic AUROCC was 0.865 for OSCC. Using ultrapure liquid chromatography (UPLC) coupled with quadrupole TOF MS and multivariate statistical analysis, valine, lactic acid, and phenylalanine were uncovered as salivary biomarkers of OSCC [79]. As a panel, the sensitivity, specificity, and AUROCC were 86.5%, 82.4%, and 0.89 in differentiating OSCC from healthy controls and 94.6%, 84.4%, and 0.97 from oral leukoplakia. UPLC-electrospray ionization MS analysis of saliva uncovered L-phenylalanine and L-leucine, which together achieved a sensitivity of 92.3% and specificity of 91.7% for early diagnosis of OSCC [80]. In a follow-up study, a panel of five biomarkers (propionylcholine, N-acetyl-L-phenylalanine, sphingosine, phytosphingosine, and S-carboxymethyl-L-cysteine) achieved a sensitivity of 100%, specificity of 96.7%, and an AUROCC of 0.997 for early OSCC detection [81]. A metabolomic analysis of both primary tumor and matched salivary samples identified 17-shared metabolites for OSCC [82]. However, a panel consisting of just two of these metabolites was accurate at OSCC detection with AUROCC of 0.827. Sridharan et al. used quadrupole TOF-LCMS coupled with MassHunter profile software to identify a number of serum metabolites altered in oral leukoplakia and OSCC [83]. Elevated levels of L-carnitine, lysine, 2-methylcitric acid, putrescine, 8-hydroxyadenine, 17-estradiol, 5,6-dihydrouridine, and 5-methylthioadenosine (MTA) could be of diagnostic utility in oral leukoplakia and OSCC. The significantly increased levels of putrescine, 8-hydroxyadenine, and 5,6-dihydrouridine in OSCC than oral leukoplakia indicated their potential role in predicting the progression of oral leukoplakia. In a follow-up study, quadrupole TOF-LCMS coupled with MassHunter profile software and Metlin database analysis uncovered a number of salivary metabolites altered in oral leukoplakia and OSCC [84]. These included significant upregulation of 1-methylhistidine, inositol 1,3,4-triphosphate, d-glycerate-2-phosphate, 4-nitroquinolone-1-oxide, 2-oxoarginine, norcocaine nitroxide, sphinganine-1-phosphate, and pseudouridine, with downregulation of L-homocysteic acid, ubiquinone, neuraminic acid, and estradiol valerate in oral leukoplakia and OSCC.

3.4 Promising Salivary Head and Neck Cancer Diagnostic Biomarkers

A meta-analysis of 15 studies inclusive of 771 cases and 740 controls concluded that salivary biomarkers have clinical utility in HNSCC detection [85]. Expectedly, single biomarkers performed less well than panel biomarkers. Single biomarker metrics have been very variable with sensitivity and specificity ranges of 14–100% and 38–100%, respectively. The panel biomarkers achieved sensitivities and specificities of 82–100% and 78–100%, respectively. Additionally, and importantly, this analysis demonstrated that salivary biomarkers were much superior at detecting early-stage HNSCC than late-stage disease. Of the 37 biomarkers examined, only 5 achieved excellent diagnostic test accuracy for HNSCC. These biomarkers include four metabolites (pipecolinic acid, choline, L-phenylalanine, and S-carboxymethyl-L-cysteine) and the most commonly studied salivary HNSCC biomarker, IL-8. As single biomarkers, L-phenylalanine achieved a sensitivity of 84.1% and specificity of 95.0% for OSCC, while S-carboxymethyl-L-cysteine performed at a sensitivity of 84.6% and specificity of 93.3% for early-stage and a sensitivity of 88.2% and specificity of 90.0% for advanced-stage OSCC detection [80, 81]. However, the diagnostic test accuracy was highest for pipecolinic acid in this meta-analysis. Another meta-analysis of biomarkers in saliva for OSCC detection included 9 articles with 340 cases and 308 controls [86]. The biomarkers that achieved the highest sensitivity were MMP9, chemerin, and a combination of choline, betaine, pipecolinic acid, and L-carnitine. The highest specificity was achieved for MMP9, chemerin, decreased miR-25b (100%), and elevated miR-136 (88%). These biomarkers therefore hold promise for OSCC detection in a noninvasive fashion.

3.5 Salivary Nasopharyngeal Carcinoma Biomarkers

Biomarkers of nasopharyngeal carcinoma (NPC) are detectable in saliva and nasopharyngeal brushes and washes from patients. While both Epstein-Barr virus (EBV) and NPC cellular alterations are present in saliva, many studies have focused on EBV targets. The utility of these biomarkers in NPC detection and management has been successfully explored.

EBV DNA copy number is much higher in nasopharyngeal brushing and swab samples from patients than non-cancer controls. Tong et al. observed a median level of 8.94 copies/actin in patients compared to 0 copies/actin in controls [87]. The sensitivity and specificity for NPC detection were 96.4% and 96.2%, respectively, and the levels increased with advancing tumor stage. The diagnostic value of EBV DNA load in nasopharyngeal brushings was examined in a prospective study [88]. EBV DNA levels were significantly much higher in patients than controls. At a defined cutoff value (mean of controls plus 3SD), sensitivity and specificity of 90% and 98%, respectively, were achieved. The diagnostic utility of nasopharyngeal EBV DNA load may be much better than other tests for early detection of NPC. In a Chinese population, similarly high levels of EBV DNA were demonstrated (mean 46,360 copies/ng DNA in patients vs. 28 copies/ng DNA in healthy controls and 50 copies/ng DNA in high-risk controls). At a cutoff value of 225 copies/ng DNA, the diagnostic sensitivity and specificity were 96% and 97%, respectively, which was much superior to the performances of plasma EBV DNA load, anti-VCA IgA antibodies, and initial biopsy [89].

Additionally, EBV nuclear antigen 1 (EBNA1) and cancer-specific BARF1 transcripts were positive in 86% and 74%, respectively, of samples from patients. Detection of EBV LMP1 and EBNA genes also demonstrates utility as noninvasive biomarkers of NPC. In a pilot study, the detection of LMP1 in nasopharyngeal swabs achieved a sensitivity and specificity of 94.7% and 100%, respectively [90]. In a follow-up study, the sensitivity was 87.3%, and specificity was 98.4% in NPC detection [91]. The sensitivity of LMP1 in nasopharyngeal swabs outperformed nasopharyngoscopy (sensitivity of 62%, specificity of 99.6%) in NPC detection. In another study, the addition of EBNA to LMP1 slightly enhanced the sensitivity (91.4%), but specificity remained unchanged at 98.3% [92].

Mass screening of NPC is frequently accomplished by serological detection of anti-EBV antibodies. But high seropositivity rates lead to false classification of many as high risk for follow-up. To help reduce the false-positive screening results, a prospective study of VCA-positive individuals was conducted and found significantly higher EBV DNA load in nasopharyngeal swabs in people who developed NPC (mean 2.8×10^6 copies/swab) than those without cancer (5.6×10^3 copies/swab) [93]. Using mean EBV DNA load of non-cancer controls plus 2SD as cutoff, the AUROCC was 0.980 compared to 0.895 for anti-VCA serology for NPC detection in this cohort. Thus, the ancillary use of EBV load in nasopharyngeal swabs could help further stratify VCA-seropositive individuals to be monitored for early detection. Though preliminary, salivary EBV DNA content appears significantly higher in advanced-stage (T3/T4) than early-stage (T1/T2) NPC patients [94, 95]. While the detection rate was lower than serology (80% vs. >90% for serology), the findings suggest complementary utility with serology in early-stage disease diagnosis and stage prediction.

EBV DNA load may modulate with treatment and hence useful for disease monitoring. A high pretreatment EBV DNA in nasopharyngeal brushings (median 9714 copies/mL) significantly reduced (median 6 copies/mL) following treatment [96].

In another study, the significantly elevated EBV DNA load in nasopharyngeal brushings and blood from cases showed significant reductions 2 months after treatment. VCA-IgA serology however failed to demonstrate this change [97]. Following radiotherapy, however, Pow et al. observed significantly higher EBV DNA in saliva than pretreatment levels [94]. In a pilot study, the combined detection of EBV genome and telomerase activity in nasopharyngeal swabs achieved a sensitivity of 100% and specificity of 92.6% in NPC detection [98].

EBV and host genetic variants may be risk prediction biomarkers of NPC. A SNP (G155391A) in EBV RPMS1 gene, as well as seven host SNPs (rs1412829, rs28421666, rs2860580, rs2894207, rs31489, rs6774494, and rs9510787), conferred elevated risk for NPC. To apply these as noninvasive diagnostic biomarkers of NPC, Cui et al. developed a single, convenient, and cost-effective salivary assay targeting all these SNPs [99]. In a pilot population-based case-control study, an NPC-risk prediction model achieved an AUROCC of 0.74.

Surface-enhanced Raman spectroscopic (SERS) analysis of saliva revealed significant differences in spectral intensities between NPC patients and healthy controls [100]. Spectral intensities at 447, 498, 635, 729, 1134, 1270, and 1448 cm^{-1} that correspond to proteins, nucleic acids, fatty acids, glycogen, and collagen were of much discriminatory value. The use of principal component and linear discriminatory analyses enabled a diagnostic sensitivity of 86.7%, specificity of 81.3%, and accuracy of 83.9% to be achieved for NPC detection.

A number of gene methylation markers have been identified for NPC. The frequencies of methylation in *DAPK, CDKN2A*, and *RASSF1A* were 50.0%, 46.4%, and 39.3%, respectively, in nasopharyngeal brushing samples from patients [87]. In another series, the methylation of at least one of *RASSF1A, DAPK, CDH1, CDKN2A*, or *CDKN2B* in nasopharyngeal swabs and mouth/throat rinsing was 63% and 50%, respectively [101]. *CDH13* was methylated at a frequency of 89.7% in primary NPC samples and, as a noninvasive diagnostic biomarker, achieved a sensitivity of 81% at a perfect specificity in detecting nasopharyngeal cancer [102]. Similarly, methylation in one of *RASSF1A, WIF1, CDKN2A, CHFR*, or *RIZ1* in nasopharyngeal brushings or paraffin tissue achieved a cancer detection rate of 98% [103]. In another analysis of multiple sample sets, methylation of *DAPK1, RASSSF1A, NIF1*, or *RARβ2* in biopsies, cell-free plasma, and nasopharyngeal brushings significantly enhanced the detection rate of stage-independent NPC and local recurrences [104].

3.6 Salivary Biomarkers of Non-head and Neck Cancer

Because a component of whole saliva is blood filtrate, biomarkers of systemic diseases can reflect in saliva. Thus, biomarkers of cancers outside the oropharyngeal cavity have been explored in saliva. Available evidence suggests the utility of such biomarkers for noninvasive early detection of lung, breast, pancreatic, and other cancers. Transcriptomic, proteomic, and metabolomic alterations in saliva have all proven as rigorous biomarkers of non-HNCs.

Transcriptomic profiling of saliva from lung cancer patients uncovered seven discriminatory transcripts (*CCNI, FGF19, FRS2, GREB1, BRAF, LZTS1,* and *EGFR*) that were validated [105]. A panel of five of these transcripts (*CCNI, FGF19, FRS2, GREB1*, and *EGFR*) achieved a sensitivity of 93.75%, specificity of 82.81% and AUROCC of 0.93 in discriminating lung cancer patients from healthy controls. In a proteomic effort, 2D-DIGE of saliva followed by MS enabled the identification of calprotectin, zinc-α-2-glycoprotein, and haptoglobin (Hp2) as lung cancer biomarkers [106]. As diagnostic biomarkers of lung cancer, the sensitivity, specificity, and AUROCC were 88.5%, 92.3%, and 0.90, respectively. The application of surface-enhanced Raman spectroscopy on saliva from lung cancer patients enabled identification of nine relevant spectral peaks with wavelengths of 822, 884, 909, 925, 1009, 1077, 1369, 1393, and 1721 cm^{-1} as lung cancer biomarkers [107]. These Raman spectra, which belong to amino acids and nucleic acid bases, had sensitivity, specificity, and an overall accuracy of 94%, 81%, and 86%, respectively, for lung cancer detection.

The breast cancer transcriptome in saliva includes alterations in *CSTA, TPT1, IGF2BP1, GRM1, GRIK1, H6PD, MDM4,* and *S100A8* that were uncovered by microarray profiling followed by RT-PCR validation [108]. The performance of these biomarkers in breast cancer detection achieved a sensitivity of 83%, specificity of 97%, and an accuracy of 92%. This study also included 2D-DIGE analyses that uncovered salivary CA6 as breast cancer biomarker. A quantitative proteomic approach with iTRAQ technology coupled with LC-MS/MS uncovered nine salivary protein biomarkers upregulated or downregulated in association with breast cancer [109]. A metabolomics profile of saliva by CE-TOF MS achieved an AUROCC of 0.97 for breast cancer detection [78].

A preliminary SELDI-TOF MS proteomic study of salivary samples from gastric cancer patients identified differential peaks between cancer patients and healthy controls [110]. A panel of four of these peaks achieved a sensitivity of 95.65% and specificity of 100% in gastric cancer detection.

Salivary transcriptomic and metabolomic signatures have been identified for pancreatic cancer. The well-designed study by Zhang et al. provided diagnostic transcriptome biomarkers that were more accurate than traditional blood tests for resectable pancreatic cancer detection [111]. Alterations in the expression of *KRAS, ACRV1, DPM1,* and *MBD3L2* achieved diagnostic sensitivity, specificity, and AUROCC of 90%, 95%, and 0.97, respectively. Of interest, these biomarkers failed to detect a confounding disease, pancreatitis. Similarly, a salivary metabolomic signature consisting of tryptophan, valine, leucine, isoleucine, phenylalanine, glutamine, glutamate, and aspartate was accurate (AUROCC of 0.99) at differentiating pancreatic cancer patients from healthy controls as well as oral and breast cancer patients [78].

3.7 Technological Platforms for Head and Neck Cancer Screening Using Saliva

Several technologies have been developed or are under development for detection and measurement of various salivary biomarkers (to help advance the concept of salivary diagnostics). Targeted conditions and devices include:

- An α-amylase biosensor for detecting stress-induced diseases
- OraQuick for HIV and HCV testing
- Cortisol level detection using label-free chemiresistor immune sensor
- Periodontal disease diagnosis using integrated microfluidic platform for peptide and metabolite measurement
- Acute myocardial infarction detection using lab-on-a-chip for measuring C-reactive protein, myoglobin, and myeloperoxidase
- Cytokine detection in asthma and chronic obstructive pulmonary disease with fiber-optic microsphere-based antibody arrays
- Diabetes by measuring salivary glucose levels with nanostructured biosensor

For cancer, an electromechanical magneto biosensor for IL-8 measurement for oral cancer and a programmable biochip system for CEA, CA125, HER2, and PSA measurement for various cancers have been developed. The microelectromechanical and nanoelectromechanical systems (MEMS/NEMS) for the measurement of DNA, RNA, proteins, electrolytes, and other small molecules are so sensitive that they can detect analyte at the single-molecule level. The prototype product of MEMS/NEMS is the oral fluid nanosensor test (OFNASET). This is a handheld automated device for salivary protein and nucleic acid detection.

These sensitive diagnostic tests will enable point-of-care detections that will form part of personalized or individualized medicine. Some of the important technologies include photometry, microfluidics, electrochemistry, and electronic noses.

Photometry was developed as a portable biosensor device for testing salivary amylase to determine individual stress level [112]. This colorimetric device could read sympathetic nervous system activity within 30 s. The technology has now been explored for using the ubiquitous smartphones in risk assessment. Based on the fact that the metal oxide semiconductors in smartphone cameras are able to detect chemiluminescence, this technology has been extended to the use of this device for biotesting of saliva and other body fluids. Thus, a chemiluminescence system in smartphones using just small amounts of saliva could quantify cortisol levels [113], and results were available within 30 min. Automated low-cost lateral flow saliva test reader with smartphones was also developed to test drug of abuse [114].

Microfluidic technology is a system that has been developed for detection of disease biomarkers including biomolecules such as DNA, RNA, proteins, hormones, drugs, metabolites, and even pathogens in several body fluids. Microfluidics involve micro-nanoscale fabrication with fluid channels that enable sample flow through while being manipulated (e.g., amplification) and analyzed with target detection and quantification. It could involve sensor array platform for multianalyte detection. Indeed, Zilberman and Sonkusale developed an optoelectronic and microfluidic system for measurement of ammonium and carbon dioxide levels in unfiltered saliva as indicative of *H. pylori*-mediated gastric cancer risk [115]. Another device was developed for salivary sample processing with a detection system that enabled identification of bacterial pathogens [116].

The electrochemical sensor detector technique is based on the Clark glucose electrode system whereby the interaction of blood glucose with glucose oxidase enables the measurement of blood glucose levels. This technology has also been explored for salivary diagnostics. It has been adopted using a smartphone for the measurement of salivary amylase, an enzyme involved in carbohydrate metabolism, with results being available within 5 min [117]. Another proof of the concept of point-of-care biomarker detection used electrochemistry and novel nanotubes to detect salivary biomarkers [118].

Electronic noses are technologically developed devices that are capable of detecting diseases and other volatile biomarkers in exhale air. Explored methodologies include mass spectrometry and use of metal oxide gas sensor. While still under refinement, electronic noses have been tested for the detection of volatile substances in sputum [119]. Their use in real-time scenario has also been tested for pathogen detection in respiratory intensive care. While still in development, their potential utility as point-of-care devices holds enormous potential, especially for the low-to-medium Human Development Index countries.

3.8 Clinical Translation of Commercial Products

Perceptronix Medical Inc., Laboratories (PMI Labs) is an anatomic pathology lab with expertise in quantitative cytologic analysis of noninvasive samples for early cancer detection. OralAdvance™ is a test developed by PMI Labs for early detection of oral cancer. It uses a painless collection kit referred to as cyto-brush kit that contains Rovers®Orcellex® Brush (Rovers Medical Devices BV). The kit is used to collect oral mucosal cells from suspicious areas and transported to PMI Labs. The samples undergo quantitative cytologic examination that includes enumeration of epithelial cell nuclei and nuclear DNA index and ploidy (plotted as a histogram). The test results are available in 2–3 days for the care provider to be used in complementary management of the patient.

3.9 Summary

- In concert with the global trend of many cancers, HNC incidence has been on the rise with an estimated 888,000 new cases diagnosed in 2018 compared to past projected estimates of 600,000.
- OSCC is the most common HNC that globally accounted for 40% of all HNSCC in 2018.

- Given the known etiologic factors of tobacco and alcohol use, as well as infections with HPV (HNSCC) and EBV (NPC), primary prevention is advocated for curtailment.
- The noninvasively collected proximal fluid of HNC, saliva, is rich in biomarkers for HNC and is also a source of biomarkers of cancers located elsewhere in the body, as well as other oral and systemic diseases.
- Promising salivary transcriptomic (and proteomic) biomarkers for OSCC include IL-8, IL-1β, SAT, OAZ1, S100P, DUSP1, and H3FP3A. Validation has been provided for SAT, IL8, IL1b, and OAZ1 for OSCC detection.
- The emerging potential of salivary noncoding RNA and extracellular vesicles remain to be explored in-depth.
- Metabolomic approaches have identified salivary pipecolinic acid, choline, L-phenylalanine, and S-carboxymethyl-L-cysteine as potentially accurate HNSCC biomarkers.
- Measurement of salivary EBV DNA load and detection of EBV genes such as LMP1, EBNA1, and BARF1 demonstrate utility in NPC detection.
- Many technologies are being developed for point-of-care salivary diagnostics.

References

1. Etter JF. A longitudinal study of cotinine in long-term daily users of e-cigarettes. Drug Alcohol Depend. 2016;160:218–21. https://doi.org/10.1016/j.drugalcdep.2016.01.003. PubMed PMID: 26804899
2. Cunningham A, Sommarstrom J, Sisodiya AS, Errington G, Prasad K. Longitudinal study of long-term smoking behaviour by biomarker-supported determination of exposure to smoke. BMC Public Health. 2014;14:348. https://doi.org/10.1186/1471-2458-14-348. PubMed PMID: 24725994; PubMed Central PMCID: PMCPMC3990006
3. Dwivedi R, Gupta YK, Singh M, Joshi R, Tiwari P, Kaleekal T, et al. Correlation of saliva and serum free valproic acid concentrations in persons with epilepsy. Seizure. 2015;25:187–90. https://doi.org/10.1016/j.seizure.2014.10.010. PubMed PMID: 25455060
4. Criado-Garcia L, Ruszkiewicz DM, Eiceman GA, Thomas CL. A rapid and non-invasive method to determine toxic levels of alcohols and gamma-hydroxybutyric acid in saliva samples by gas chromatography-differential mobility spectrometry. J Breath Res. 2016;10(1):017101. https://doi.org/10.1088/1752-7155/10/1/017101. PubMed PMID: 26744364
5. Cone EJ, Clarke J, Tsanaclis L. Prevalence and disposition of drugs of abuse and opioid treatment drugs in oral fluid. J Anal Toxicol. 2007;31(8):424–33. PubMed PMID: 17988455
6. Zloczower M, Reznick AZ, Zouby RO, Nagler RM. Relationship of flow rate, uric acid, peroxidase, and superoxide dismutase activity levels with complications in diabetic patients: can saliva be used to diagnose diabetes? Antioxid Redox Signal. 2007;9(6):765–73. https://doi.org/10.1089/ars.2007.1515. PubMed PMID: 17511593
7. Greabu M, Battino M, Mohora M, Totan A, Didilescu A, Spinu T, et al. Saliva – a diagnostic window to the body, both in health and in disease. J Med Life. 2009;2(2):124–32. PubMed PMID: 20108531; PubMed Central PMCID: PMCPMC3018981
8. Goncalves AC, Marson FA, Mendonca RM, Ribeiro JD, Ribeiro AF, Paschoal IA, et al. Saliva as a potential tool for cystic fibrosis diagnosis. Diagn Pathol. 2013;8:46. https://doi.org/10.1186/1746-1596-8-46. PubMed PMID: 23510227; PubMed Central PMCID: PMCPMC3621375

9. Hu S, Wang J, Meijer J, Ieong S, Xie Y, Yu T, et al. Salivary proteomic and genomic biomarkers for primary Sjogren's syndrome. Arthritis Rheum. 2007;56(11):3588–600. https://doi.org/10.1002/art.22954. PubMed PMID: 17968930; PubMed Central PMCID: PMCPMC2856841
10. Punyadeera C, Dimeski G, Kostner K, Beyerlein P, Cooper-White J. One-step homogeneous C-reactive protein assay for saliva. J Immunol Methods. 2011;373(1–2):19–25. https://doi.org/10.1016/j.jim.2011.07.013. PubMed PMID: 21821037
11. Floriano PN, Christodoulides N, Miller CS, Ebersole JL, Spertus J, Rose BG, et al. Use of saliva-based nano-biochip tests for acute myocardial infarction at the point of care: a feasibility study. Clin Chem. 2009;55(8):1530–8. https://doi.org/10.1373/clinchem.2008.117713. PubMed PMID: 19556448
12. Mirzaii-Dizgah I, Hejazi SF, Riahi E, Salehi MM. Saliva-based creatine kinase MB measurement as a potential point-of-care testing for detection of myocardial infarction. Clin Oral Investig. 2012;16(3):775–9. https://doi.org/10.1007/s00784-011-0578-z. PubMed PMID: 21681388
13. Mirzaii-Dizgah I, Riahi E. Salivary high-sensitivity cardiac troponin T levels in patients with acute myocardial infarction. Oral Dis. 2013;19(2):180–4. https://doi.org/10.1111/j.1601-0825.2012.01968.x. PubMed PMID: 22834943
14. Mirzaii-Dizgah I, Riahi E. Salivary troponin I as an indicator of myocardial infarction. Indian J Med Res. 2013;138(6):861–5. PubMed PMID: 24521627; PubMed Central PMCID: PMCPMC3978973
15. Masters JM, Noyce AJ, Warner TT, Giovannoni G, Proctor GB. Elevated salivary protein in Parkinson's disease and salivary DJ-1 as a potential marker of disease severity. Parkinsonism Relat Disord. 2015;21(10):1251–5. https://doi.org/10.1016/j.parkreldis.2015.07.021. PubMed PMID: 26231472
16. Al-Nimer MS, Mshatat SF, Abdulla HI. Saliva alpha-synuclein and a high extinction coefficient protein: a novel approach in assessment biomarkers of Parkinson's disease. N Am J Med Sci. 2014, 6;(12):633–7. https://doi.org/10.4103/1947-2714.147980. PubMed PMID: 25599051; PubMed Central PMCID: PMCPMC4290052
17. Mougeot JL, Hirsch MA, Stevens CB, Mougeot F. Oral biomarkers in exercise-induced neuroplasticity in Parkinson's disease. Oral Dis. 2016;22(8):745–53. https://doi.org/10.1111/odi.12463. PubMed PMID: 26878123
18. Mair YH, Jhamb T, Visser MB, Aguirre A, Kramer JM. Sera and salivary matrix metalloproteinases are elevated in patients with vesiculoerosive disease: a pilot study. Oral Surg Oral Med Oral Pathol Oral Radiol. 2016;121(5):520–9. https://doi.org/10.1016/j.oooo.2016.01.002. PubMed PMID: 26948018
19. Masayesva BG, Mambo E, Taylor RJ, Goloubeva OG, Zhou S, Cohen Y, et al. Mitochondrial DNA content increase in response to cigarette smoking. Cancer Epidemiol Biomark Prev. 2006;15(1):19–24. https://doi.org/10.1158/1055-9965.EPI-05-0210. PubMed PMID: 16434581
20. Kim MM, Clinger JD, Masayesva BG, Ha PK, Zahurak ML, Westra WH, et al. Mitochondrial DNA quantity increases with histopathologic grade in premalignant and malignant head and neck lesions. Clin Cancer Res. 2004;10(24):8512–5. https://doi.org/10.1158/1078-0432.CCR-04-0734. PubMed PMID: 15623632
21. Jiang WW, Masayesva B, Zahurak M, Carvalho AL, Rosenbaum E, Mambo E, et al. Increased mitochondrial DNA content in saliva associated with head and neck cancer. Clin Cancer Res. 2005;11(7):2486–91. https://doi.org/10.1158/1078-0432.CCR-04-2147. PubMed PMID: 15814624
22. Jiang WW, Rosenbaum E, Mambo E, Zahurak M, Masayesva B, Carvalho AL, et al. Decreased mitochondrial DNA content in posttreatment salivary rinses from head and neck cancer patients. Clin Cancer Res. 2006;12(5):1564–9. https://doi.org/10.1158/1078-0432.CCR-05-1471. PubMed PMID: 16533782

23. Zhou S, Kachhap S, Sun W, Wu G, Chuang A, Poeta L, et al. Frequency and phenotypic implications of mitochondrial DNA mutations in human squamous cell cancers of the head and neck. Proc Natl Acad Sci U S A. 2007;104(18):7540–5. https://doi.org/10.1073/pnas.0610818104. PubMed PMID: 17456604; PubMed Central PMCID: PMCPMC1863503
24. Fliss MS, Usadel H, Caballero OL, Wu L, Buta MR, Eleff SM, et al. Facile detection of mitochondrial DNA mutations in tumors and bodily fluids. Science. 2000;287(5460):2017–9. PubMed PMID: 10720328
25. Mithani SK, Smith IM, Zhou S, Gray A, Koch WM, Maitra A, et al. Mitochondrial resequencing arrays detect tumor-specific mutations in salivary rinses of patients with head and neck cancer. Clin Cancer Res. 2007;13(24):7335–40. https://doi.org/10.1158/1078-0432.CCR-07-0220. PubMed PMID: 18094415
26. Rosas SL, Koch W, da Costa Carvalho MG, Wu L, Califano J, Westra W, et al. Promoter hypermethylation patterns of p16, O6-methylguanine-DNA-methyltransferase, and death-associated protein kinase in tumors and saliva of head and neck cancer patients. Cancer Res. 2001;61(3):939–42. PubMed PMID: 11221887
27. Viet CT, Jordan RC, Schmidt BL. DNA promoter hypermethylation in saliva for the early diagnosis of oral cancer. J Calif Dent Assoc. 2007;35(12):844–9. PubMed PMID: 18240747
28. Schussel J, Zhou XC, Zhang Z, Pattani K, Bermudez F, Jean-Charles G, et al. EDNRB and DCC salivary rinse hypermethylation has a similar performance as expert clinical examination in discrimination of oral cancer/dysplasia versus benign lesions. Clin Cancer Res. 2013;19(12):3268–75. https://doi.org/10.1158/1078-0432.CCR-12-3496. PubMed PMID: 23637120; PubMed Central PMCID: PMCPMC3687013
29. Guerrero-Preston R, Soudry E, Acero J, Orera M, Moreno-Lopez L, Macia-Colon G, et al. NID2 and HOXA9 promoter hypermethylation as biomarkers for prevention and early detection in oral cavity squamous cell carcinoma tissues and saliva. Cancer Prev Res (Phila). 2011;4(7):1061–72. https://doi.org/10.1158/1940-6207.CAPR-11-0006. PubMed PMID: 21558411; PubMed Central PMCID: PMCPMC3131432
30. Nagata S, Hamada T, Yamada N, Yokoyama S, Kitamoto S, Kanmura Y, et al. Aberrant DNA methylation of tumor-related genes in oral rinse: a noninvasive method for detection of oral squamous cell carcinoma. Cancer. 2012;118(17):4298–308. https://doi.org/10.1002/cncr.27417. PubMed PMID: 22252571
31. Ovchinnikov DA, Cooper MA, Pandit P, Coman WB, Cooper-White JJ, Keith P, et al. Tumor-suppressor gene promoter hypermethylation in saliva of head and neck cancer patients. Transl Oncol. 2012;5(5):321–6. PubMed PMID: 23066440; PubMed Central PMCID: PMCPMC3468923
32. Arantes LM, de Carvalho AC, Melendez ME, Centrone CC, Gois-Filho JF, Toporcov TN, et al. Validation of methylation markers for diagnosis of oral cavity cancer. Eur J Cancer. 2015;51(5):632–41. https://doi.org/10.1016/j.ejca.2015.01.060. PubMed PMID: 25686481
33. Rettori MM, de Carvalho AC, Bomfim Longo AL, de Oliveira CZ, Kowalski LP, Carvalho AL, et al. Prognostic significance of TIMP3 hypermethylation in post-treatment salivary rinse from head and neck squamous cell carcinoma patients. Carcinogenesis. 2013;34(1):20–7. https://doi.org/10.1093/carcin/bgs311. PubMed PMID: 23042095
34. Huang MF, Chang YC, Liao PS, Huang TH, Tsay CH, Chou MY. Loss of heterozygosity of p53 gene of oral cancer detected by exfoliative cytology. Oral Oncol. 1999;35(3):296–301. PubMed PMID: 10621851
35. Liao PH, Chang YC, Huang MF, Tai KW, Chou MY. Mutation of p53 gene codon 63 in saliva as a molecular marker for oral squamous cell carcinomas. Oral Oncol. 2000;36(3):272–6. PubMed PMID: 10793330
36. Mewara A, Gadbail AR, Patil S, Chaudhary M, Chavhan SD. C-deletion mutation of the p53 gene at exon 4 of codon 63 in the saliva of oral squamous cell carcinoma in Central India: a preliminary study. J Investig Clin Dent. 2010;1(2):108–13. https://doi.org/10.1111/j.2041-1626.2010.00014.x. PubMed PMID: 25427266

37. Sethi S, Benninger MS, Lu M, Havard S, Worsham MJ. Noninvasive molecular detection of head and neck squamous cell carcinoma: an exploratory analysis. Diagn Mol Pathol. 2009;18(2):81–7. https://doi.org/10.1097/PDM.0b013e3181804b82. PubMed PMID: 19430297; PubMed Central PMCID: PMCPMC2693294
38. Nunes DN, Kowalski LP, Simpson AJ. Detection of oral and oropharyngeal cancer by microsatellite analysis in mouth washes and lesion brushings. Oral Oncol. 2000;36(6):525–8. PubMed PMID: 11036246
39. Spafford MF, Koch WM, Reed AL, Califano JA, Xu LH, Eisenberger CF, et al. Detection of head and neck squamous cell carcinoma among exfoliated oral mucosal cells by microsatellite analysis. Clin Cancer Res. 2001;7(3):607–12. PubMed PMID: 11297256
40. El-Naggar AK, Mao L, Staerkel G, Coombes MM, Tucker SL, Luna MA, et al. Genetic heterogeneity in saliva from patients with oral squamous carcinomas: implications in molecular diagnosis and screening. J Mol Diagn. 2001;3(4):164–70. https://doi.org/10.1016/S1525-1578(10)60668-X. PubMed PMID: 11687600; PubMed Central PMCID: PMCPMC1906964
41. Okami K, Imate Y, Hashimoto Y, Kamada T, Takahashi M. Molecular detection of cancer cells in saliva from oral and pharyngeal cancer patients. Tokai J Exp Clin Med. 2002;27(3):85–9. PubMed PMID: 12701646
42. Li Y, St John MA, Zhou X, Kim Y, Sinha U, Jordan RC, et al. Salivary transcriptome diagnostics for oral cancer detection. Clin Cancer Res. 2004;10(24):8442–50. https://doi.org/10.1158/1078-0432.CCR-04-1167. PubMed PMID: 15623624
43. Brinkmann O, Wong DT. Salivary transcriptome biomarkers in oral squamous cell cancer detection. Adv Clin Chem. 2011;55:21–34. PubMed PMID: 22126022
44. Li Y, Elashoff D, Oh M, Sinha U, St John MA, Zhou X, et al. Serum circulating human mRNA profiling and its utility for oral cancer detection. J Clin Oncol. 2006;24(11):1754–60. https://doi.org/10.1200/JCO.2005.03.7598. PubMed PMID: 16505414
45. Spielmann N, Ilsley D, Gu J, Lea K, Brockman J, Heater S, et al. The human salivary RNA transcriptome revealed by massively parallel sequencing. Clin Chem. 2012;58(9):1314–21. https://doi.org/10.1373/clinchem.2011.176941. PubMed PMID: 22773539
46. Brinkmann O, Kastratovic DA, Dimitrijevic MV, Konstantinovic VS, Jelovac DB, Antic J, et al. Oral squamous cell carcinoma detection by salivary biomarkers in a Serbian population. Oral Oncol. 2011;47(1):51–5. https://doi.org/10.1016/j.oraloncology.2010.10.009. PubMed PMID: 21109482; PubMed Central PMCID: PMCPMC3032819
47. Elashoff D, Zhou H, Reiss J, Wang J, Xiao H, Henson B, et al. Prevalidation of salivary biomarkers for oral cancer detection. Cancer Epidemiol Biomark Prev. 2012;21(4):664–72. https://doi.org/10.1158/1055-9965.EPI-11-1093. PubMed PMID: 22301830; PubMed Central PMCID: PMCPMC3319329
48. Michailidou E, Tzimagiorgis G, Chatzopoulou F, Vahtsevanos K, Antoniadis K, Kouidou S, et al. Salivary mRNA markers having the potential to detect oral squamous cell carcinoma segregated from oral leukoplakia with dysplasia. Cancer Epidemiol. 2016;43:112–8. https://doi.org/10.1016/j.canep.2016.04.011. PubMed PMID: 27263493
49. Stott-Miller M, Houck JR, Lohavanichbutr P, Mendez E, Upton MP, Futran ND, et al. Tumor and salivary matrix metalloproteinase levels are strong diagnostic markers of oral squamous cell carcinoma. Cancer Epidemiol Biomark Prev. 2011;20(12):2628–36. https://doi.org/10.1158/1055-9965.EPI-11-0503. PubMed PMID: 21960692; PubMed Central PMCID: PMCPMC3237810
50. Lallemant B, Evrard A, Combescure C, Chapuis H, Chambon G, Raynal C, et al. Clinical relevance of nine transcriptional molecular markers for the diagnosis of head and neck squamous cell carcinoma in tissue and saliva rinse. BMC Cancer. 2009;9:370. https://doi.org/10.1186/1471-2407-9-370. PubMed PMID: 19835631; PubMed Central PMCID: PMCPMC2767357
51. Weber JA, Baxter DH, Zhang S, Huang DY, Huang KH, Lee MJ, et al. The microRNA spectrum in 12 body fluids. Clin Chem. 2010;56(11):1733–41. https://doi.org/10.1373/

clinchem.2010.147405. PubMed PMID: 20847327; PubMed Central PMCID: PMCPMC4846276

52. Patel RS, Jakymiw A, Yao B, Pauley BA, Carcamo WC, Katz J, et al. High resolution of microRNA signatures in human whole saliva. Arch Oral Biol. 2011;56(12):1506–13. https://doi.org/10.1016/j.archoralbio.2011.05.015. PubMed PMID: 21704302; PubMed Central PMCID: PMCPMC3189266
53. Gallo A, Alevizos I. Isolation of circulating microRNA in saliva. Methods Mol Biol. 2013;1024:183–90. https://doi.org/10.1007/978-1-62703-453-1_14. PubMed PMID: 23719951
54. Ogawa Y, Taketomi Y, Murakami M, Tsujimoto M, Yanoshita R. Small RNA transcriptomes of two types of exosomes in human whole saliva determined by next generation sequencing. Biol Pharm Bull. 2013;36(1):66–75. PubMed PMID: 23302638
55. Bahn JH, Zhang Q, Li F, Chan TM, Lin X, Kim Y, et al. The landscape of microRNA, Piwi-interacting RNA, and circular RNA in human saliva. Clin Chem. 2015;61(1):221–30. https://doi.org/10.1373/clinchem.2014.230433. PubMed PMID: 25376581; PubMed Central PMCID: PMCPMC4332885
56. Park NJ, Zhou H, Elashoff D, Henson BS, Kastratovic DA, Abemayor E, et al. Salivary microRNA: discovery, characterization, and clinical utility for oral cancer detection. Clin Cancer Res. 2009;15(17):5473–7. https://doi.org/10.1158/1078-0432.CCR-09-0736. PubMed PMID: 19706812; PubMed Central PMCID: PMCPMC2752355
57. Langevin SM, Stone RA, Bunker CH, Grandis JR, Sobol RW, Taioli E. MicroRNA-137 promoter methylation in oral rinses from patients with squamous cell carcinoma of the head and neck is associated with gender and body mass index. Carcinogenesis. 2010;31(5):864–70. https://doi.org/10.1093/carcin/bgq051. PubMed PMID: 20197299; PubMed Central PMCID: PMCPMC2864416
58. Wiklund ED, Gao S, Hulf T, Sibbritt T, Nair S, Costea DE, et al. MicroRNA alterations and associated aberrant DNA methylation patterns across multiple sample types in oral squamous cell carcinoma. PLoS One. 2011;6(11):e27840. https://doi.org/10.1371/journal.pone.0027840. PubMed PMID: 22132151; PubMed Central PMCID: PMCPMC3222641
59. Liu CJ, Kao SY, Tu HF, Tsai MM, Chang KW, Lin SC. Increase of microRNA miR-31 level in plasma could be a potential marker of oral cancer. Oral Dis. 2010;16(4):360–4. https://doi.org/10.1111/j.1601-0825.2009.01646.x. PubMed PMID: 20233326
60. Liu CJ, Lin SC, Yang CC, Cheng HW, Chang KW. Exploiting salivary miR-31 as a clinical biomarker of oral squamous cell carcinoma. Head Neck. 2012;34(2):219–24. https://doi.org/10.1002/hed.21713. PubMed PMID: 22083872
61. Salazar C, Nagadia R, Pandit P, Cooper-White J, Banerjee N, Dimitrova N, et al. A novel saliva-based microRNA biomarker panel to detect head and neck cancers. Cell Oncol (Dordr). 2014;37(5):331–8. https://doi.org/10.1007/s13402-014-0188-2. PubMed PMID: 25156495
62. Momen-Heravi F, Trachtenberg AJ, Kuo WP, Cheng YS. Genomewide study of salivary MicroRNAs for detection of oral cancer. J Dent Res. 2014;93(7 Suppl):86S–93S. https://doi.org/10.1177/0022034514531018. PubMed PMID: 24718111; PubMed Central PMCID: PMCPMC4107544
63. Wang Z, Zhang J, Guo Y, Wu X, Yang W, Xu L, et al. A novel electrically magnetic-controllable electrochemical biosensor for the ultra sensitive and specific detection of attomolar level oral cancer-related microRNA. Biosens Bioelectron. 2013;45:108–13. https://doi.org/10.1016/j.bios.2013.02.007. PubMed PMID: 23455049
64. Tian X, Chen Z, Shi S, Wang X, Wang W, Li N, et al. Clinical diagnostic implications of body fluid MiRNA in Oral squamous cell carcinoma: a Meta-analysis. Medicine (Baltimore). 2015;94(37):e1324. https://doi.org/10.1097/MD.0000000000001324. PubMed PMID: 26376377; PubMed Central PMCID: PMCPMC4635791
65. Tang H, Wu Z, Zhang J, Su B. Salivary lncRNA as a potential marker for oral squamous cell carcinoma diagnosis. Mol Med Rep. 2013;7(3):761–6. https://doi.org/10.3892/mmr.2012.1254. PubMed PMID: 23292713

66. He QY, Chen J, Kung HF, Yuen AP, Chiu JF. Identification of tumor-associated proteins in oral tongue squamous cell carcinoma by proteomics. Proteomics. 2004;4(1):271–8. https://doi.org/10.1002/pmic.200300550. PubMed PMID: 14730689
67. Chen J, He QY, Yuen AP, Chiu JF. Proteomics of buccal squamous cell carcinoma: the involvement of multiple pathways in tumorigenesis. Proteomics. 2004;4(8):2465–75. https://doi.org/10.1002/pmic.200300762. PubMed PMID: 15274141
68. St John MA, Li Y, Zhou X, Denny P, Ho CM, Montemagno C, et al. Interleukin 6 and interleukin 8 as potential biomarkers for oral cavity and oropharyngeal squamous cell carcinoma. Arch Otolaryngol Head Neck Surg. 2004;130(8):929–35. https://doi.org/10.1001/archotol.130.8.929. PubMed PMID: 15313862
69. Roesch Ely M, Nees M, Karsai S, Magele I, Bogumil R, Vorderwulbecke S, et al. Transcript and proteome analysis reveals reduced expression of calgranulins in head and neck squamous cell carcinoma. Eur J Cell Biol. 2005;84(2–3):431–44. https://doi.org/10.1016/j.ejcb.2005.01.003. PubMed PMID: 15819419
70. Arellano-Garcia ME, Hu S, Wang J, Henson B, Zhou H, Chia D, et al. Multiplexed immunobead-based assay for detection of oral cancer protein biomarkers in saliva. Oral Dis. 2008;14(8):705–12. https://doi.org/10.1111/j.1601-0825.2008.01488.x. PubMed PMID: 19193200; PubMed Central PMCID: PMCPMC2675698
71. Hu S, Yu T, Xie Y, Yang Y, Li Y, Zhou X, et al. Discovery of oral fluid biomarkers for human oral cancer by mass spectrometry. Cancer Genomics Proteomics. 2007;4(2):55–64. PubMed PMID: 17804867
72. de Jong EP, Xie H, Onsongo G, Stone MD, Chen XB, Kooren JA, et al. Quantitative proteomics reveals myosin and actin as promising saliva biomarkers for distinguishing pre-malignant and malignant oral lesions. PLoS One. 2010;5(6):e11148. https://doi.org/10.1371/journal.pone.0011148. PubMed PMID: 20567502; PubMed Central PMCID: PMCPMC2887353
73. Csosz E, Labiscsak P, Kallo G, Markus B, Emri M, Szabo A, et al. Proteomics investigation of OSCC-specific salivary biomarkers in a Hungarian population highlights the importance of identification of population-tailored biomarkers. PLoS One. 2017;12(5):e0177282. https://doi.org/10.1371/journal.pone.0177282. PubMed PMID: 28545132; PubMed Central PMCID: PMCPMC5436697
74. Franzmann EJ, Reategui EP, Pereira LH, Pedroso F, Joseph D, Allen GO, et al. Salivary protein and solCD44 levels as a potential screening tool for early detection of head and neck squamous cell carcinoma. Head Neck. 2012;34(5):687–95. https://doi.org/10.1002/hed.21810. PubMed PMID: 22294418; PubMed Central PMCID: PMCPMC3323768
75. Jou YJ, Lin CD, Lai CH, Chen CH, Kao JY, Chen SY, et al. Proteomic identification of salivary transferrin as a biomarker for early detection of oral cancer. Anal Chim Acta. 2010;681(1–2):41–8. https://doi.org/10.1016/j.aca.2010.09.030. PubMed PMID: 21035601
76. Jou YJ, Lin CD, Lai CH, Tang CH, Huang SH, Tsai MH, et al. Salivary zinc finger protein 510 peptide as a novel biomarker for detection of oral squamous cell carcinoma in early stages. Clin Chim Acta. 2011;412(15–16):1357–65. https://doi.org/10.1016/j.cca.2011.04.004. PubMed PMID: 21497587
77. Sun G, Ping FY. Application of saliva protein fingerprints in the diagnosis of oral squamous cell cancer by surface enhanced laser desorption ionization time of flight mass. Zhonghua Kou Qiang Yi Xue Za Zhi. 2009;44(11):664–7. PubMed PMID: 20079267
78. Sugimoto M, Wong DT, Hirayama A, Soga T, Tomita M. Capillary electrophoresis mass spectrometry-based saliva metabolomics identified oral, breast and pancreatic cancer-specific profiles. Metabolomics. 2010;6(1):78–95. https://doi.org/10.1007/s11306-009-0178-y. PubMed PMID: 20300169; PubMed Central PMCID: PMCPMC2818837
79. Wei J, Xie G, Zhou Z, Shi P, Qiu Y, Zheng X, et al. Salivary metabolite signatures of oral cancer and leukoplakia. Int J Cancer. 2011;129(9):2207–17. https://doi.org/10.1002/ijc.25881. PubMed PMID: 21190195
80. Wang Q, Gao P, Cheng F, Wang X, Duan Y. Measurement of salivary metabolite biomarkers for early monitoring of oral cancer with ultra performance liquid chromatography-mass spec-

trometry. Talanta. 2014;119:299–305. https://doi.org/10.1016/j.talanta.2013.11.008. PubMed PMID: 24401418

81. Wang Q, Gao P, Wang X, Duan Y. The early diagnosis and monitoring of squamous cell carcinoma via saliva metabolomics. Sci Rep. 2014;4:6802. https://doi.org/10.1038/srep06802. PubMed PMID: 25354816; PubMed Central PMCID: PMCPMC4213796
82. Ishikawa S, Sugimoto M, Kitabatake K, Sugano A, Nakamura M, Kaneko M, et al. Identification of salivary metabolomic biomarkers for oral cancer screening. Sci Rep. 2016;6:31520. https://doi.org/10.1038/srep31520. PubMed PMID: 27539254; PubMed Central PMCID: PMCPMC4990923
83. Sridharan G, Ramani P, Patankar S. Serum metabolomics in oral leukoplakia and oral squamous cell carcinoma. J Cancer Res Ther 2017;13(3):556–561. https://doi.org/10.4103/jcrt.JCRT_1233_16. PubMed PMID: 28862226.
84. Sridharan G, Ramani P, Patankar S, Vijayaraghavan R. Evaluation of salivary metabolomics in oral leukoplakia and oral squamous cell carcinoma. J Oral Pathol Med. 2019; https://doi.org/10.1111/jop.12835. PubMed PMID: 30714209
85. Guerra EN, Acevedo AC, Leite AF, Gozal D, Chardin H, De Luca Canto G. Diagnostic capability of salivary biomarkers in the assessment of head and neck cancer: a systematic review and meta-analysis. Oral Oncol 2015;51(9):805–818. https://doi.org/10.1016/j.oraloncology.2015.06.010. PubMed PMID: 26170140.
86. Hema Shree K, Ramani P, Sherlin H, Sukumaran G, Jeyaraj G, Don KR, et al. Saliva as a diagnostic tool in oral squamous cell carcinoma – a systematic review with Meta analysis. Pathol Oncol Res. 2019; https://doi.org/10.1007/s12253-019-00588-2.
87. Tong JH, Tsang RK, Lo KW, Woo JK, Kwong J, Chan MW, et al. Quantitative Epstein-Barr virus DNA analysis and detection of gene promoter hypermethylation in nasopharyngeal (NP) brushing samples from patients with NP carcinoma. Clin Cancer Res. 2002;8(8):2612–9. PubMed PMID: 12171892
88. Stevens SJ, Verkuijlen SA, Hariwiyanto B, Harijadi, Paramita DK, Fachiroh J, et al. Noninvasive diagnosis of nasopharyngeal carcinoma: nasopharyngeal brushings reveal high Epstein-Barr virus DNA load and carcinoma-specific viral BARF1 mRNA. Int J Cancer. 2006;119(3):608–14. https://doi.org/10.1002/ijc.21914. PubMed PMID: 16572427
89. Zheng XH, Lu LX, Li XZ, Jia WH. Quantification of Epstein-Barr virus DNA load in nasopharyngeal brushing samples in the diagnosis of nasopharyngeal carcinoma in southern China. Cancer Sci. 2015;106(9):1196–201. https://doi.org/10.1111/cas.12718. PubMed PMID: 26082292; PubMed Central PMCID: PMCPMC4582989
90. Lin SY, Tsang NM, Kao SC, Hsieh YL, Chen YP, Tsai CS, et al. Presence of Epstein-Barr virus latent membrane protein 1 gene in the nasopharyngeal swabs from patients with nasopharyngeal carcinoma. Head Neck. 2001;23(3):194–200. PubMed PMID: 11428449
91. Hao SP, Tsang NM, Chang KP. Screening nasopharyngeal carcinoma by detection of the latent membrane protein 1 (LMP-1) gene with nasopharyngeal swabs. Cancer. 2003;97(8):1909–13. https://doi.org/10.1002/cncr.11312. PubMed PMID: 12673717
92. Hao SP, Tsang NM, Chang KP, Ueng SH. Molecular diagnosis of nasopharyngeal carcinoma: detecting LMP-1 and EBNA by nasopharyngeal swab. Otolaryngol Head Neck Surg. 2004;131(5):651–4. https://doi.org/10.1016/j.otohns.2004.04.013. PubMed PMID: 15523443
93. Chen Y, Zhao W, Lin L, Xiao X, Zhou X, Ming H, et al. Nasopharyngeal Epstein-Barr virus load: an efficient supplementary method for population-based nasopharyngeal carcinoma screening. PLoS One. 2015;10(7):e0132669. https://doi.org/10.1371/journal.pone.0132669. PubMed PMID: 26151639; PubMed Central PMCID: PMCPMC4495031
94. Pow EH, Law MY, Tsang PC, Perera RA, Kwong DL. Salivary Epstein-Barr virus DNA level in patients with nasopharyngeal carcinoma following radiotherapy. Oral Oncol. 2011;47(9):879–82. https://doi.org/10.1016/j.oraloncology.2011.06.507. PubMed PMID: 21767975

95. Shan J, Pow EH, Tsang PC, Perera RA, Kwong DL. Comparison of two laboratory extraction techniques for the detection of Epstein-Barr virus in the saliva of nasopharyngeal carcinoma patients. J Investig Clin Dent. 2014;5(2):104–8. https://doi.org/10.1111/jicd.12078. PubMed PMID: 24574317
96. Makitie AA, Reis PP, Zhang T, Chin SF, Gullane P, Siu LL, et al. Epstein-Barr virus DNA measured in nasopharyngeal brushings in patients with nasopharyngeal carcinoma: pilot study. J Otolaryngol. 2004;33(5):299–303. PubMed PMID: 15931814
97. Adham M, Greijer AE, Verkuijlen SA, Juwana H, Fleig S, Rachmadi L, et al. Epstein-Barr virus DNA load in nasopharyngeal brushings and whole blood in nasopharyngeal carcinoma patients before and after treatment. Clin Cancer Res. 2013;19(8):2175–86. https://doi.org/10.1158/1078-0432.CCR-12-2897. PubMed PMID: 23493345
98. Kerekhanjanarong V, Sitawarin S, Sakdikul S, Saengpanich S, Chindavijak S, Supiyaphun P, et al. Telomerase assay and nested polymerase chain reaction from nasopharyngeal swabs for early noninvasive detection of nasopharyngeal carcinoma. Otolaryngol Head Neck Surg. 2000;123(5):624–9. https://doi.org/10.1067/mhn.2000.109368. PubMed PMID: 11077353
99. Cui Q, Feng FT, Xu M, Liu WS, Yao YY, Xie SH, et al. Nasopharyngeal carcinoma risk prediction via salivary detection of host and Epstein-Barr virus genetic variants. Oncotarget. 2017;8(56):95066–74. https://doi.org/10.18632/oncotarget.11144. PubMed PMID: 29221111; PubMed Central PMCID: PMCPMC5707005
100. Qiu S, Xu Y, Huang L, Zheng W, Huang C, Huang S, et al. Non-invasive detection of nasopharyngeal carcinoma using saliva surface-enhanced Raman spectroscopy. Oncol Lett. 2016;11(1):884–90. https://doi.org/10.3892/ol.2015.3969. PubMed PMID: 26870300; PubMed Central PMCID: PMCPMC4727062
101. Chang HW, Chan A, Kwong DL, Wei WI, Sham JS, Yuen AP. Evaluation of hypermethylated tumor suppressor genes as tumor markers in mouth and throat rinsing fluid, nasopharyngeal swab and peripheral blood of nasopharyngeal carcinoma patient. Int J Cancer. 2003;105(6):851–5. https://doi.org/10.1002/ijc.11162. PubMed PMID: 12767073
102. Sun D, Zhang Z, Van do N, Huang G, Ernberg I, Hu L. Aberrant methylation of CDH13 gene in nasopharyngeal carcinoma could serve as a potential diagnostic biomarker. Oral Oncol. 2007;43(1):82–7. https://doi.org/10.1016/j.oraloncology.2006.01.007. PubMed PMID: 16807071
103. Hutajulu SH, Indrasari SR, Indrawati LP, Harijadi A, Duin S, Haryana SM, et al. Epigenetic markers for early detection of nasopharyngeal carcinoma in a high risk population. Mol Cancer. 2011;10(48) https://doi.org/10.1186/1476-4598-10-48. PubMed PMID: 21535891; PubMed Central PMCID: PMCPMC3114786
104. Yang X, Dai W, Kwong DL, Szeto CY, Wong EH, Ng WT, et al. Epigenetic markers for noninvasive early detection of nasopharyngeal carcinoma by methylation-sensitive high resolution melting. Int J Cancer. 2015;136(4):E127–35. https://doi.org/10.1002/ijc.29192. PubMed PMID: 25196065
105. Zhang L, Xiao H, Zhou H, Santiago S, Lee JM, Garon EB, et al. Development of transcriptomic biomarker signature in human saliva to detect lung cancer. Cell Mol Life Sci. 2012;69(19):3341–50. https://doi.org/10.1007/s00018-012-1027-0. PubMed PMID: 22689099; PubMed Central PMCID: PMCPMC4121486
106. Xiao H, Zhang L, Zhou H, Lee JM, Garon EB, Wong DT. Proteomic analysis of human saliva from lung cancer patients using two-dimensional difference gel electrophoresis and mass spectrometry. Mol Cell Proteomics. 2012;11(2):M111 012112. https://doi.org/10.1074/mcp.M111.012112. PubMed PMID: 22096114; PubMed Central PMCID: PMCPMC3277759
107. Li X, Yang T, Lin J. Spectral analysis of human saliva for detection of lung cancer using surface-enhanced Raman spectroscopy. J Biomed Opt. 2012;17(3):037003. https://doi.org/10.1117/1.JBO.17.3.037003. PubMed PMID: 22502575
108. Zhang L, Xiao H, Karlan S, Zhou H, Gross J, Elashoff D, et al. Discovery and preclinical validation of salivary transcriptomic and proteomic biomarkers for the non-invasive detection of

breast cancer. PLoS One. 2010;5(12):e15573. https://doi.org/10.1371/journal.pone.0015573. PubMed PMID: 21217834; PubMed Central PMCID: PMCPMC3013113

109. Cao MQ, Wu ZZ, Wu WK. Identification of salivary biomarkers in breast cancer patients with thick white or thick yellow tongue fur using isobaric tags for relative and absolute quantitative proteomics. Zhong Xi Yi Jie He Xue Bao. 2011;9(3):275–80. PubMed PMID: 21419079
110. Wu ZZ, Wang JG, Zhang XL. Diagnostic model of saliva protein finger print analysis of patients with gastric cancer. World J Gastroenterol. 2009;15(7):865–70. PubMed PMID: 19230049; PubMed Central PMCID: PMCPMC2653388
111. Zhang L, Farrell JJ, Zhou H, Elashoff D, Akin D, Park NH, et al. Salivary transcriptomic biomarkers for detection of resectable pancreatic cancer. Gastroenterology. 2010;138(3):949–57 e1-7. https://doi.org/10.1053/j.gastro.2009.11.010. PubMed PMID: 19931263; PubMed Central PMCID: PMCPMC2831159
112. Shetty V, Zigler C, Robles TF, Elashoff D, Yamaguchi M. Developmental validation of a point-of-care, salivary alpha-amylase biosensor. Psychoneuroendocrinology. 2011;36(2):193–9. https://doi.org/10.1016/j.psyneuen.2010.07.008. PubMed PMID: 20696529; PubMed Central PMCID: PMCPMC2996479
113. Zangheri M, Cevenini L, Anfossi L, Baggiani C, Simoni P, Di Nardo F, et al. A simple and compact smartphone accessory for quantitative chemiluminescence-based lateral flow immunoassay for salivary cortisol detection. Biosens Bioelectron. 2015;64:63–8. https://doi.org/10.1016/j.bios.2014.08.048. PubMed PMID: 25194797
114. Carrio A, Sampedro C, Sanchez-Lopez JL, Pimienta M, Campoy P. Automated low-cost smartphone-based lateral flow saliva test reader for drugs-of-abuse detection. Sensors (Basel). 2015;15(11):29569–93. https://doi.org/10.3390/s151129569. PubMed PMID: 26610513; PubMed Central PMCID: PMCPMC4701349
115. Zilberman Y, Sonkusale SR. Microfluidic optoelectronic sensor for salivary diagnostics of stomach cancer. Biosens Bioelectron. 2015;67:465–71. https://doi.org/10.1016/j.bios.2014.09.006. PubMed PMID: 25223554
116. Chen Z, Mauk MG, Wang J, Abrams WR, Corstjens PL, Niedbala RS, et al. A microfluidic system for saliva-based detection of infectious diseases. Ann N Y Acad Sci. 2007;1098:429–36. https://doi.org/10.1196/annals.1384.024. PubMed PMID: 17435147
117. Zhang L, Yang W, Yang Y, Liu H, Gu Z. Smartphone-based point-of-care testing of salivary alpha-amylase for personal psychological measurement. Analyst. 2015;140(21):7399–406. https://doi.org/10.1039/c5an01664a. PubMed PMID: 26415134
118. Lee PT, Compton RG. Selective thiol detection in authentic biological samples with the use of screen-printed electrodes. Anal Sci. 2015;31(7):685–91. https://doi.org/10.2116/analsci.31.685. PubMed PMID: 26165292
119. Fend R, Kolk AH, Bessant C, Buijtels P, Klatser PR, Woodman AC. Prospects for clinical application of electronic-nose technology to early detection of Mycobacterium tuberculosis in culture and sputum. J Clin Microbiol. 2006;44(6):2039–45. https://doi.org/10.1128/JCM.01591-05. PubMed PMID: 16757595; PubMed Central PMCID: PMCPMC1489436

Chapter 4
Lung Cancer Biomarkers in Proximal Fluids

4.1 Introduction

For decades, lung cancer (LnCa) has remained a challenge in oncology and cancer research by being the highest in both incidence and mortality. The 2018 global incidence, mortality, and 5-year prevalence were 2,093,876; 1,761,007; and 2,129,964, respectively (GLOBOCAN 2018). Sadly, the vast majority of cases occur in the resource-poor parts of the world. Added to this unfavorable statistic are the dismal survival rates, with many deaths occurring in the developing world. Globally, LnCa is the leading cause of cancer-related deaths. Even more worrisome is the fact that the global incident rate of 2,093,876 mirrors the 5-year prevalence of 2,129,964. While first in both incidence and mortality, LnCa is fourth in reference to the 5-year prevalence (led by breast, colorectal, and prostate cancers), which is partly due to the high case fatality coupled with the lack of regional variability in survival rates. A disturbing changing trend in regard to sex was observed in GLOBOCAN 2018 analysis and stated, "one of the key concerns raised by the IARC is that lung cancer is the leading cause of death globally and its prevalence is rising amongst women, surpassing breast cancer in 28 countries."

The aforementioned dismal statistics of LnCa is due to a number of factors. First is the lack of evidence-based screening modalities (imaging or biochemical markers) even for those at elevated risk above the general population, such as smokers. Second, because of the lack of recommended screening guidelines, the vast majority of patients are diagnosed with late- and advanced-stage disease, when the prognosis is poor. If detected early, the 5-year survival rate could be as high as 70%. However, this rate is about 20% for stage IIIb and 5% for stage IV LnCa. Improved imaging and treatment have enabled some progress to be made over the past several decades in the 5-year survival rates. Third, patients with late-stage disease are subjected to chemotherapy and various targeted therapies. However, lack of response and evolution of resistant clones lead to disease relapse. Additionally, field cancerization accounts for some relapses due to the emergence of second primary tumors.

G. D. Dakubo, *Cancer Biomarkers in Body Fluids*,
https://doi.org/10.1007/978-3-030-24725-6_4

Finally, although LnCa is histopathologically dichotomized into non-small cell LnCa (NSCLC – 80% of all cases) and small cell LnCa (SCLC – the remaining 20%), the disease is very heterogeneous at the molecular level, thus hampering efficient targeted therapy delivery.

Lifestyle choices, as well as environmental and occupational exposures to carcinogens, are the primary causes of LnCa, which is probably the best evidence of the role of carcinogens in cancer. Not surprisingly, LnCa is probably the most studied cancer with regard to environmental exposures. Cessation of active and passive smoking, elimination of environmental and occupational exposures, and avoidance of indoor air pollution are key primary prevention measures. Clearly, early detection and diagnosis of LnCa is key to improving the dismal 5-year survival outcome. The need for validated biomarkers and molecular imaging techniques that can be deployed at the point-of-care is urgent. Of even more importance will be biomarkers that can be assayed noninvasively in body fluids for LnCa screening, diagnosis, treatment stratification, longitudinal monitoring for treatment response, detection of early recurrences, and the study of tumor evolution over time so as to inform clinical decision-making. Thus, various investigators are diligently pursuing these biomarkers, and this chapter provides a synthesis of these findings in proximal fluids of the lung.

4.2 Pulmonary Anatomy and Histology

The pulmonary tree is part of the respiratory system. The system extends from the nostrils to the alveolar and includes the nasal cavities, paranasal sinuses, nasopharynx, the trachea, bronchi, bronchioles, alveolar ducts, and sacs. The trachea divides repeatedly into primary or main bronchi, then secondary or lobar bronchi, and tertiary or segmental bronchi (Fig. 4.1). The segmental bronchi divide into smaller bronchioles (no cartilage in walls) and finally into terminal or respiratory bronchioles that also divide into several alveolar ducts, alveolar sacs, and their associated alveoli. The alveoli are the regions of gaseous exchange. The respiratory epithelium, from which many lung cancers arise, changes in structure from the bronchi to the bronchioles. The primary bronchi are lined by pseudostratified columnar epithelium with many goblet cells. The secondary and tertiary bronchi demonstrate reducing pseudostratification of the epithelium, becoming tall columnar in structure. Goblet cells are also reduced in number. Ciliated columnar cells and few goblet cells line the bronchioles. The terminal and respiratory bronchioles have no goblet cells but, instead, contain Clara cells and ciliated cuboidal epithelium. Flattened epithelial cells referred to as pneumocytes line the alveoli. There are two types of pneumocytes: type 1 and type 2 pneumocytes. Type 1 pneumocytes are flat squamous cells and hence occupy most of the alveolar surface. They form part of the gaseous diffusion barrier. Type 2 pneumocytes, however, are rounded in shape and, though they form about 60% of the alveolar cells, occupy just a little portion of the alveolar surface. They, together with Clara cells, secrete surfactant that helps reduce

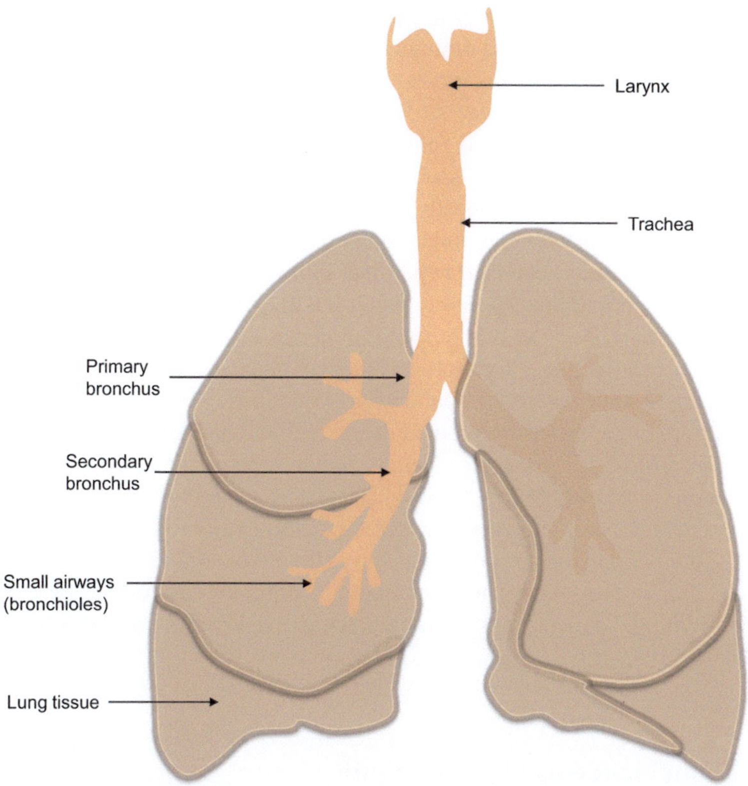

Fig. 4.1 Anatomy of the lung

pulmonary tension during respiration. The proximal fluids of the lung, including sputum, bronchial fluid, and exhaled breath condensate that harbor LnCa biomarkers, emanate from these respiratory structures.

4.3 Sputum

Sputum or expectorate is the material produced by cells lining the respiratory tract. It is acquired either spontaneously or by induction and is coughed, spat out, and collected. Thus, sputum tends to contain some saliva, but sputum of near purity can be obtained through separation from saliva.

Sputum collection follows standard operating procedures (SOPs) of the organization or institution. To collect sputum, the client or patient is instructed on how to optimally produce sputum. Usually they place hands on their hips and forcefully cough to produce sputum that is carefully spat into a well-labeled container. For biomarker analysis, sputum is processed and stored at −20 °C or −80 °C for subsequent analysis. For proteome analysis, sputum can be vortexed and incubated at 37 °C for 10 min and filtered through 50 um nylon filter before centrifugation at 3000 rpm for 10 min at 4 °C. Supernatant and cells can then be aliquoted and stored for later use.

Sputum can also be collected following induction. Because many adults can spontaneously produce sufficient sputum for analysis, this may not be necessary in LnCa studies because they are mostly disease of the adult. Children are often poor sputum producers, for whom an induction is often needed. For this procedure, the client or patient inhales nebulized hypertonic saline (concentration of 3%) solution for about 15–30 min to liquefy airway secretions and enhance coughing and expectoration of sputum. Because this procedure induces coughing into the air, precautions to prevent infection by airborne pathogens must be observed. In asthmatic patients, people with severely impaired lung functions (FEV1 < 1 l) or likely to develop severe bronchospasms, premedication with salbutamol (or other bronchodilators) is recommended prior to induction. Sputum induction is contraindicated in patients with severe respiratory pathologies such as acute respiratory distress, pulmonary embolism, and pneumothorax. Many investigators follow a four-step process for sputum induction and collection: bronchodilator administration; delivery of nebulized hypertonic saline; chest percussion or vibration performed by a technician; and sample collection by spontaneous expectoration or suction via the nasopharynx.

4.4 Bronchoalveolar Lavage Fluid

Bronchoalveolar lavage fluid (BALF) is fluid obtained by washing the respiratory tract and alveolar. It is a diagnostic procedure whereby a fiber-optic bronchoscope is introduced through either the mouth or nostrils into the specific region of the airway. Sterile 0.9% saline solution is then squirted in to fill the airway distal to the tip of the bronchoscope. The fluid is then recollected and kept on ice prior to processing. The fluid therefore contains materials (primarily cells), from the epithelial lining of the bronchial tree and alveolar surface, and soluble factors of interest in diagnostic examination. The cells are mainly white blood cells, epithelial cells, and microbes that can be used for microbiome studies. In smokers, total cell counts are increased about fourfold primarily due to macrophages. In addition, the proportion of the various cells changes with lung diseases. Much of the soluble factors in BALF are serum proteins. Others are surfactants, urea, markers of collagen metabolism, fibronectin, cytokines, and mediators of inflammation, as well as angiotensin-converting enzyme (ACE).

4.5 Exhaled Breath Condensate

Exhaled breath condensate (EBC) is another noninvasive lung proximal fluid that has been extensively explored for LnCa and other lung disease biomarkers. As the name indicates, EBC is a condensate of expired air from the respiratory tree as it comes into a cold interface. Hence it contains biomolecules from alveoli and other epithelial lining of the respiratory tree.

4.5.1 Constituents of Exhaled Breath Condensate

Exhaled breath condensate contains three defined components: water from exhaled air (>99%), water-soluble volatile compounds, and variable-sized particles aerosolized from alveolar lining fluid (ALF). The volatile compounds include oxygen, carbon dioxide, nitric oxide, ethane, and pentane; the nonvolatile compounds include nucleic acids, small organic ions, organic acids, urea, amino acids, peptides, proteins, surfactants, and macromolecules usually from microbes [1]. Levels of aerosolized particles range from 0.1 to 4 particles per cm^{-3}, with mean diameter of about 0.3 um [2]. The volatile compounds and aerosolized ALF components serve as biomarkers of respiratory diseases including LnCa. This source of biomarkers differs from those in sputum and BALF because they lack cellular components. However, EBC biomarkers are derived from the ALF and hence are derivative of cells of the respiratory tree [3, 4]. Indeed, miRNAs have been detected in exosomes from EBC [5].

The ALF consists of a watery or sol phase that contains soluble components of bronchial origin and serum proteins, as well as a mucus or gel phase made up of glycoproteins from the bronchial wall and serum proteins. Component and anatomic analyses indicate that phospholipids (80%), cholesterol (10%), proteins (10%), and small amounts of carbohydrates emanate from the respiratory bronchioles, alveolar ducts, and alveoli [6]. The presence of prostaglandins and cytokines indicates sampling from the central and peripheral air passages, while the presence of surfactants suggests biomarkers from alveoli.

4.5.2 Collection of Exhaled Breath Condensate

EBC is a noninvasive process of collecting ALF for various uses. Collection is simple, requiring tidal (normal) breathing by the subject. The process involves cooling of exhaled air in a specialized device. The American Thoracic and European Respiratory Societies (ATS/ERS) have published guidelines for the collection of EBC for biomarker analysis [7]. However, there is still interlaboratory variability in EBC collection procedures.

Different types of commercial and custom-made devices are available for collecting EBC. The commercial devices include EcoScreen [8], EcoScreen 2 [9], EcoScreen Turbo [8], RTube™ [8], RTubeVOC™, Anacon [10, 11], and TURBO-DECCS [12]. Modifications to some of the commercial devices enable their utility on infants [13], children [14], and patients on mechanical ventilation [15, 16]. The basic principle of EBC collection is cooling of exhaled air; however, the various devices differ in regard to design, cooling methods, and material used for cooling. The choice of device is important because the design can significantly affect the levels of different biomarkers.

EBC devices contain a one-way inspiratory valve to prevent the subject from inspiring the condensed cold air during inspiration and also to prevent condensation of ambient air in the device. The commercial devices use different cooling systems including refrigerated cooling chamber (EcoScreen series, Anacon, and TURBO-DECCS) or a pre-cooled aluminum-condensing sleeve (RTube™). Custom-made EBC collection devices consist of a mouthpiece with a one-way inspiratory valve connected to a collecting system in a coolant made of dry ice, salted ice, ice, or liquid nitrogen.

The exhaled air condenses at 4 °C or lower temperatures. The cooling temperature affects the consistency of the condensate, which could be liquid, frozen ice, or a mixture of both. Moreover, the temperature employed for cooling affects the relative concentration of some biomarkers in the condensate. Supposedly, collection at lower temperatures (< – 10 °C) increases the volume of EBC compared to wet ice (4 °C) cooling systems [17, 18]. The effect of cooling temperatures on biomarker concentration needs further evaluation.

The volume and concentration of biomarkers in EBC is affected by the duration of collection and respiratory patterns during the collection process. Several studies have reported collecting EBC over 10–15 min duration, although a few have used very short (3 min) or prolonged (60 min) collection times [7, 19]. Ten minutes is sufficient to collect 1–2 ml of EBC. This volume of EBC can be generated at a rate of 100 ul min^{-1} (range 40–300 ul min^{-1}) at a tidal respiratory rate of 15–20 breaths min^{-1} [20, 21]. The volume of expired air is linearly correlated with the volume of EBC collected from healthy volunteers. The ATS/ERS recommend a collection time of at least 10 min and reporting of collection time [7]. Breathing patterns also affect both the volume and biomarker concentration of EBC. Increased tidal volume and/or minute ventilation, hyperventilation, and mechanical ventilation are associated with increased volume of EBC [22–24]. Reasons offered for this include increased expiratory volume, increased aerosolization of ALF as a result of increased turbulent airflow, and increased alveoli recruitment [24–26]. The recommendation by the ATS/ERS Task Force is to collect EBC during tidal breathing [7].

Although mainly from the central parts of the lung, EBC also originate from smaller airways and alveoli [27]. Thus, biomarkers in EBC differ based on the anatomic region of the lung where they are mostly generated. Respiratory airflow influences biomarkers from large bronchi, but not those from alveoli because air movement is minimal in alveoli [28].

4.5.3 *Testing for Oropharyngeal Contamination of Exhaled Breath Condensate*

Given that EBC collection requires passage of exhaled air through the upper aerodigestive tract, oropharyngeal contamination is possible. This is more problematic when analysis involves volatile organic biomarkers. For instance, bacterial degradation of urea is suggested to contribute to the levels of ammonia in EBC [29]. Moreover, nitrite levels in EBC are partly from oropharyngeal bacteria microbiota, because levels decrease following oral rinses with chlorhexidine prior to sample collection [30]. While not required by ATS/ERS because many investigators find no evidence of salivary contamination, others recommend analysis of salivary amylase (constitutes 10–20% of total salivary proteins) to determine the level of salivary contamination in EBC [4, 31]. Noteworthy, salivary amylase has been detected in EBC collected from the lower airways, suggesting it lacks exclusivity to the oropharynx [32, 33]. Another suggested marker for detecting salivary contamination in EBC is measurement of phosphate levels [32]. There are measures that can be used to mitigate salivary contamination of EBC. The recommendation by the ATS/ERS Task Force is to use a nose clip to exclude sample loss via the nose and to be wary of the potential effects of nasal airflow on biomarkers. Sampling methods as to the route of airflow and use of nose clip are ought to be reported [7]. Other precautionary measures used to minimize salivary contamination include use of swan neck-shaped tube design, saliva trap, prior mouthwashes, and periodic swallowing of saliva during the collection process [34].

4.5.4 *Processing and Storage of Exhaled Breath Condensate*

Of note, much of EBC consist of condensed water vapor. Biomarkers exist in the medium at extremely diluted levels. This variability in biomarker concentration is a potential source of heterogeneity in various studies and hence has been a major obstacle in data reproducibility. Thus, for macromolecular (e.g., protein) analysis, samples tend to be pooled and concentrated, which could confound biomarker discovery because of individual marker variability unless multiple samples are pooled from the same subject.

Freeze-drying (lyophilization) and vacuum centrifugation to remove free water without excessive sample drying have been applied to concentrate biomarkers in EBC [35]. Many investigators have found lyophilization to be optimal for biomarker concentration. For example, lyophilization could concentrate cytokines up to 33 times for analysis [36–38]. Similar to all biological samples for biomarker studies, immediate analysis is preferable, but this is not always possible. It is recommended to store EBC samples at −70 °C or −80 °C and to check for the stability of biomarkers during the storage window [7, 39]. One study found no relationship in the concentration of cytokines in EBC for up to 1-year storage at −80 °C [40]. To minimize biomarker degradation due to repetitive freeze-thaw cycles, aliquots should be made before freezing.

4.6 Malignant Pleural Effusion

The serous membrane that covers the thoracic cavity is called the pleura. The parts covering the chest wall and lung are named parietal and visceral pleura, respectively, and the space in between the two constitutes the pleural cavity or space. The physiological imbalances in oncotic and hydrostatic pressures in capillary and lymphatic vessels of the pleurae usually produce little normal fluid in this space in healthy individuals. This physiologic fluid is not easily accessible to sampling.

However, a pathophysiologic disturbance in this fluid formation and rate of absorption leads to increased fluid accumulation in the pleural cavity. Such effusions can result from compromised cardiopulmonary system, inflammatory conditions of the chest, and malignancy (primary or secondary). Malignant effusion can result from primary lung cancer (mostly), pleural mesothelioma, or lung metastasis from other sites such as the breast, gastrointestinal tract, or ovaries. Accurate diagnosis of malignant effusion is hence important for subsequent management. In a large number of cases (about 40%) involving malignancy, cytologic evaluation is negative for cancer cells, thus suggesting the need for ancillary diagnostic procedures. Biomarkers for such uses have been explored.

4.7 Proximal Fluid Lung Cancer Biomarkers

Lung cancer is a disease of epigenetic and genetics, and hence several alterations in biomolecules are potential clinical biomarkers. These genetic and epigenetic changes impinge on cellular regulatory pathways such as apoptosis, proliferation, and senescence. Aberrant effects of proto-oncogenes and tumor suppressor genes primarily mediate development of both SCLC and NSCLC. Thus, methylation of a number of genes including *CDKN2A*, *RASSF1A*, *APC*, *DAPK*, *MGMT*, *GSTP1*, *CDH1*, and *CDH13* characterizes LnCa. *CDKN2A* methylation is detectable in 100% of sputum samples and 63% of serum, *MGMT* is methylated in about 66% of sputum and serum samples, and *APC* is methylated in 95% of tumors but detectable in about 50% of serum samples. Low levels of *MGMT* and *APC* methylation are associated with better survival. Similarly, *DAPK* and *RASSF1A* promoter methylation have prognostic implications. LnCa also demonstrates methylation and loss of imprinting in *IGF2* and *H19*, which promote tumor development. Chromosomal structural and numeric instabilities are common in lung cancer. These include nonreciprocal translocations and deletions involving tumor suppressor genes, amplifications of oncogenes, and aneuploidy. Allelic losses at 3p, 4p, 4q, 5q, 8p, 10q, 13q,

17p, and 22q are common in SCLC, while losses at 3p, 6q, 8p, 9p, 13p, 17p, and 19q are associated with NSCLC. Microsatellite instability is observed in about 35% of SCLC and about 22% of NSCLC. Efforts to use microsatellite instability (MSI) in early detection using body fluids and sputum have been encouraging.

Traditional serum biomarkers of lung cancer include CEA, CYFRA21-1, NSE, squamous cell carcinoma antigen (SCCA, for NSCLC), and progastrin-releasing peptide (ProGRP, for SCLC). Several other novel epigenomic, genomic, proteomic, and metabolomic biomarkers have been explored in proximal lung fluids.

4.7.1 Lung Cancer Biomarkers in Sputum

Because it is acquired virtually in a noninvasive fashion, sputum has been an attractive sample for LnCa biomarker development. Thus, this proximal fluid has been extensively evaluated for such biomarkers.

4.7.1.1 Lung Cancer Methylation Biomarkers in Sputum

DNA methylation is an attractive biomarker target in sputum because it can stably be measured. In view of this, numerous studies have examined diagnostic accuracies of several methylated genes in sputum from LnCa patients in comparison to healthy controls. Some studies had available primary tumor tissue for comparison with methylated genes in sputum. Belinsky et al. found that gene methylation was more commonly found in sputum from cancer patients than controls [41]. The frequencies of methylated *MGMT*, *RAS effector homologue 1*, *DAPK*, and *PAX5α* were higher in cancer patients than control never smokers, and the odds of three or more methylated genes in sputum was 6.2-fold greater in patients than controls. Of 165 individuals exposed to coal emissions, 58 developed cancer with the remaining without cancer. As early warning signs, methylation of *CDKN2A* was commonly detected in sputum from non-cancer patients (51.4%), and this was much higher than methylation in *RASSF1A* (29.9%), *MGMT* (17.8%), and *DAPK* (15.9%) [42]. As a cancer biomarker, *CDKN2A* methylation was even detected at a much higher frequency in sputum from cancer (70.7%) than non-cancer (51.7%) individuals. Thus, gene methylation is an early biomarker of lung carcinogenesis.

Meta-analytical studies have examined the possible utility of sputum methylated biomarkers for LnCa detection. A meta-analytical study conducted in 2014 included 22 studies that met the inclusion criteria [43]. The combined sensitivity, specificity, diagnostic odds ratio (DOR), and area under the receiver operating characteristic curve (AUROCC) were 62%, 73%, 10.3, and 0.78, respectively. Because of the suboptimal accuracy, the authors concluded this was not satisfactory for detection of NSCLC in the average at risk population. In another meta-analysis that considered studies up to the end of 2016, 33 studies involving 2238 cases and 2563 controls satisfied inclusion criteria for analysis [44]. In total, 32 methylated genes were analyzed in the sputum samples. The overall sensitivity was 46% (range, 41–50%), and specificity was 83% (range, 80–86%). The top performers as LnCa methylated genes in sputum were *SOX17* (sensitivity, 84%; specificity, 88%), *CDO1* (sensitivity, 78%; specificity, 67%), *ZFP42* (sensitivity, 87%; specificity, 63%), and *TAC1* (sensitivity, 86%; specificity, 75%). Methylations of *FAM19A4*, *FHIT*, *MGMT*, *CDKN2A/p16*, and *RASSF1A* were also identified as potential LnCa biomarkers.

4.7.1.2 Chromosomal Alterations as Lung Cancer Biomarkers in Sputum

Fluorescent in situ hybridization (FISH) has been applied to analysis of sputum for chromosomal aneusomy, rearrangement, and copy number changes. In one study, while copy number gains in sputum did not significantly differ between high-risk and low-risk never smokers, targeting deletions in *HYAL2* and *FHIT* in sputum achieved a sensitivity and specificity of 76% and 92%, respectively, for LnCa detection [45]. Notwithstanding this finding, the overall FISH sensitivity of 58% is comparable to cytology of 53% in enriched sputum [46]. However, it appears that FISH can improve the sensitivity of cytology when combined [47]. Microsatellite alteration (MSA) including loss of heterozygosity (LOH) and microsatellite instability (MSI) has also been examined in sputum from LnCa patients. LOH is reported in 26–55% of LnCa patients and 0–11% of non-cancer controls [48–51]. The frequencies of MSI in sputum are rather low, being demonstrated in 4–35% of LnCa patients and 0–5% of controls.

4.7.1.3 Lung Cancer DNA Mutation Biomarkers in Sputum

DNA mutation detection in sputum is another attractive LnCa biomarker that has been extensively evaluated. Both nuclear and mitochondrial DNA mutations have been demonstrated in sputum from LnCa patients. While the roles of nuclear gene mutations in LnCa are well established, those of mtDNA have yet to be determined. For example, 50% of LnCa harbors mutations or deletions in *TP53*, 20–30% (mostly adenocarcinoma) are characterized by oncogenic *KRAS* mutations, and 3–6% of adenocarcinoma harbor oncogenic *EML4-ALK* fusion gene that is responsive to ALK TKIs. Additionally, mutations in tyrosine kinase domain of *EGFR* are found in LnCa that also respond to TKIs. Thus, sputum as a noninvasive sample has been interrogated for these and other gene mutations.

A number of pilot studies have uncovered *KRAS* and *TP53* mutations in sputum from LnCa patients. *KRAS* mutations were detectable in 79% of sputum samples from mutant *KRAS*-positive LnCa patients, but not in healthy controls [52]. Indeed, *KRAS* mutation has been detected in sputum 1 year prior to LnCa diagnosis [53]. Because of possible dilution of mutant cells by nonmutant and other component of sputum, Keohavong et al. used laser-capture microdissection to sample epithelial cells in sputum for *KRAS* and *TP53* mutation analysis [54]. This approach enabled detection of mutations in sputum from 46.7% of patients (five patients with *TP53*, one with *KRAS*, and one with mutations in both genes). Baryshnikova et al. performed the first large-scale study of sputum obtained from a screening cohort [55]. This study involved 803 asymptomatic heavy smokers undergoing low-dose computed tomography (LDCT) screening for LnCa. The sputum was analyzed for *TP53* and *KRAS* mutations, as well as promoter methylation of *CDKN2A/INK2A*, *RASSF1A*, and *NORE1A*. Consistent with *TP53* mutations being more prevalent than *KRAS* mutations in LnCa, 15 of the 803 participants (2%) harbored *TP53* mutations, of which 1 developed early-stage LnCa on follow-up. Although a very sensitive mutation detection method (detects 1 mutant copy on a background of 1000 wild-type copies) was used to detect *KRAS* mutations, none of the 18 subjects who developed LnCa on follow-up demonstrated detectable *KRAS* mutations in sputum. These findings suggest *KRAS* mutation detection in sputum may not be useful for risk assessment in this high-risk population. However, patients positive for *TP53* mutation in sputum may require close surveillance for early cancer detection. Further studies are, however, required to establish this conclusion. In another prospective screening cohort, *EML4-ALK* fusion gene was detected in 4 of 35 (11%) sputum samples [56]. *EGFR* mutations have been detected in 3 of 25 sputum samples that were positive for malignant cells by cytology [57–59].

Mitochondrial genome changes have also been detected in sputum from LnCa patients. In a study by Jakupciak et al., whereby whole mitochondrial genome was sequenced in lung, bladder, and renal cancer, sputum from heavy smokers were included in the analysis. Mutations in mtDNA were detected in 17% of the sputum samples. In a region of China (Xuan Wei) where LnCa rates are above the national average due to use of smoky coal carcinogen as fuel, mtDNA alterations were studied in 122 LnCa patients and 121 controls. Increased sputum mtDNA content above 157 copies per cell were associated with elevated LnCa risk (OR = 1.8; 95% CI = 1.0–3.2). This risk was associated with older cancer patients [60]. The increased mtDNA content might be due to increased mtDNA deletions that will be associated with increased smaller deleted genomes that replicate faster to increase cellular content of mtDNA.

4.7.1.4 Lung Cancer mRNA Biomarkers in Sputum

While less attractive than miRNA as a body fluid biomarker because of ease of degradation, gene transcripts have been analyzed in sputum from LnCa patients. In a study of 134 cases and 140 controls, sputum analysis of *MAGEA1-6* transcripts achieved a sensitivity of 54% and specificity of 98% in LnCa detection [61]. In another study targeting transcripts of *APRIL* in sputum from 71 cases and 62 controls, a sensitivity and specificity of 82% and 97%, respectively, was achieved [62]. These encouraging performances deserve further evaluation.

4.7.1.5 Lung Cancer miRNA Biomarkers in Sputum

Analyses of miRNAs in sputum demonstrate discriminatory potential for LnCa screening. Reported sputum miRNAs with diagnostic potential include miR-21, miR-31, miR-126, miR-139, miR-143, miR-155, miR-200b, miR-205, miR-210, miR-372, miR-375, miR-429, miR-486, and miR-708. Sensitivity has ranged from 61% (for miR-31 and miR-210) to 100% (for miR-21, miR-143, miR-155, miR-210, and miR-375), and specificity has also been as high as 80% (for miR-21, miR-200b, miR-375, and miR-486) to 100% (for miR-21 and miR-155) [63].

Levels of miR-21 were elevated in sputum from LnCa patients compared to controls, and this achieved a sensitivity of 70% for LnCa detection, which was superior to cytology sensitivity of 48% [64]. Several studies have used panel miRNAs as diagnostic biomarkers. Sputum miR-205, miR-210, and miR-708 as a panel could differentiate squamous cell lung cancer form controls at a sensitivity and specificity of 73% and 96%, respectively [65]. For differentiating lung adenocarcinoma from controls, combined sputum miR-21, miR-200b, miR-375, and miR-486 achieved a sensitivity of 81% and specificity of 92%. These miRNAs are suggested to be early detection biomarkers because of their lack of association with disease stage. Various studies using panel miRNAs have demonstrated modest diagnostic accuracies for LnCa detection with sensitivities of 61.5–100% and specificities of 80–100%.

Meta-analyses of the various sputum miRNA alterations in LnCa diagnosis have been conducted. A meta-analysis performed in 2014 included 8 studies involving 514 cases and 491 controls [66]. The pooled sensitivity, specificity, and AUROCC were 70%, 89%, and 0.83, respectively. Significant heterogeneity in the specificity was attributed to miRNA profiles. Another meta-analysis of sputum miRNA for NSCLC included 6 more studies (total of 14 studies) with 1009 patients and 1006 controls [67]. The pooled sensitivity, specificity, positive likelihood ratio (PLR), negative likelihood ratio (NLR), and DOR were 75%, 88%, 5.70, 0.30, and 22.43, respectively. The summarized AUROCC (SAUROCC) was 0.8917, indicating the potential of sputum miRNA analysis as diagnostic biomarkers of LnCa. Two other meta-analytical studies of miRNA for noninvasive diagnosis of NSCLC included other body fluids [68, 69]. Both analyses concluded that miRNA analysis in blood was more superior to sputum for LnCa detection. Moreover, panel biomarkers performed better than single miRNAs. The SAUROCC was 0.89 vs. 0.81 for panel vs. single biomarkers in both studies. Subgroup analysis from the Chen et al. study achieved a pooled sensitivity, specificity, and AUROCC of 78%, 80%, and 0.85, respectively, for blood and 66%, 79%, and 0.79, respectively, for sputum [68]. In the other study, the corresponding performances were 78%, 80%, and 0.86 for blood and 69%, 80%, and 0.81 for sputum [69].

4.7.1.6 Lung Cancer Protein Biomarkers in Sputum

A number of studies have targeted traditional LnCa serum biomarkers including CEA, NSE, and CYFRA-21, as well as other candidate LnCa proteins including APRIL and complement factor H in sputum as potential LnCa biomarkers. As a screening biomarker, performances have been variable due to study design, methodologies, and selected targets. Sensitivity has ranged from 57% (CEA) to 86% (CYFRA-21), while specificity has ranged from 75% (CYFRA-21) to 97% (APRIL) [70–72].

4.7.1.7 Other Analyses of Lung Cancer Biomarkers in Sputum

Repeated exposure to air pollution and inhalation of smoke or coal dust can lead to carbon pigment deposition on bronchi (known as anthracosis), which is a risk factor for LnCa. In one study, mean anthracotic index in sputum was significantly higher in LnCa patients than healthy controls, and this was independent of tobacco smoke [73]. Fourier transform-infrared (FTIR) spectroscopy has been used in a pilot study to analyze biochemical changes in sputum [74]. The biochemical changes, which show as absorbance levels of infrared wave numbers were able to distinguish between sputum from cancer patients and controls.

4.7.2 Lung Cancer Biomarkers in Bronchoalveolar Lavage Fluid

Mostly targeted in BAL fluid (BALF) are protein biomarkers. Also examined are gene methylations, mutations, miRNAs, metabolites, oxidative stress, and microbiome biomarkers of LnCa.

Protein biomarkers have demonstrated diagnostic and prognostic utility in LnCa management. BALF analysis uncovered significantly elevated levels of VEGFC and NSE (but not CEA and CYFRA21-1) in squamous cell carcinoma than benign disease patients. At a cutoff value of 2.06 ng/ml, the sensitivity and specificity were 72.9% and 69.2% for NSE in detecting malignant pulmonary masses [75]. In a prospective study of BALF from patients presenting with solitary lung nodules, the levels of VEGF and sVEGFR1 were measured. Only VEGF showed significant elevation in patients with cancer compared to control patients with benign masses. At a cutoff value of 214 pg/ml, the diagnostic sensitivity and specificity were 81.8% and 84.2%, respectively, in predicting the presence of malignancy [76]. Levels of CEA, NSE, and CYFRA21-1 in BALF were higher in cancer than controls. Specifically, NSE concentration was highest in SCLC, CYRA21-1 in squamous cell carcinoma, and CEA in lung adenocarcinoma subgroups [77]. CEA, SCC antigen, CYFRA21-1, and NSE levels in BALF from patients with peripheral LnCa and controls uncovered the diagnostic potential of CYFRA21-1 and CEA. In cancer patients, BALF were obtained from tumor-bearing bronchus and corresponding opposite healthy lung bronchus. While all biomarkers were significantly elevated in cancer vs. controls, CYFRA21-1 with sensitivities of 76–86% and specificity of 91% was the best biomarker. The diagnostic performance was increased to 93% when CYFRA21-1 was combined with SCC antigen and NSE and 86% when CEA was combined [78]. Significant difference was uncovered in BALF proteins from patients with peripheral LnCa compared to controls. The biomarkers uncovered included ubiquitin-specific peptidase 8 (USP8), chitinase 3-like 1 (YKL40), HSP90a, GSTP1, CEA, NSE, and CYFRA21-1. The diagnostic performances were superior for USP8, YKL40, and HSP90a over CYFRA21-1 and NSE, with CEA being the lowest [79].

The prognostic role of VEGF and VEGFR2 in serum and bronchial washes has been uncovered. Lower levels of VEGF in serum and bronchial washes correlated with best chemotreatment response. High VEGF levels and VEGF/VEGFR2 ratio in bronchial washes were associated with worse overall survival (OS) and progression-free survival (PFS). In multivariate analysis, VEGFR2 levels in serum and bronchial washes were independent predictors of OS [80]. Measurement of soluble HLA-G in BALF from LnCa patients was averaged at 49.04 ng/ml. Significant differences in levels were associated with histologic types, especially metastatic cancers. Overall patient status according to the Karnofsky scale showed a significant inverse relationship to BALF sHLA-G [81]. While levels of HGF and IL-22 were higher in serum samples from NSCLC patients than controls, they were on the contrary lower in BALF from patients. As prognostic biomarkers, increased serum HGF levels and increased BALF IL-22 levels were linked to shorter OS [82].

Oxidative stress markers in BALF have shown potential as LnCa biomarkers. A statistically significant increase in the total antioxidant status and glutathione (GSH) was observed in BALF from LnCa patients compared to controls, and a total antioxidant status significantly correlated with IL-1α and TNFα levels [83]. Because LnCa and chronic obstructive pulmonary disease (COPD) commonly coexist, and COPD is a risk factor for developing LnCa, proteomic approach was used to uncover oxidative stress biomarkers for these conditions in BALF. 2D-PAGE followed by MALDI-TOF MS uncovered differential levels of 16 oxidative stress-related proteins between cases and healthy controls that could be involved in the pathogenesis of LnCa and COPD [84].

Mass spectrometric technologies have uncovered potential diagnostic biomarkers of LnCa in BALF. SELDI-TOT MS analysis uncovered protein peaks in BALF of diagnostic relevance for LnCa. Of 8 peaks that were significantly higher in cancer than controls, peaks with m/z 7976 and 11,809 were selected for construction of a classification tree model. This model achieved a diagnostic sensitivity and specificity of 86% and 72%, respectively, and in a blind screen, a sensitivity and specificity of 90% each for LnCa detection. The performance was perfect at 100% when combined with a serum peak with m/z 5639 [85].

Potential N-glycoprotein biomarkers for LnCa were identified in BALF using solid-phase extraction of N-glycoproteins, iTRAQ labeling, and tandem LCMS. The glycoproteins that were elevated over twofold in cancer BALF were neutrophil elastase, integrin α-M, cullin-4B, naspin A (validated by ELISA), lysosome-associated membrane protein 2 (LAMP2), cathepsin D, BPI fold-containing family B member 2, and neutrophil gelactinase-associated lipocalin [86]. In a separate study, naspin A levels in epithelial lining fluid obtained by bronchoscopic microsampling from nodule site and contralateral non-disease site were higher in tumor-associated samples. In this cohort of lung adenocarcinoma patients, 18 patients undiagnosed by bronchoscopy but were finally diagnosed by surgery harbored equally high naspin A levels in bronchial lining fluid, indicating its superior sensitivity to bronchoscopy. The AUROCC was 0.84 for naspin A in detecting lung adenocarcinoma [87].

Proteomic analysis of BALF uncovered overexpression of complement network activation in lung adenocarcinoma. Other potential LnCa biomarkers in BALF included GSTP1, haptoglobin, and complement C4-A [88]. LCMS analysis of BALF samples from patients with lung adenocarcinoma and non-cancer controls uncovered 1100 differential protein levels, of which 33 were consistently elevated in cancer patient samples. The elevated proteins included annexin A1, annexin A2, S100-A8, thymidine phosphorylase, and transglutaminase 2 [89]. In a separate study, Biaoxue et al. measured annexin A1 levels by immunohistochemistry (IHC) and enzyme immunoassays of BALF from LnCa patients and demonstrated higher levels than control group of patients [90]. The elevated levels correlated with lymphatic invasion and disease progression. The performance of BALF annexin A1 achieved a sensitivity and specificity of 94% and 90.2%, respectively, in detecting LnCa.

In a prospective cohort of patients, proteomic analysis of BALF samples identified 133 potential biomarkers with differential levels between cancer and non-cancer controls. Samples from 13 LnCa patients diagnosed during a 2-year follow-up clustered with the cases diagnosed at the time of sample collection, suggestive of early diagnosis using LCMS data [91]. Label-free MS analysis of BALF samples uncovered differential protein levels between lung adenocarcinoma and squamous cell carcinoma patients vs. controls. Cystatin-C, TIMP1, lipocalin 2, and HSP70/HSPA1A were selected from the discovery BALF MS analysis and tested in a larger cohort of plasma samples. TIMP1, lipocalin 2, and cystatin C were significantly elevated in plasma from lung adenocarcinoma and squamous cell carcinoma patients [92].

Metabolomic analysis of BALF from LnCa patients and controls with partial least square discriminant analysis (PLS-DA) uncovered 42 altered metabolites in LnCa patient samples. Mainly involved were glutamate and glutamine metabolic pathways. AUROCC analysis uncovered glycerol and phosphoric acid as potential diagnostic and prognostic biomarkers [93]. In a follow-up study, GCMS and PLS-DA uncovered 16 metabolites in BALF that differed between LnCa and non-cancer controls. Using pathway analysis, several of these metabolites were noticed to be involved in amino acid metabolism.

Immune-mediated and angiogenic factors in BALF appear as useful biomarkers for LnCa. Complement factor H was quantified in BALF supernatants from LnCa and control benign lung disease patients. LnCa patients had significantly higher levels of complement factor H, and the diagnostic sensitivity and specificity were 82% and 77%, respectively, which were confirmed in an independent set of patients. Of interest, 70% and 45% of BALF samples from the central and peripheral tumors, respectively, that were negative by cytology could be reclassified as positive by complement factor H levels [72]. Measurement of C4d-containing complement degradation fragments that were significantly elevated in BALF supernatants from LnCa patients uncovered its diagnostic value. In a cohort of smaller and larger samples, the AUROCC was 0.8 (for the smaller sample cohort) and 0.67 (for the larger samples) for LnCa detection. Additionally, BALF levels of C4d fragments improved the sensitivity of bronchoscopy in LnCa detection. Of interest, levels in sputum also achieved AUROCC of 0.70 for LnCa detection [94]. Regulatory T-cell (Treg) levels in BALF were significantly higher in LnCa patients than in peripheral blood. The altered levels in BALF may be useful in selecting patients for immunotherapies [95].

BALF profile of cancerous inflammation has been uncovered. Significantly higher percentage of neutrophils and lower percentages of macrophages characterized LnCa and nonspecific inflammation. Lung adenocarcinoma was associated with high percentage of lymphocytes, while CD163-positive macrophages were more prevalent in BALF from squamous cell carcinoma patients. LnCa BALF had high IL-8 and VEGF levels [96]. CCL-1 and IL-11 in BALF were higher in lung adenocarcinoma with or without COPD. At a cutoff value of 42 pg/ml, IL-11 achieved a sensitivity, specificity, and AUROCC of 90%, 86%, and 0.93, respectively, while CCL-1 at 39.5 pg/ml had sensitivity, specificity, and AUROCC of 83%, 74%, and 0.83, respectively. Both biomarkers were significantly correlated and, in combination, improved diagnostic accuracy to 96.1% [97]. Levels of TGFβ and HMGB1 in BALF from LnCa patients prior to chemotherapy were compared to control healthy group and those with sarcoidosis. TGFβ levels were significantly higher in NSCLC patients than healthy controls but lower than sarcoidosis patient samples. HMGB1 levels were associated with distant metastasis. In stage IIIB patients, a positive correlation of HMGB1 and TGFβ with OS was uncovered [98].

Gene methylation, mutation, and transcript alterations in LnCa BALF have been demonstrated. A panel of methylated *SHOX2* and *RASSF1A* in BALF achieved a sensitivity and specificity of 81% and 97.4%, respectively, in LnCa detection in prospectively collected samples. This performance was much superior to LnCa detection by other methods such as cytology (sensitivity of 68.3%, specificity of 97.4%) and serum CEA (sensitivity of 30.6%, specificity of 100%). The combination of the methylated genes with cytology improved diagnostic accuracy [99]. Comparison of mutations in *KRAS* and *TP53* in BALF from patients with peripheral NSCLC and benign lung diseases achieved a combined diagnostic sensitivity of 66%, which was superior to cytology and histology on first bronchoscopy (38%). BALF gene mutations were the same as in primary tumor tissues [100]. Extracellular vesicle (EV)-derived DNA from BALF proved successful for analysis of *EGFR* mutations in NSCLC patients. There was mutational concordance between BALF EV-derived and biopsy samples, and BALF EV DNA was more efficient than rebiopsy for detecting p.T790 M mutations in patients resistant to EGFR-TKIs [101]. It is possible to detect anaplastic lymphoma kinase (ALK) translocations in cytologic samples from LnCa patients. By RT-PCR, detection was successful in 99% with 3% positive samples. The positive cytologic samples were confirmed by IHC and FISH analysis [102]. The transcripts of survivin and livin are significantly higher in bronchial aspirates from cancer patients than controls. The diagnostic sensitivity and specificity were, respectively, 83% and 96% for survivin and 63% and 96% for livin [103].

Alterations in miRNA and microbiome have also been demonstrated in BALF from LnCa patients. Dysregulated miRNAs in LnCa are measurable in BALF samples. Pooled samples were used to uncover differential levels of extracellular miRNAs in bronchial lavage from patients and controls. These were then confirmed in different sample sets. The miRNA microarray identified eight miRNAs that showed differential levels between cancer and controls, but five (U6 snRNA, miR-1285, miR-1303, miR-29a-5p, and miR-650) were significantly different by RT-PCR analyses [104]. Select miRNAs altered in lung adenocarcinoma were assayed in exosomes isolated from BALF. miR-126 and Let-7a levels were significantly higher in cancer than controls, and these changes were similar to findings in primary tumor and normal lung tissues [105]. 16s rRNA-based next-generation sequencing analysis of the microbiome in BALF samples in a prospective cohort of patients presenting with lung masses uncovered potential disease biomarkers. Abundance of two phyla (*Firmicutes* and TM7) was significantly increased in LnCa patients. As well, two genera (*Veillonella* and *Megasphaera*) were abundant. The sensitivity and specificity were, respectively, 95% and 75% for *Veillonella* and 70% and 100% for *Megasphaera*, and the AUROCC for the combined genera was 0.88 in LnCa detection [106].

4.7.3 Lung Cancer Biomarkers in Exhaled Breath Condensate

Exhaled breath is simply the air expelled from the lungs. It is a practically easy and noninvasive sample to obtain for disease detection and management. Even very sick people are able to provide such samples for analysis. Constituents of exhaled breath come from both endogenous and exogenous sources. The exogenous compounds do not indicate disease states but merely an acute exposure. Thus, altered endogenous substances have been explored as LnCa biomarkers in EBC.

4.7.3.1 Lung Cancer Volatile Organic Compound Biomarkers in Exhaled Breath Condensate

Exhaled breath contains important gaseous and nongaseous substances that reflect body physiologic and metabolic processes, and hence altered normal cellular functions (disease) produce a different spectral patterns and specific volatile organic compounds (VOCs). These compounds can be measured for disease detection. Over a thousand compounds, both volatile and nonvolatile are demonstrated in exhaled breath. VOCs have been categorized into three main groups. While this categorization is important to know for diagnostic purposes, several studies rely on profiles of VOCs rather than specific compounds.

Gordon et al. pioneered the possible utility of VOCs in LnCa detection [107]. Using GCMS in the analysis of just 12 samples from NSCLC patients and 9 control subjects, 4 VOC peaks were identified and appeared specific to LnCa because none of the control subjects had them. This initial encouraging data raised hopes in the use of VOCs in exhaled breath for early detection of lung cancer. Since then several studies addressing the use of VOCs in exhaled breath in LnCa detection have been performed. Reported performances have ranged in sensitivity and specificity from 72–100% to 72–94%, respectively. Primarily the differences in performances are due to sample sizes used in studies, methodologies used, as well as the use of specific panels of VOCs as predictive models for cancer detection. Conclusively, there is merit in translation of the detection of VOCs in LnCa management.

Methods for detection of VOCs in exhaled breath include the original GCMS by Gordon and colleagues [107], infrared spectroscopy, laser absorption spectrometry, ion flow tube mass spectrometry, coated quartz crystal microbalance sensors, and polymer-coated surface acoustic wave sensors. Problems with these methods are that they are slow to perform, thus requiring longer times and use of complex expensive instruments and expertise. A group from Israel has developed an easy, cost-effective, and fast nano-device capable of early LnCa detection [108]. The device is composed of arrays and networks of chemiresistors of functionalized gold nanoparticles. The different nanoparticles have specific or identifiable organic substances that react to various VOCs in exhaled breath. This array of gold nanoparticle sensors coupled with pattern recognition algorithm enabled early lung cancer detection. Initial selection of 42 LnCa VOC biomarkers enabled this team to focus on a few for discrete discrimination between cancer and normal samples. Using 4 of the 42 VOCs to train and optimize sensor arrays, LnCa could be accurately differentiated from normal lung in exhaled breath. More intriguingly, this device could as well separate various subtypes of LnCa. In spite of the promise, there are technical and analytical difficulties associated with use of VOCs in disease management. However, some commercial companies are making breakthroughs to make their use in clinics a routine.

4.7.3.2 Lung Cancer Epigenetic and Genetic Biomarkers in Exhaled Breath Condensate

Discriminatory LnCa epigenetic biomarkers have been demonstrated in EBC. As a pilot study, promoter methylation of *RASSF1A*, *DAPK*, and *PAX5B* was analyzed in EBC from LnCa patients and non-cancer controls including smokers and nonsmokers [109]. The density of methylation in *RASSF1A* promoter was significantly higher in former than current smokers. Of importance, methylation status at specific CpG loci uncovered relevant associations with cancer. Methylation of *PAX5A* at CpG +52 and *DAPK* at CpG −63 were both significantly related to LnCa. *CDKN2A* methylation has also been studied in EBC from LC patients [110].

Khyshiktyev et al. first recognized the LnCa diagnostic utility of EBC [111], following which Gessner et al. demonstrated microsatellite alterations (MSA) of *TP53* in EBC that were in association with tobacco use [112]. A direct survival effect of chromosome 3p instability in EBC has been recognized as well. Carpagnano and colleagues are the primary group that has studied MSA in EBC from LnCa patients [113]. The frequency of MSA in EBC DNA was significantly higher in NSCLC patients than healthy controls. Of interest, these alterations were similar to MSA profile in matched tumor tissues. A prognostic relevance of EBC MSA was suggested because they were associated with patient survival [113–115]. This same group also examined MSA in the long arm of chromosome 19 in EBC. While nonsmokers exhibited no MSA in EBC, 16% of healthy smokers and 25% of NSCLC patients demonstrated MSA in EBC [116]. This group tested the LnCa origin of MSA in EBC. To this end, MSA in EBC from LnCa patients with pleural effusion were significantly higher than patients with pleural effusions due to metastasis from non-LnCa [117].

Established LnCa mutations have been demonstrated in EBC from patients. In 2004, Gessner et al. analyzed EBC from LnCa patients and healthy controls for *TP53* mutations [112]. Amplification of β-actin (*ACTB*) was used to ascertain the presence of DNA in the EBC. Of the 18 NSCLC patients, 11 were positive for *ACTB* of which 4 (36%) were also positive for *TP53* mutations. No mutation was demonstrated in EBC from controls. There were no matching mutations in corresponding primary tumor biopsies. However, in a smoker with squamous cell LnCa, *EGFR* exon 19 deletion detected in EBC matched mutation in transbronchial biopsy of the primary tumor [118]. In a large-scale study conducted between 2007 and 2011, 134 LnCa patients and 57 controls were examined for *KRAS* codon 12 mutation in EBC [119]. The mutation was detected in EBC from 57 patients (46 with NSCLC and 11 with benign lung lesions) and in 26 controls. In the patient cohort, tumor tissue, normal-looking pulmonary parenchyma, and EBC collected on day 7 and 30 after surgery were also tested for the mutation. The mutation was present in all tumor tissues that were positive for the mutation in EBC and 28% of normal-looking lung parenchyma (evidence of field cancerization). The authors quantified wild-type and mutant *KRAS* and computed a ratio of mutant to wild type (mut/wild *KRAS*). This ratio was highest in tumor tissue, followed by pre-surgical EBC, with the lowest in normal-looking lung parenchymal samples. Moreover, in control individuals positive for *KRAS* mutation in EBC, the ratio was low, being <0.09. Additionally, in tumor tissues, pre-surgical EBC, and normal-looking lung parenchyma, the ratio was significantly higher in samples from NSCLC patients than those with benign lesions. Consistent with lung lesion being the source of the mutation, the ratio significantly decreased after tumor removal in all patients, with ten NSCLC patients demonstrating no *KRAS* mutation in EBC on day 30 post-surgery. *CDKN2A* exons 1 and 2 mutations were detected in 15% of EBC from 58 NSCLC patients, with none found in EBC from controls [120]. Mutated *CDKN2A* in EBC demonstrated statistically significant differences associated with tumor stages that were unattainable with clinicopathological variables including pathologic tumor type, smoking history, and presence or absence of nodal spread.

MiRNAs, viral DNA, and mtDNA have also been detected in EBC from LnCa patients. miR-21 and miR-486 have been examined in EBC and tumor tissues from NSCLC patients [121]. Levels of miR-21 were significantly higher in EBC from cancer patients than controls and correlated positively with the levels in tumor tissues. Also, the levels of miR-486 were significantly lower in EBC from patients than controls. Because HPV infection is implicated in the pathogenesis of some LnCa, Carpagnano et al. examined EBC from LnCa patients for HPV DNA [122]. They demonstrated the presence of HPV DNA in EBC, bronchial brushings, and tumor tissues from patients. In this cohort, HPV infection was present in 16.4% of the NSCLC patients, but not in healthy controls. EBC from LnCa patients, smokers, and nonsmokers have been analyzed for mtDNA mutations [123]. The prevalence of mitochondrial genome D-loop mutations was higher in LnCa patients than healthy controls. While the mutations were higher in heavy than light smokers, this failed to reach statistical significance.

4.7.3.3 Lung Cancer Protein Biomarkers in Exhaled Breath Condensate

Because of several hurdles needed to overcome for efficient proteomic applications in EBC, protein analyses of EBC from LnCa patients have focused on single or a few panel proteins analyzed simultaneously. The potential of proteomic approaches for discovery of novel biomarkers is currently being explored. For specific single or panel multiplex LnCa biomarkers in EBC, cytokines and keratins have been mostly studied.

Cytokines have been analyzed in EBC from LnCa patients as potential biomarkers. Mostly studied are IL-6, IL-8, TNFα, VEGF, and sICAM-1. IL-6 levels in EBC were elevated in patients with NSCLC compared to controls, and the elevated levels significantly correlated with increasing tumor stage [124]. In an independent study, increased EBC IL-6, IL-17, TNFα, and VEGF were all significantly associated with tumor diameter [125]. EBC IL-2, TNFα, and leptin were increased in stages I and II NSCLC patients compared to healthy previous smokers [126]. In another series, elevated EBC TNFα and VEGF were associated with stages III and IV NSCLC [127]. Preoperative levels of TNFα and sICAM-1 in EBC were significantly elevated in patients with bronchial carcinoma than control group comprised of patients who underwent thoracoscopy with minimal wedge resection [128]. Simultaneous detection of multiples cytokines in EBC has been possible. An antibody microarray targeting 120 cytokines enabled multiplex analysis of EBC cytokines in LnCa patients [129]. Because of the low abundance of proteins in EBC, the investigators lyophilized, resuspended, and pooled the EBC samples to increase the concentration of protein for analysis. Cytokine profiles were different between LnCa patients and controls irrespective of smoking history, airway inflammation, and lung functional status. Ten cytokines, including IL-10, FGF, macrophage inflammatory protein 3, and eotaxin, demonstrated over twofold differences between cases and controls. However, other methods of protein detection failed to reproduce these findings, which may be due to technical factors including sample pooling. An eminent issue with inflammatory cytokine biomarkers is the lack of specificity for cancer. Other pulmonary inflammatory conditions as well as invasive procedures associated with inflammation could equally cause alterations of these biomarkers.

Keratins (KRTs) have also been detected in EBC from LnCa patients. Levels of KRTs 14, 16, and 17 in EBC were significantly different between NSCLC patients and healthy controls. But due to the variability in their expression in respiratory tract between individuals, their specificity for LnCa will require establishment of normal levels or diagnostic threshold for LnCa.

4.7.4 Lung Cancer Biomarkers in Malignant Pleural Effusion

Malignant pleural effusion (MPE) could be from pulmonary or extrapulmonary metastatic cancers, although LnCa is the most common cause. The accumulation of fluid in the pleural cavity is an important cause of cancer-related morbidity and mortality. The median survival after diagnosis is only 4–9 months, because none of the therapeutic approaches is more effective than symptomatic relief. Thus, prompt and accurate early diagnosis using minimally invasive tests is important to potentially optimize therapeutic efficacy. Similar to cytologic analysis of other cancer-associated body fluids, cytology is the gold standard and an important feature in MPE diagnostic algorithms, but the limited sensitivity (30–60%) hampers its usefulness. Therefore, many patients need to undergo invasive diagnostic tests such as thoracoscopic pleural biopsy for definite diagnosis. This calls for the need to validate additional biomarkers to augment cytologic analysis. Current gene methylation, genomic, transcriptomic, and proteomic studies of pleural effusions have yielded novel molecular biomarkers that demonstrate potential in enhancing the diagnostic accuracy of cytologic evaluation of MPEs. Similar to many discovery biomarkers, clinical translation requires biomarker validation in well-designed prospective, randomized, and cost-effective studies.

Genes commonly methylated in several cancers including *MGMT*, *RASSF1A*, *DAPK*, *RARβ*, and *CDKN2A/INK4A* have been assayed in MPE and found to have complementary utility with cytology. Combined with cytology, epigenetic analysis increases the sensitivity of detection and the NPV. However, several studies have evaluated protein biomarkers for the differential diagnosis of MPE in general, while others have focused on differentiating between effusions from mesothelioma and metastatic cancers. The plethora of protein biomarker studies has been subjected to numerous meta-analytical studies that are summarized hereinafter.

A number of tumor markers including CEA, cancer antigens (CAs), NSE, and CYFRA21-1 among others have been examined for differential diagnosis of malignant and benign effusions. Systematic review and meta-analysis of CEA and

CYFRA21-1 in differential diagnosis of pleural effusion included 19 studies involving 3228 subjects [130]. The pooled sensitivity and specificity were, respectively, 45.9% and 97.0% for CEA and 47.3% and 91.8% for CYFRA21-1. Observed heterogeneity was due to variable assay methods. In another meta-analytical study, Liang et al. achieved pooled sensitivities and specificities, respectively, of 48% and 85% for CA125, 51% and 96% for CA15-3, 25% and 96% for CA19-9, and 55% and 91% for CYFRA21-1 [131]. Consistent with the previous study, this analysis revealed dismal performances for any of these single biomarkers as useful for the differential diagnosis of MPE. However, it was suggested that panel biomarkers might increase the sensitivity. Another analysis by this group that considered only CEA in diagnosing MPE included 45 studies [132]. The pooled sensitivity, specificity, PLR, NLR, and DOR were 54%, 94%, 9.52, 0.49, and 22.5, respectively. Eleven studies were further analyzed to identify biomarkers for ruling out the diagnosis of mesothelioma. Levels of CEA exceeding a defined cutoff achieved a sensitivity and specificity of 97% and 60%, respectively. Thus, pleural effusion levels of CEA could confirm MPE and help rule out mesothelioma, but the dismal sensitivity precludes routine clinical utility. In another analysis that included a large number (49) of studies, the pooled sensitivities and specificities were, respectively, 54.9% and 96.2% for CEA, 50.7% and 98.3% for CA15-3, 37.6% and 98.0% for CA19-9, 57.5% and 92.8% for CA125, 62.5% and 93.2% for CYFRA21-1, and 61.3% and 88.4% for NSE. Again, the performances as individual biomarkers showed high specificities, but their low sensitivities preclude clinical utility [133]. Feng et al. performed a validation study and meta-analysis of CEA, CYFRA21-1, and CA19-9 in detecting MPE from lung adenocarcinoma [134]. In the validation study, the optimal cutoff values and AUROCC were, respectively, 4.55 ng/ml and 0.93 for CEA, 43.10 ug/ml and 0.85 for CYFRA21-1, and 12.89 U/ml and 0.81 for CA19-9. The combination of the three biomarkers increased the sensitivity to 95.06% with AUROCC of 0.95. In a meta-analysis that included eight studies, CEA was the best biomarker with pooled sensitivity, specificity, PLR, NLR, DOR, and AUROCC of 75%, 96%, 16.01, 0.23, 81.49, and 0.93, respectively. The improved performance of the panel biomarkers in the validation study might have stimulated another meta-analysis of these biomarker combinations in diagnosis of MPE [135]. This analysis, which included 20 studies, examined combinations of biomarkers using more than 3 studies. The sensitivities and specificities of the combined biomarkers were, respectively, 65% and 98% for CEA and CA125, 64% and 98% for CEA and CA15-3, 58% and 98% for CEA and CA19-9, 82% and 92% for CEA and CYFRA21-1, and 88% and 95% for CA15-3 and CYFRA21-1. This analysis uncovered the superiority of CEA and CYFRA21-2 and CA15-3 and CYFRA21-1 in detecting MPE.

The diagnostic accuracies of NSE, epithelial membrane antigen (EMA), sVEGF, endostatin, and survivin have been tested by meta-analytical studies. A validation study and meta-analysis of NSE were conducted on malignant and benign effusions [136]. The sensitivity and specificity were 59.56% and 83.33%, respectively, at a cutoff value of 8.92 ng/ml. The meta-analysis inclusive of 14 studies and 1896 subjects achieved pooled sensitivity, specificity, PLR, NLR, DOR, and AUROCC of 53%, 85%, 3.54, 0.56, 6.39, and 0.78. This evidence failed to support its clinical utility. The diagnostic usefulness of epithelial membrane antigen (EMA) was examined by meta-analysis involving 11 studies [137]. The pooled sensitivity, specificity, PLR, NLR, DOR, and AUROCC were 90%, 87%, 5.8, 0.15, 52.63, and 0.88, respectively. The sensitivity and specificity maximum joint point on a ROC (Q-value) was 0.94. Pleural effusion EMA demonstrates potential for diagnosing MPE. The levels of sVEGF are more elevated in MPE than benign pleural effusion (BPE). A systematic review of 20 and meta-analysis of 11 studies revealed MPE VEGF to be increased by 1.98 ng/ml in comparison to levels in BPE, indicating a diagnostic potential for VEGF. Tian et al. performed a study and meta-analysis of endostatin for diagnosis of MPE [138]. At a cutoff value of 79.7 ng/ml, the sensitivity and specificity were 51.92% and 82.94%, respectively, with AUROCC of 0.747. Inclusive of this study with eight other studies for meta-analysis achieved pooled sensitivity, specificity, PLR, NLR, DOR, and AUROCC of 69%, 78%, 3.16, 0.4, 7.89, and 0.79, respectively. While the levels were significantly elevated in MPE, the diagnostic performance was dismal with low sensitivity. This group also performed another clinical study and meta-analysis of survivin in pleural effusions [139]. Survivin levels were significantly higher in MPE (844.17 pg/ml) than BPE (508.05 pg/ml). At a cutoff value of 683.2 pg/ml, the sensitivity and specificity were 57.5% and 88.89%, respectively. A meta-analysis of six studies achieved pooled sensitivity, specificity, PLR, NLR, DOR, and AUROCC of 74%, 85%, 4.79, 0.31, 15.50, and 0.86, respectively. This preliminary study uncovers moderate diagnostic potential for survivin.

Mesothelioma develops from mesothelial coverings of internal organs. However, they commonly develop from the pleural coverings of the lung and chest wall. The majority (60–70%) of patients (mostly men) will have been exposed to asbestos. While smoking increases LnCa development in people exposed to asbestos, it does not mediate the etiology of mesothelioma. Screening is not recommended because it is not known to improve survival. However, because of its origin from the lining of the lung, pleural effusion commonly develops and requires differential diagnosis from other causes of MPE. The performances of calretinin and fibulin-3 in differentiating MPE from mesothelioma and metastatic cancers have been evaluated by meta-analysis [140, 141]. Analysis of 18 studies of calretinin achieved pooled sensitivity, specificity, PLR, NLR, DOR, AUROCC, and Q-value of 91%, 96%, 14.42, 0.1, 163.03, 0.97, and 0.92, respectively. The analysis of fibulin-3 included eight studies, and the pooled sensitivity, specificity, and AUROCC were 73%, 80%, and 0.83, respectively. The peripheral circulating levels of fibulin-3 achieved a better performance with sensitivity of 87%, specificity of 89%, and SAUROCC of 0.94. Thus, calretinin and fibulin-3 have potential in confirming MPE from mesothelioma.

4.8 Clinical Translation of Commercial Products

4.8.1 LungSign™

A complementary test to current efforts at early LnCa detection is that developed by Perceptronix Medical Inc. (PMI) called LungSign™. This noninvasive test is indicated for individuals at risk for LnCa, namely, people over 50 years, heavy smokers, people exposed to industrial carcinogens including asbestos, and those with persistent cough or shortness of breath suggestive of lung pathology. Patients in any of these categories who require the test will have to make a request through their physician. A kit is then obtained and used at home to collect sputum. Included in the kit is a lung flute device from (Medical Acoustics) to aid in sputum production. Collected sputum is transported to PMI laboratory where it is analyzed and results are returned to the physician in about a week's period. At the PMI laboratory, the sputum is smeared on glass slides and undergoes DNA staining followed by automated image cytometry that includes measurement of DNA amount, texture, and conformation. A proprietary algorithm is then used to generate a risk score that indicates the likelihood of cancer. Similar to the test being developed by Allegro Diagnostics Inc. (see below), the LungSign™ test utilizes the "field effect concept" of lung carcinogenesis, which is that malignant-associated changes are observed in normal-appearing cells that coexist with cancer in the lung. Pneumothorax, flu-like symptoms, recent thoracic surgery, asthmatic attack, or exacerbations of chronic obstructive pulmonary disease are contraindications for the test.

4.8.2 Breath Methylated Alkane Contour

Menssana Research Inc. has a focus on disease detection using molecular analysis of exhaled breath. The company has overcome the technical difficulty of breath chemical analysis by developing a portable breath collection apparatus (BCA), which is currently approved by the FDA for clinical trials involving heart transplant rejection. Breath scanners developed by this company analyze VOCs of oxidative stress by GCMS and have a sensitivity of detection at the picomolar level. A constellation of biomarkers produced as a consequence of lipid peroxidation, referred to as breath methylated alkane contour (BMAC), constitute proprietary diagnostic marker for several diseases. BMAC is a 3-D plot of alveolar gradients of C2-C20 methylated alkanes. Clinical studies are ongoing in evaluating the effectiveness of these BMAC biomarkers in diseases such as heart transplant rejection, ischemic heart disease, diabetes, renal diseases, pulmonary tuberculosis, as well as breast and lung cancers.

4.8.3 Nanotechnology Electronic Noses

Nanomix Inc. is a nanotechnology company with a proprietary technology that enables detection of a wide range of molecules and gaseous substances applying different chemistries. Their technology is equivalent to "smelling lung cancer using nanotechnology electronic noses." Their proprietary sensation technology using electrical conductance of carbon nanotubes enabled the production of a device small in size but with ultra-sensitivity and specificity that could be used at the point of care. Currently the technology is used to measure nitric oxide (NO) levels implicated in asthmatic inflammation. This device targets both the doctors' office and home use. Conceivably, measurement of exhaled breath biomarkers of LnCa can be developed using such nanotechnology.

4.8.4 Allegro Diagnostics Inc.

Founded in 2006 by Drs. Jerome Brody and Avrum Spira of Boston University, the company retrieves lung epithelial cells for gene expression analysis for the early detection of LnCa and other diseases. Specifically, the company explores the concept of field cancerization by analyzing genetic signatures in normal-appearing epithelial cells that signal the presence or otherwise of cancer. This enables early cancer detection and prognostication. The LnCa test under development will determine expression profiles on non-cancerous epithelial cells from high-risk individuals to enable the confirmation of the presence or absence of LnCa and also help characterize the disease.

4.8.5 Epigenomics AG

Epi *pro*Lung BL Reflex Assay is a reflex test on bronchoalveolar lavage samples obtained during routine investigational procedure for LnCa. Admittedly, up to 50% of people at risk for LnCa who undergo bronchoscopic sampling for histopathologic evaluation for LnCa return false-negative results. Epi *pro*Lung is therefore a complementary diagnostic test to bronchoscopic workflow of patients at risk for LnCa. The Epi *pro*Lung BL Reflex Assay is based on the analysis of *SHOX2* methylation in bronchial lavage samples. Evidence accrued so far indicates strong association between LnCa and methylation of this gene. Because methylation events occur early in carcinogenesis, a positive Epi *pro*Lung test could indicate early and impending disease in high-risk individuals, even if other tests are negative for cancer. In a CE validation study, this assay performed very well in LnCa detection with a sensitivity of 81% and a specificity of 95%. Additionally, the assay is very robust and reproducible, obviating these inherent problems associated with many such tests. The Epi *pro*Lung test involves three assay kits provided by Epigenomics AG:

- A DNA preparation kit is used for cell lysis, bisulfite conversion of genomic DNA, as well as extraction and purification of DNA from fixed bronchial lavage samples. Thus, the assay does not interfere with the routine histopathologic evaluation process of such samples.
- An Epi proLung BL real-time PCR assay kit is next employed for quantitative measurement of *SHOX2* methylation.
- As required for a good clinical assay, the third component of the assay, named Epi *pro*Lung BL Work Flow Control Kit, entails positive and negative control reagents and samples that monitor the successful execution of the entire assay, from cell lysis, bisulfite conversion, DNA purification, target amplification to signal detection, which enhances the quality control of the test.

4.9 Summary

- LnCa remains the most commonly diagnosed cancer in the world.
- The prognosis of LnCa is poor due to late diagnosis, thus also making it the leading cause of cancer-related deaths globally.
- Being a disease of environmental and lifestyle exposures, primary prevention remains a choice to reverse the current statistics.
- In addition, early detection using biomarkers in proximal lung fluids, especially for screening of the above-average-risk population, should improve the dismal survival outcomes.
- Sputum and EBC samples harbor LnCa biomarkers easily amenable to population screening purposes.
- Accurate biomarkers in MPE are needed for accurate differential diagnosis so as to inform clinical decision-making on appropriate patient management.
- Uptake and reimbursement of commercially available biomarker detection technologies and leveraging these for point-of-care screening of people in low-to-medium Human Development Index countries should help curb the current dismal global statistics of LnCa.

References

1. Horvath I. The exhaled biomarker puzzle: bacteria play their card in the exhaled nitric oxide-exhaled breath condensate nitrite game. Thorax. 2005;60:179–80.
2. Mutlu GM, Garey KW, Robbins RA, et al. Collection and analysis of exhaled breath condensate in humans. Am J Respir Crit Care Med. 2001;164:731–7.
3. Balbi B, Pignatti P, Corradi M, et al. Bronchoalveolar lavage, sputum and exhaled clinically relevant inflammatory markers: values in healthy adults. Eur Respir J. 2007;30:769–81.
4. Jackson AS, Sandrini A, Campbell C, et al. Comparison of biomarkers in exhaled breath condensate and bronchoalveolar lavage. Am J Respir Crit Care Med. 2007;175:222–7.
5. Sinha A, Yadav AK, Chakraborty S, et al. Exosome-enclosed microRNAs in exhaled breath hold potential for biomarker discovery in patients with pulmonary diseases. J Allergy Clin Immunol. 2013;132:219–22.
6. Ng AW, Bidani A, Heming TA. Innate host defense of the lung: effects of lung-lining fluid pH. Lung. 2004;182:297–317.
7. Horvath I, Hunt J, Barnes PJ, et al. Exhaled breath condensate: methodological recommendations and unresolved questions. Eur Respir J. 2005;26:523–48.
8. Hoffmeyer F, Weiss T, Lehnert M, et al. Increased metal concentrations in exhaled breath condensate of industrial welders. J Environ Monit. 2011;13:212–8.
9. Hoffmeyer F, Raulf-Heimsoth M, Harth V, et al. Comparative analysis of selected exhaled breath biomarkers obtained with two different temperature-controlled devices. BMC Pulm Med. 2009;9:48.
10. Czebe K, Barta I, Antus B, et al. Influence of condensing equipment and temperature on exhaled breath condensate pH, total protein and leukotriene concentrations. Respir Med. 2008;102:720–5.
11. Romero PV, Rodriguez B, Martinez S, et al. Analysis of oxidative stress in exhaled breath condensate from patients with severe pulmonary infections. Arch Bronconeumol. 2006;42:113–9.
12. Mutti A, Corradi M, Goldoni M, et al. Exhaled metallic elements and serum pneumoproteins in asymptomatic smokers and patients with COPD or asthma. Chest. 2006;129:1288–97.
13. Moeller A, Franklin P, Hall GL, et al. Measuring exhaled breath condensates in infants. Pediatr Pulmonol. 2006;41:184–7.
14. Rosias PP, Robroeks CM, van de Kant KD, et al. Feasibility of a new method to collect exhaled breath condensate in pre-school children. Pediatr Allergy Immunol. 2010;21:e235–44.
15. Carter SR, Davis CS, Kovacs EJ. Exhaled breath condensate collection in the mechanically ventilated patient. Respir Med. 2012;106:601–13.
16. Gessner C, Dihazi H, Brettschneider S, et al. Presence of cytokeratins in exhaled breath condensate of mechanical ventilated patients. Respir Med. 2008;102:299–306.
17. Vyas A, Zhang Q, Gunaratne S, et al. The effect of temperature on exhaled breath condensate collection. J Breath Res. 2012;036002:6.
18. Goldoni M, Caglieri A, Andreoli R, et al. Influence of condensation temperature on selected exhaled breath parameters. BMC Pulm Med. 2005;5:10.
19. Vaughan J, Ngamtrakulpanit L, Pajewski TN, et al. Exhaled breath condensate pH is a robust and reproducible assay of airway acidity. Eur Respir J. 2003;22:889–94.
20. Eberini I, Gianazza E, Pastorino U, Sirtori C. Assessment of individual lung cancer risk by the proteomic analysis of exhaled breath condensate. Expert Opin Med Diagn. 2008;2:1309–15.

21. Chapman EA, Thomas PS, Yates DH. Breath analysis in asbestos-related disorders: a review of the literature and potential future applications. J Breath Res. 2010;4:034001.
22. Huttmann EM, Greulich T, Hattesohl A, et al. Comparison of two devices and two breathing patterns for exhaled breath condensate sampling. PLoS One. 2011;6:e27467.
23. Borrill ZL, Roy K, Vessey RS, et al. Non-invasive biomarkers and pulmonary function in smokers. Int J Chron Obstruct Pulmon Dis. 2008;3:171–83.
24. Liu J, Conrad DH, Chow S, et al. Collection devices influence the constituents of exhaled breath condensate. Eur Respir J. 2007;30:807–8.
25. Carraro S, Corradi M, Zanconato S, et al. Exhaled breath condensate cysteinyl leukotrienes are increased in children with exercise-induced bronchoconstriction. J Allergy Clin Immunol. 2005;115:764–70.
26. Ahmadzai H, Huang S, Hettiarachchi R, et al. Exhaled breath condensate: a comprehensive update. Clin Chem Lab Med. 2013;51:1343–61.
27. Bondesson E, Jansson LT, Bengtsson T, Wollmer P. Exhaled breath condensate-site and mechanisms of formation. J Breath Res. 2009;3:016005.
28. Montuschi P. Analysis of exhaled breath condensate in respiratory medicine: methodological aspects and potential clinical applications. Ther Adv Respir Dis. 2007;1:5–23.
29. Vass G, Huszar E, Barat E, et al. Comparison of nasal and oral inhalation during exhaled breath condensate collection. Am J Respir Crit Care Med. 2003;167:850–5.
30. Zetterquist W, Marteus H, Kalm-Stephens P, et al. Oral bacteria--the missing link to ambiguous findings of exhaled nitrogen oxides in cystic fibrosis. Respir Med. 2009;103:187–93.
31. Effros RM, Hoagland KW, Bosbous M, et al. Dilution of respiratory solutes in exhaled condensates. Am J Respir Crit Care Med. 2002;165:663–9.
32. Griese M, Noss J, von Bredow C. Protein pattern of exhaled breath condensate and saliva. Proteomics. 2002;2:690–6.
33. Zweifel M, Rechsteiner T, Hofer M, Boehler A. Detection of pulmonary amylase activity in exhaled breath condensate. J Breath Res. 2013;7:046007.
34. Rosias PP, Dompeling E, Hendriks HJ, et al. Exhaled breath condensate in children: pearls and pitfalls. Pediatr Allergy Immunol. 2004;15:4–19.
35. Grob NM, Aytekin M, Dweik RA. Biomarkers in exhaled breath condensate: a review of collection, processing and analysis. J Breath Res. 2008;2:037004.
36. Gessner C, Scheibe R, Wotzel M, et al. Exhaled breath condensate cytokine patterns in chronic obstructive pulmonary disease. Respir Med. 2005;99:1229–40.
37. Gessner C, Rechner B, Hammerschmidt S, et al. Angiogenic markers in breath condensate identify non-small cell lung cancer. Lung Cancer. 2010;68:177–84.
38. Konstantinidi EM, Lappas AS, Tzortzi AS, Behrakis PK. Exhaled breath condensate: technical and diagnostic aspects. ScientificWorldJournal. 2015;2015:435160.
39. Conrad DH, Goyette J, Thomas PS. Proteomics as a method for early detection of cancer: a review of proteomics, exhaled breath condensate, and lung cancer screening. J Gen Intern Med. 2008;23(Suppl 1):78–84.
40. Robroeks CM, van de Kant KD, Jobsis Q, et al. Exhaled nitric oxide and biomarkers in exhaled breath condensate indicate the presence, severity and control of childhood asthma. Clin Exp Allergy. 2007;37:1303–11.
41. Belinsky SA, Liechty KC, Gentry FD, et al. Promoter hypermethylation of multiple genes in sputum precedes lung cancer incidence in a high-risk cohort. Cancer Res. 2006;66:3338–44.
42. Liu Y, Lan Q, Shen M, et al. Aberrant gene promoter methylation in sputum from individuals exposed to smoky coal emissions. Anticancer Res. 2008;28:2061–6.
43. Wang X, Ling L, Su H, et al. Aberrant methylation of genes in sputum samples as diagnostic biomarkers for non-small cell lung cancer: a meta-analysis. Asian Pac J Cancer Prev. 2014;15:4467–74.
44. Liu D, Peng H, Sun Q, et al. The indirect efficacy comparison of DNA methylation in sputum for early screening and auxiliary detection of lung cancer: a meta-analysis. Int J Environ Res Public Health. 2017;23:14.

45. Li R, Todd NW, Qiu Q, et al. Genetic deletions in sputum as diagnostic markers for early detection of stage I non-small cell lung cancer. Clin Cancer Res. 2007;13:482–7.
46. Qiu Q, Todd NW, Li R, et al. Magnetic enrichment of bronchial epithelial cells from sputum for lung cancer diagnosis. Cancer. 2008;114:275–83.
47. Katz RL, Zaidi TM, Fernandez RL, et al. Automated detection of genetic abnormalities combined with cytology in sputum is a sensitive predictor of lung cancer. Mod Pathol. 2008;21:950–60.
48. Arvanitis DA, Papadakis E, Zafiropoulos A, Spandidos DA. Fractional allele loss is a valuable marker for human lung cancer detection in sputum. Lung Cancer. 2003;40:55–66.
49. Castagnaro A, Marangio E, Verduri A, et al. Microsatellite analysis of induced sputum DNA in patients with lung cancer in heavy smokers and in healthy subjects. Exp Lung Res. 2007;33:289–301.
50. Hsu HS, Chen TP, Wen CK, et al. Multiple genetic and epigenetic biomarkers for lung cancer detection in cytologically negative sputum and a nested case-control study for risk assessment. J Pathol. 2007;213:412–9.
51. Wang YC, Lu YP, Tseng RC, et al. Inactivation of hMLH1 and hMSH2 by promoter methylation in primary non-small cell lung tumors and matched sputum samples. J Clin Invest. 2003;111:887–95.
52. Destro A, Bianchi P, Alloisio M, et al. K-ras and p16(INK4A)alterations in sputum of NSCLC patients and in heavy asymptomatic chronic smokers. Lung Cancer. 2004;44:23–32.
53. Somers VA, Pietersen AM, Theunissen PH, Thunnissen FB. Detection of K-ras point mutations in sputum from patients with adenocarcinoma of the lung by point-EXACCT. J Clin Oncol. 1998;16:3061–8.
54. Keohavong P, Gao WM, Zheng KC, et al. Detection of K-ras and p53 mutations in sputum samples of lung cancer patients using laser capture microdissection microscope and mutation analysis. Anal Biochem. 2004;324:92–9.
55. Baryshnikova E, Destro A, Infante MV, et al. Molecular alterations in spontaneous sputum of cancer-free heavy smokers: results from a large screening program. Clin Cancer Res. 2008;14:1913–9.
56. Soda M, Isobe K, Inoue A, et al. A prospective PCR-based screening for the EML4-ALK oncogene in non-small cell lung cancer. Clin Cancer Res. 2012;18:5682–9.
57. Boldrini L, Gisfredi S, Ursino S, et al. Mutational analysis in cytological specimens of advanced lung adenocarcinoma: a sensitive method for molecular diagnosis. J Thorac Oncol. 2007;2:1086–90.
58. Takano T, Ohe Y, Tsuta K, et al. Epidermal growth factor receptor mutation detection using high-resolution melting analysis predicts outcomes in patients with advanced non small cell lung cancer treated with gefitinib. Clin Cancer Res. 2007;13:5385–90.
59. Tanaka T, Matsuoka M, Sutani A, et al. Frequency of and variables associated with the EGFR mutation and its subtypes. Int J Cancer. 2010;126:651–5.
60. Bonner MR, Shen M, Liu CS, et al. Mitochondrial DNA content and lung cancer risk in Xuan Wei, China. Lung Cancer. 2009;63:331–4.
61. Jheon S, Hyun DS, Lee SC, et al. Lung cancer detection by a RT-nested PCR using MAGE A1--6 common primers. Lung Cancer. 2004;43:29–37.
62. Sun B, Wang H, Wang X, et al. A proliferation-inducing ligand: a new biomarker for non-small cell lung cancer. Exp Lung Res. 2009;35:486–500.
63. Gyoba J, Shan S, Roa W, Bedard EL. Diagnosing lung cancers through examination of micro-RNA biomarkers in blood, plasma, serum and sputum: a review and summary of current literature. Int J Mol Sci. 2016;17:494.
64. Xie Y, Todd NW, Liu Z, et al. Altered miRNA expression in sputum for diagnosis of non-small cell lung cancer. Lung Cancer. 2010;67:170–6.
65. Xing L, Todd NW, Yu L, et al. Early detection of squamous cell lung cancer in sputum by a panel of microRNA markers. Mod Pathol. 2010;23:1157–64.

66. Liao QB, Guo JQ, Zheng XY, et al. Test performance of sputum microRNAs for lung cancer: a meta-analysis. Genet Test Mol Biomarkers. 2014;18:562–7.
67. Zhang X, Wang Q, Zhang S. MicroRNAs in sputum specimen as noninvasive biomarkers for the diagnosis of nonsmall cell lung cancer: an updated meta-analysis. Medicine (Baltimore). 2019;98:e14337.
68. Chen L, Jin H. MicroRNAs as novel biomarkers in the diagnosis of non-small cell lung cancer: a meta-analysis based on 20 studies. Tumour Biol. 2014;35:9119–29.
69. Wang H, Wu S, Zhao L, et al. Clinical use of microRNAs as potential non-invasive biomarkers for detecting non-small cell lung cancer: a meta-analysis. Respirology. 2015;20:56–65.
70. Kalomenidis I, Dimakou K, Kolintza A, et al. Sputum carcinoembryonic antigen, neuron-specific enolase and cytokeratin fragment 19 levels in lung cancer diagnosis. Respirology. 2004;9:54–9.
71. Hillas G, Moschos C, Dimakou K, et al. Carcinoembryonic antigen, neuron-specific enolase and cytokeratin fragment 19 (CYFRA 21-1) levels in induced sputum of lung cancer patients. Scand J Clin Lab Invest. 2008;68:542–7.
72. Pio R, Garcia J, Corrales L, et al. Complement factor H is elevated in bronchoalveolar lavage fluid and sputum from patients with lung cancer. Cancer Epidemiol Biomark Prev. 2010;19:2665–72.
73. Konno S, Morishita Y, Fukasawa M, et al. Anthracotic index and DNA methylation status of sputum contents can be used for identifying the population at risk of lung carcinoma. Cancer. 2004;102:348–54.
74. Lewis PD, Lewis KE, Ghosal R, et al. Evaluation of FTIR spectroscopy as a diagnostic tool for lung cancer using sputum. BMC Cancer. 2010;10:640.
75. Cao C, Chen ZB, Sun SF, et al. Evaluation of VEGF-C and tumor markers in bronchoalveolar lavage fluid for lung cancer diagnosis. Sci Rep. 2013;3:3473.
76. Cao C, Sun SF, Lv D, et al. Utility of VEGF and sVEGFR-1 in bronchoalveolar lavage fluid for differential diagnosis of primary lung cancer. Asian Pac J Cancer Prev. 2013;14:2443–6.
77. Wang H, Zhang X, Liu X, et al. Diagnostic value of bronchoalveolar lavage fluid and serum tumor markers for lung cancer. J Cancer Res Ther. 2016;12:355–8.
78. Li J, Chen P, Mao CM, et al. Evaluation of diagnostic value of four tumor markers in bronchoalveolar lavage fluid of peripheral lung cancer. Asia Pac J Clin Oncol. 2014;10:141–8.
79. Zhang S, Zhao YF, Zhang MZ, Wu XL. The diagnostic value of tumor markers in bronchoalveolar lavage fluid for the peripheral pulmonary carcinoma. Clin Respir J. 2017;11:481–8.
80. Charpidou A, Gkiozos I, Konstantinou M, et al. Bronchial washing levels of vascular endothelial growth factor receptor-2 (VEGFR2) correlate with overall survival in NSCLC patients. Cancer Lett. 2011;304:144–53.
81. Montilla D, Perez M, Borges L, et al. Soluble human leukocyte antigen-G in the Bronchoalveolar lavage of lung Cancer patients. Arch Bronconeumol. 2016;52:420–4.
82. Naumnik W, Naumnik B, Niklinska W, et al. Clinical implications of hepatocyte growth factor, interleukin-20, and interleukin-22 in serum and bronchoalveolar fluid of patients with non-small cell lung cancer. Adv Exp Med Biol. 2016;952:41–9.
83. Kontakiotis T, Katsoulis K, Hagizisi O, et al. Bronchoalveolar lavage fluid alteration in antioxidant and inflammatory status in lung cancer patients. Eur J Intern Med. 2011;22:522–6.
84. Pastor MD, Nogal A, Molina-Pinelo S, et al. Identification of oxidative stress related proteins as biomarkers for lung cancer and chronic obstructive pulmonary disease in bronchoalveolar lavage. Int J Mol Sci. 2013;14:3440–55.
85. Zhou JH, Liu GN, Huang SM, et al. Comparative study of protein markers in serum and bronchoalveolar lavage fluid from patients with lung cancer by surface-enhanced laser desorption ionization time of flight mass spectrometry. Zhonghua Jie He He Hu Xi Za Zhi. 2011;34:274–7.
86. Li QK, Shah P, Li Y, et al. Glycoproteomic analysis of bronchoalveolar lavage (BAL) fluid identifies tumor-associated glycoproteins from lung adenocarcinoma. J Proteome Res. 2013;12:3689–96.

87. Uchida A, Samukawa T, Kumamoto T, et al. Napsin A levels in epithelial lining fluid as a diagnostic biomarker of primary lung adenocarcinoma. BMC Pulm Med. 2017;17:195.
88. Ortea I, Rodriguez-Ariza A, Chicano-Galvez E, et al. Discovery of potential protein biomarkers of lung adenocarcinoma in bronchoalveolar lavage fluid by SWATH MS data-independent acquisition and targeted data extraction. J Proteome. 2016;138:106–14.
89. Almatroodi SA, McDonald CF, Collins AL, et al. Quantitative proteomics of bronchoalveolar lavage fluid in lung adenocarcinoma. Cancer Genomics Proteomics. 2015;12:39–48.
90. Biaoxue R, Xiguang C, Hua L, et al. Increased level of annexin A1 in bronchoalveolar lavage fluid as a potential diagnostic indicator for lung cancer. Int J Biol Markers. 2017;32:e132–40.
91. Carvalho AS, Cuco CM, Lavareda C, et al. Bronchoalveolar lavage proteomics in patients with suspected lung Cancer. Sci Rep. 2017;7:42190.
92. Hmmier A, O'Brien ME, Lynch V, et al. Proteomic analysis of bronchoalveolar lavage fluid (BALF) from lung cancer patients using label-free mass spectrometry. BBA Clin. 2017;7:97–104.
93. Callejon-Leblic B, Garcia-Barrera T, Gravalos-Guzman J, et al. Metabolic profiling of potential lung cancer biomarkers using bronchoalveolar lavage fluid and the integrated direct infusion/ gas chromatography mass spectrometry platform. J Proteome. 2016;145:197–206.
94. Ajona D, Razquin C, Pastor MD, et al. Elevated levels of the complement activation product C4d in bronchial fluids for the diagnosis of lung cancer. PLoS One. 2015;10:e0119878.
95. Osinska I, Stelmaszczyk-Emmel A, Polubiec-Kownacka M, et al. CD4+/CD25(high)/FoxP3+/CD127- regulatory T cells in bronchoalveolar lavage fluid of lung cancer patients. Hum Immunol. 2016;77:912–5.
96. Chen L, Li Q, Zhou XD, et al. Increased pro-angiogenic factors, infiltrating neutrophils and CD163(+) macrophages in bronchoalveolar lavage fluid from lung cancer patients. Int Immunopharmacol. 2014;20:74–80.
97. Pastor MD, Nogal A, Molina-Pinelo S, et al. IL-11 and CCL-1: novel protein diagnostic biomarkers of lung adenocarcinoma in bronchoalveolar lavage fluid (BALF). J Thorac Oncol. 2016;11:2183–92.
98. Jakubowska K, Naumnik W, Niklinska W, Chyczewska E. Clinical significance of HMGB-1 and TGF-beta level in serum and BALF of advanced non-small cell lung cancer. Adv Exp Med Biol. 2015;852:49–58.
99. Zhang C, Yu W, Wang L, et al. DNA methylation analysis of the SHOX2 and RASSF1A panel in bronchoalveolar lavage fluid for lung cancer diagnosis. J Cancer. 2017;8:3585–91.
100. Li J, Hu YM, Wang Y, et al. Gene mutation analysis in non-small cell lung cancer patients using bronchoalveolar lavage fluid and tumor tissue as diagnostic markers. Int J Biol Markers. 2014;29:e328–36.
101. Hur JY, Kim HJ, Lee JS, et al. Extracellular vesicle-derived DNA for performing EGFR genotyping of NSCLC patients. Mol Cancer. 2018;17:15.
102. Nakamichi S, Seike M, Miyanaga A, et al. RT-PCR for detecting ALK translocations in cytology samples from lung cancer patients. Anticancer Res. 2017;37:3295–9.
103. Li J, Chen P, Li XQ, et al. Elevated levels of survivin and livin mRNA in bronchial aspirates as markers to support the diagnosis of lung cancer. Int J Cancer. 2013;132:1098–104.
104. Rehbein G, Schmidt B, Fleischhacker M. Extracellular microRNAs in bronchoalveolar lavage samples from patients with lung diseases as predictors for lung cancer. Clin Chim Acta. 2015;450:78–82.
105. Kim JE, Eom JS, Kim WY, et al. Diagnostic value of microRNAs derived from exosomes in bronchoalveolar lavage fluid of early-stage lung adenocarcinoma: a pilot study. Thorac Cancer. 2018;9:911–5.
106. Lee SH, Sung JY, Yong D, et al. Characterization of microbiome in bronchoalveolar lavage fluid of patients with lung cancer comparing with benign mass like lesions. Lung Cancer. 2016;102:89–95.
107. Gordon SM, Szidon JP, Krotoszynski BK, et al. Volatile organic compounds in exhaled air from patients with lung cancer. Clin Chem. 1985;31:1278–82.

108. Peng G, Tisch U, Adams O, et al. Diagnosing lung cancer in exhaled breath using gold nanoparticles. Nat Nanotechnol. 2009;4:669–73.
109. Han W, Wang T, Reilly AA, et al. Gene promoter methylation assayed in exhaled breath, with differences in smokers and lung cancer patients. Respir Res. 2009;10:86.
110. Xiao P, Chen JR, Zhou F, et al. Methylation of P16 in exhaled breath condensate for diagnosis of non-small cell lung cancer. Lung Cancer. 2014;83:56–60.
111. Khyshiktyev BS, Khyshiktueva NA, Ivanov VN, et al. Diagnostic value of investigating exhaled air condensate in lung cancer. Vopr Onkol. 1994;40:161–4.
112. Gessner C, Kuhn H, Toepfer K, et al. Detection of p53 gene mutations in exhaled breath condensate of non-small cell lung cancer patients. Lung Cancer. 2004;43:215–22.
113. Carpagnano GE, Foschino-Barbaro MP, Mule G, et al. 3p microsatellite alterations in exhaled breath condensate from patients with non-small cell lung cancer. Am J Respir Crit Care Med. 2005;172:738–44.
114. Carpagnano GE, Spanevello A, Carpagnano F, et al. Prognostic value of exhaled microsatellite alterations at 3p in NSCLC patients. Lung Cancer. 2009;64:334–40.
115. Carpagnano GE, Foschino-Barbaro MP, Spanevello A, et al. 3p microsatellite signature in exhaled breath condensate and tumor tissue of patients with lung cancer. Am J Respir Crit Care Med. 2008;177:337–41.
116. Carpagnano GE, Spanevello A, Beghe B, et al. Microsatellite alterations suggestive of organ-specific asthma and atopy in exhaled breath condensate. Allergy. 2010;65:404–5.
117. Carpagnano GE, Costantino E, Palladino GP, et al. Microsatellite alterations and cell-free DNA analysis: could they increase the cytology sensitivity in the diagnosis of malignant pleural effusion? Rejuvenation Res. 2012;15:265–73.
118. Zhang D, Takigawa N, Ochi N, et al. Detection of the EGFR mutation in exhaled breath condensate from a heavy smoker with squamous cell carcinoma of the lung. Lung Cancer. 2011;73:379–80.
119. Kordiak J, Szemraj J, Hamara K, et al. Complete surgical resection of lung tumor decreases exhalation of mutated KRAS oncogene. Respir Med. 2012;106:1293–300.
120. Chen JL, Chen JR, Huang FF, et al. Analysis of p16 gene mutations and their expression using exhaled breath condensate in non-small-cell lung cancer. Oncol Lett. 2015;10:1477–80.
121. Mozzoni P, Banda I, Goldoni M, et al. Plasma and EBC microRNAs as early biomarkers of non-small-cell lung cancer. Biomarkers. 2013;18:679–86.
122. Carpagnano GE, Koutelou A, Natalicchio MI, et al. HPV in exhaled breath condensate of lung cancer patients. Br J Cancer. 2011;105:1183–90.
123. Yang Ai SS, Hsu K, Herbert C, et al. Mitochondrial DNA mutations in exhaled breath condensate of patients with lung cancer. Respir Med. 2013;107:911–8.
124. Carpagnano GE, Resta O, Foschino-Barbaro MP, et al. Interleukin-6 is increased in breath condensate of patients with non-small cell lung cancer. Int J Biol Markers. 2002;17:141–5.
125. Brussino L, Culla B, Bucca C, et al. Inflammatory cytokines and VEGF measured in exhaled breath condensate are correlated with tumor mass in non-small cell lung cancer. J Breath Res. 2014;8:027110.
126. Carpagnano GE, Spanevello A, Curci C, et al. IL-2, TNF-alpha, and leptin: local versus systemic concentrations in NSCLC patients. Oncol Res. 2007;16:375–81.
127. Dalaveris E, Kerenidi T, Katsabeki-Katsafli A, et al. VEGF, TNF-alpha and 8-isoprostane levels in exhaled breath condensate and serum of patients with lung cancer. Lung Cancer. 2009;64:219–25.
128. Jungraithmayr W, Frings C, Zissel G, et al. Inflammatory markers in exhaled breath condensate following lung resection for bronchial carcinoma. Respirology. 2008;13:1022–7.
129. Kullmann T, Barta I, Csiszer E, et al. Differential cytokine pattern in the exhaled breath of patients with lung cancer. Pathol Oncol Res. 2008;14:481–3.
130. Gu P, Huang G, Chen Y, et al. Diagnostic utility of pleural fluid carcinoembryonic antigen and CYFRA 21-1 in patients with pleural effusion: a systematic review and meta-analysis. J Clin Lab Anal. 2007;21:398–405.

131. Liang QL, Shi HZ, Qin XJ, et al. Diagnostic accuracy of tumour markers for malignant pleural effusion: a meta-analysis. Thorax. 2008;63:35–41.
132. Shi HZ, Liang QL, Jiang J, et al. Diagnostic value of carcinoembryonic antigen in malignant pleural effusion: a meta-analysis. Respirology. 2008;13:518–27.
133. Nguyen AH, Miller EJ, Wichman CS, et al. Diagnostic value of tumor antigens in malignant pleural effusion: a meta-analysis. Transl Res. 2015;166:432–9.
134. Feng M, Zhu J, Liang L, et al. Diagnostic value of tumor markers for lung adenocarcinoma-associated malignant pleural effusion: a validation study and meta-analysis. Int J Clin Oncol. 2017;22:283–90.
135. Yang Y, Liu YL, Shi HZ. Diagnostic accuracy of combinations of tumor markers for malignant pleural effusion: an updated meta-analysis. Respiration. 2017;94:62–9.
136. Zhu J, Feng M, Liang L, et al. Is neuron-specific enolase useful for diagnosing malignant pleural effusions? Evidence from a validation study and meta-analysis. BMC Cancer. 2017;17:590.
137. Lin W, Liu X, Cen Y. Diagnostic accuracy of epithelial membrane antigen for malignant effusions: a meta-analysis. Int J Biol Markers. 2016;31:e11–6.
138. Tian P, Shen Y, Feng M, et al. Diagnostic accuracy of endostatin for malignant pleural effusion: a clinical study and meta-analysis. Postgrad Med. 2015;127:529–34.
139. Tian P, Shen Y, Wan C, et al. Diagnostic value of survivin for malignant pleural effusion: a clinical study and meta-analysis. Int J Clin Exp Pathol. 2014;7:5880–7.
140. Li D, Wang B, Long H, Wen F. Diagnostic accuracy of calretinin for malignant mesothelioma in serous effusions: a meta-analysis. Sci Rep. 2015;5:9507.
141. Ren R, Yin P, Zhang Y, et al. Diagnostic value of fibulin-3 for malignant pleural mesothelioma: a systematic review and meta-analysis. Oncotarget. 2016;7:84851–9.

Chapter 5
Gastric, Pancreatic, and Hepatobiliary Cancer Biomarkers in Proximal Fluids

5.1 Introduction

Cancers of the upper gastrointestinal system including gastric, pancreatic, and hepatobiliary cancers differ in anatomic structural involvement, epidemiology, etiology, and clinicopathologic features; however, they share a common feature of dismal prognosis due to late diagnosis.

Gastric cancer (GasCa) remains among the top five most commonly diagnosed cancers and is also one of the leading causes of cancer-related deaths worldwide. The 2018 incidence, mortality, and 5-year prevalence were 1,033,701, 728,685, and 1,589,752, respectively. However, Asia-Pacific, Latin America, and Eastern Europe are some geographic regions with the highest incidence and prevalence rates in the world. For example, the age-standardized incident rates reveal high geographic regions such as Korea, Japan, and China with rates >20/100,000; intermediate regions including Singapore, Taiwan, and Malaysia with rates between 11 and 19/100,000; and low-risk areas such as Northern India, Thailand, Australia, and New Zealand with rates below 10/100,000. There are also pockets of relatively high incidences in the developed world. Los Angeles Korean men with age-standardized incident rates of >40/100,000 and Alaskan natives with age-standardized incident rates of about 36/100,000 are among the highest in the world. These figures imply the need for interventional measures to curtail mortalities from GasCa in these high-risk populations. There are various risk factors that predispose an individual to developing GasCa, and these risks relate to the major subtypes of GasCa. Primarily genetic defects underlie the development of diffuse-type GasCa, while environmental and lifestyle factors such as diet and *Helicobacter pylori* gastritis are known risk factors of intestinal-type GasCa. Gastric cancer is a major cause of cancer-related deaths globally, partly because of late diagnosis. The 5-year survival is only 30–50% for advanced stage disease even after curative-intent surgery with lymph node dissection. Local and distant recurrences are common, suggesting ineffective therapeutic targeting of residual disease. Early detection and effective treatment is key to

G. D. Dakubo, *Cancer Biomarkers in Body Fluids*,
https://doi.org/10.1007/978-3-030-24725-6_5

improving the prognosis of GasCa. Because the outlook is good when diagnosed early, there are intensive screening programs in areas with high incidence and prevalence rates. Noninvasive, cost-effective early detection and other companion diagnostic biomarkers will complement these efforts.

Pancreatic cancer (PanCa) was the 12th most diagnosed cancer and 7th leading cause of cancer-related deaths globally in 2018. The 2018 global estimated incidence, mortality, and 5-year prevalence were 458,918, 432,242, and 282,574, respectively. Notice the high case fatality and hence low prevalence. The global age-standardized incidence and mortality are 3.9/100,000 and 3.7/100,000, respectively. Thus, the incidence is similar to the mortality rate, and this has remained so for several decades. Indeed, mortality from many cancers such as breast, prostate, and colorectal cancers is declining over the past decades, but those from PanCa have remained the same or are increasing, especially in the elderly (>70 years). The reason for this poor outcome is the absence of screening programs for the general population at low-to-medium risk, and thus many tumors are diagnosed at an advanced stage, which are not amenable to surgery, and yet there is no effective alternative therapy. While there is no consensus on who, when, or how often screening should be done, several centers use their own discretion, with many urged to only screen those with a relative risk score of above 10 (out of 14.3). Because many people at risk are excluded from screening, over 80% of cases are detected at an advanced unresectable state, often associated with distant metastasis. In view of such late presentations, the majority (>74%) of patients die within 12 months of initial diagnosis, and up to 94% die within 5 years. However, the 5-year survival rate could be as high as 75% when small tumors (<1 cm) are detected. Indeed, a screening program of high-risk individuals can potentially lead to early detection of all patients, with associated excellent cure rates. Thus, early detection of organ-confined small tumors should improve the outlook for PanCa patients. Additionally, PanCa is a latent disease that develops over several years after acquiring the initial genetic alterations. Modeling of sequencing data from primary and metastatic PanCa suggests it takes about 17 years for a cell to progress from initiation to metastasis. There is thus a wide window of opportunity for early detection, using molecular biomarkers in body fluids. The need for noninvasive early detection biomarkers is thus eminent, and there are potential targets worthy of validation for product development.

Hepatocellular carcinoma (HCC) is the most common primary liver cancer. Globally, HCC remains high in incidence and a major cause of cancer-related deaths. The 2018 global incidence, mortality, and 5-year prevalence were 841,080, 781,631, and 675,210, respectively. The low prevalence is consistent with the high mortality rate of HCC, suggestive of the need for early detection and effective treatment. Validated biomarkers in body fluids should help revert this dismal statistic. The majority of HCC (about 80%) occur in Eastern and Southeastern Asia (where over half of the cases are diagnosed) and sub-Saharan Africa, due to the increased prevalence of known risk factors in these regions. The incidence is equally rising in the Western world due to the increasing incidences of hepatitis C viral (HCV) infections. The established risk factors for HCC include chronic hepatitis B and C viral infections, cirrhosis from any cause, and high-level exposure to aflatoxin-b1 (AFB1). Additional factors that modestly elevate the risk include diabetes, nonalcoholic fatty liver disease, obesity, and smoking. Liver resection and transplantation are useful treatment strategies for tumors detected early, while advanced stage disease patients are subjected to chemotherapy and other targeted therapies. The 5-year survival rate for patients with HCC in general is about 40%, but when detected early, this could be as high as 60–70% and hence the need for screening programs, especially in endemic areas. Imaging modalities are generally used in the developed parts of the world for HCC screening. However, serum biomarkers that offer a cost-effective means of early detection are the screening methods of choice in the less privileged parts of the world such as Asia. But the alpha-fetoprotein (AFP) serum biomarker for HCC suffers from sensitivity and specificity. Even when combined with des-γ-carboxyprothrombin in a panel, sensitivity ranges from 48% to 94% with equally variable specificities of 53–99% for early HCC detection. The need for more accurate early detection biomarkers in body fluids is obvious and being pursued.

Gallbladder cancer and biliary tract cancers (also known as cholangiocarcinoma) are rare but are associated with poor prognosis due to late diagnosis. The 2018 global incidence, mortality, and 5-year prevalence of gallbladder cancer were 233,820, 165,087, and 219,420, respectively. While this incidence may appear low globally, there are sex and geographic variations. The female to male ratio is about 2.6:1. High incidence rates are also observed in Southeastern Asia and among Native Americans, although the overall incidence in the USA is low. For example, exceptionally high rates are noted among Native American women in New Mexico. The gallbladder cancer incidence rate of 3.3/100,000 among American Indians contrasts with the rate of 0.4–1.5/100,000 in non-Native Americans. Other high incidence areas include Poland (14/100,000), Northern India (female rate of 21.5/100,000), south Pakistan (11.3/100,000), Japan (7/100,000), and Israel (5/100,000). Numerous risk factors have been associated with gallbladder cancer. These include chronic gallstones and cholangitis, porcelain gallbladder, bile reflux, gallbladder polyps, environmental toxins such as aflatoxins and increased capsaicin consumption, obesity, and poor socioeconomic status. The high female incidence rate is causally linked to elevated and prolonged estrogen exposure. Irrespective of these controversial risk factors, early detection saves lives, and body fluid biomarkers deployed in people at above-average risk should help improve prognosis.

All these cancers of the upper gastrointestinal system share in common late diagnosis associated with poor prognosis. Several factors may account for this, but the lack of screening or surveillance among people at high risk can be a major contributing factor. While conceivably accurate, biomarkers from all these anatomic structures will be present in stool, but the dilution effect from this body fluid hampers accurate biomarker discovery. Thus, tissue-associated body fluids such as gastric and pancreatic juices and bile are suitable media for biomarker exploration. While minimally invasive, technologies have been explored for sampling these body fluids for early cancer detection.

5.2 Upper Gastrointestinal Proximal Fluids

The proximal fluids of the upper gastrointestinal system include gastric juice, pancreatic juice, and bile.

5.2.1 *Gastric Juice*

Collectively, the gastric glands secrete about 2 l of physiologic fluid in every 24 h. This is a considerable amount of fluid amenable to biomolecular analysis, when appropriately sampled. The gastric fluid is composed of:

- Pepsinogen/pepsin that is produced by the chief (zymogen) cells and functions in protein digestion.
- Hydrochloric acid (HCl), produced by the parietal (oxyntic) cells under the control of hormones such as gastrin. HCl is required for the conversion of pepsinogen to the active enzyme pepsin.
- The parietal cells also produce an intrinsic factor needed for vitamin B12 absorption in the small intestines (ileum).
- Hormones such as gastrin, produced by enteroendocrine cells scattered within the gastric glands.
- Of interest to biomarker analysis, the gastric fluid also contains exfoliated cells, nucleic acids, proteins, glycans, and metabolites.

There are several ways by which biomarkers from the gastric epithelium are released into gastric fluid. The surface gastric mucous cells undergo continuous renewal every 3–5 days, being shed into the lumen, and are replaced by newly differentiated mucus cells from the stem cells. Additionally, the mechanical churning action of the gastric muscularis to breakdown food into chyme causes the release of cells into gastric secretion. Exfoliated cells and other biomolecules are hence expected to be abundant in gastric juice.

5.2.2 *Pancreatic Juice*

As acidic chyme from the stomach enters the duodenum, chemoreceptors are stimulated to cause the release of secretin. Secretin, as well as the actions of the autonomic nervous system, induces pancreatic acinar and ductal cells to secrete pancreatic juice. This juice is rich in enzymes including chymotrypsinogen, trypsinogen, elastase, pancreatic lipase, carboxypeptidase, nucleases, and amylase, all of which are involved in continuous food digestion. Because chyme is acidic, and yet the pancreatic enzymes function in alkaline environment, the pancreatic ductal cells secrete large amounts of bicarbonate into the juice to help neutralize the acidic pH. Secretions from duodenal or Bruner's glands further neutralize chyme. In addition to this physiologic composition, pancreatic proximal fluid is rich in disease biomarkers that have been investigated.

5.2.3 Bile

Bile is a dark green or yellowish-brown complex fluid secreted by hepatocytes and modified by bile ductal cell secretions. Compositionally, bile contains water, electrolytes, and organic compounds including cholesterol, bile acids, phospholipids, and bilirubin. Bile also contains disease biomarkers. For example, 5–7% of the dry weight of bile is protein, which should contain important biomarkers. The adult human produces 400–800 ml of bile daily. The initial bile secreted by hepatocytes into the hepatic canaliculi is rich in bile acids, cholesterol, and other organic compounds. As bile passes through the bile duct, ductal epithelial cells secrete water and bicarbonate to modify its composition, which is then delivered to the gallbladder to be concentrated during fasting state. Bile acids are amphipathic, i.e., they have both hydrophobic and hydrophilic faces. This feature enables bile acids to perform their important functions. Bile acids emulsify fats enabling easy digestion by lipases. They also solubilize lipids to enable their transport in aqueous solution. This function is important in the transport and absorption of fat-soluble vitamins. The majority (about 95%) of bile acid is absorbed at the ileum and returned to the liver via the portal circulation. Cholecystokinin (CCK) stimulates the release of bile from the gallbladder into the duodenum. When food, especially fatty food, reaches the duodenum, it stimulates the release of CCK, which in turn stimulates contraction of the gallbladder and common bile duct to release and deliver bile to the duodenum.

5.3 Sampling of Upper Gastrointestinal Proximal Fluids

There are a number of ways to sample juices from the upper gastrointestinal tract. These include endoscopy, endogastric capsule, absorbent string device, and the entero-test device for sampling bile.

5.3.1 Upper Gastrointestinal Endoscopy

Esophagogastroduodenoscopy is performed in high-risk individuals for definite diagnosis of gastric pathology via direct visualization and biopsy (Fig. 5.1). This procedure also enables the sampling of gastric juice. Being invasive, endoscopic sampling of gastric fluid is unsuitable for general screening of the healthy population. The need for noninvasive upper gastrointestinal fluid sampling has resulted in

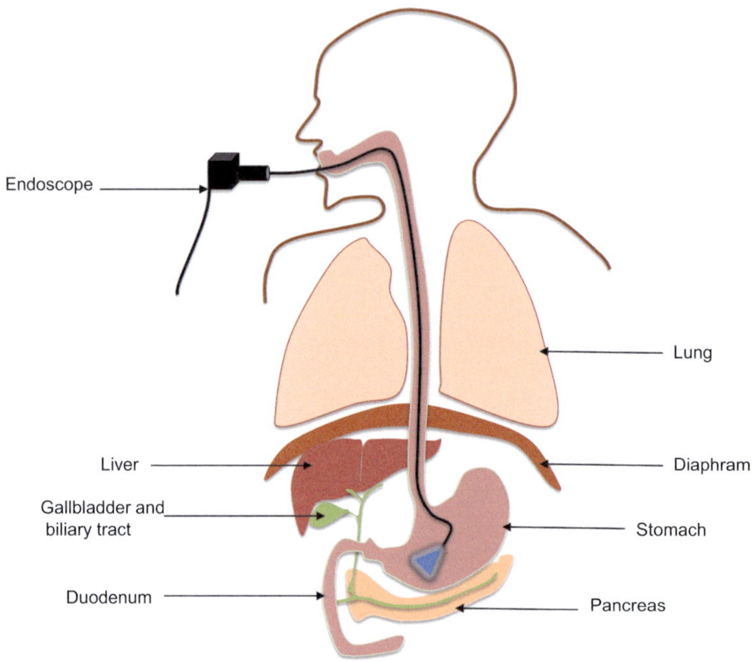

Fig. 5.1 Anatomy of the upper gastrointestinal system with illustration of upper gastrointestinal endoscopy

the development of novel devices and procedures such as an absorbent string and endogastric capsule deployment into the stomach.

5.3.2 *Endogastric Capsule*

A noninvasive mode of sampling gastric juice for biomarker analysis was conceived by P. Muretto and developed by Quercetti, Turin, Italy. The device, named endogastric capsule, is composed of a 5 × 14 mm external gelatinous envelope, which encapsulates a 4 × 13 mm internal perforated inert plastic capsule that houses a rolled-up piece of absorbent paper. The other component is a nylon string of about 45–50 cm long, attached to the plastic capsule at one end with the other end connected to a small button. The process of gastric juice sampling by this capsule is similar to the gastro-entero string device (see below). After an overnight fasting, the capsule is swallowed with small amount of water with the nylon thread fastened between two adjacent teeth. The capsule remains in the stomach for about an hour, during which the gelatin capsule is digested, and the absorbent paper gets saturated with gastric juice. Once removed by pulling on the nylon string, the absorbent paper is unrolled and can be processed in a number of ways for analysis:

- A slide smear enables direct cytological examination for abnormal cells.
- The paper can be washed into saline solution (~1 ml) and neutralized in 0.2 M sodium acetate and the resulting solution used for nucleic acid extraction for analysis.

This capsule has been used successfully for the analysis of CEA and CA19-9 by radioimmunoassay, as well as *CDH1* methylation status in gastric juices [1, 2].

5.3.3 Absorbent String Device

Two nylon string devices developed for sampling of gastrointestinal juices and cells are the gastro- and entero-test devices. Although developed for intended use to examine microbial organisms such as *H. pylori* and parasites, as well as gastrointestinal disorders such as bleeding or altered gastric pH, these devices have been successfully used to assay both gastric juices and bile. The device comprises of a highly absorbent nylon string or cotton floss of about 90 cm in length, coiled within a gelatin capsule (about 8 × 23 mm). With the free end taped to the cheek, the capsule is swallowed with the help of water. In the stomach, the gelatin is digested to expose the string to absorb gastric juice. For gastric juice sampling, the device is left in place for about 10–30 min before removal. It is estimated that every 10 cm of the string can absorb up to 0.5 ml of gastric juice, providing sufficient sample for analysis.

5.3.4 The Entero-test Device

The entero-test device is adapted for the noninvasive sampling of bile in the duodenum. To ensure entry of the string into the duodenum, the capsule is attached to a weighted nylon string of about 140 cm long. After the gelatinous capsule is digested in the stomach, the weight carries the string into the duodenum. The device is administered for between 4 and 6 h before removal and examination for bilious stain. Once in the duodenum, gallbladder contraction could be stimulated to facilitate bile release.

5.4 Gastric Cancer Biomarkers of Field Cancerization

The stomach (Fig. 5.2) is exposed to the same carcinogen that causes the "proband" cancer. The entire gastric epithelium is primed to eventual development of cancer. Thus, gastric cancer is characterized by extensive "field cancerization" that is evidenced by the:

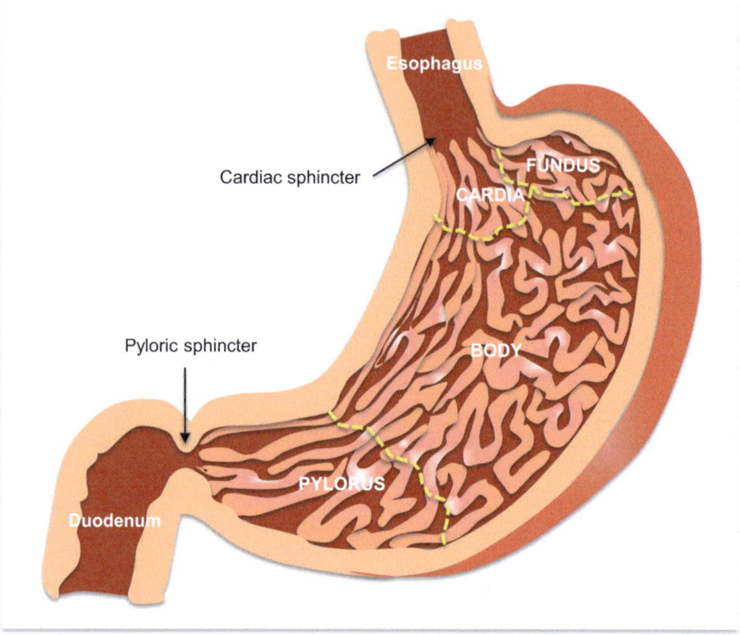

Fig. 5.2 Parts of the stomach

- Progressive nature of intestinal-type cancer
- Genetic risk predisposition in diffuse-type GasCa
- Increased risk of metachronous cancers following endoscopic mucosal resection (EMR) and endoscopic submucosal dissection (ESD)
- Increased risk of metachronous cancer development in patients with multiple initial GasCa.

The field defect is composed of nongenetic, epigenetic, genetic, and other molecular alterations in gastric cancer. These defects have important clinical utility. The nongenetic alterations are currently used to develop tests such as the serum pepsinogen test for the detection of people at high and low risk for gastric cancer. Endoscopic biopsies of equivocal nature and those from mucosa with patchy lesions can be stratified into benign and "field cancerized" mucosae. Also well-established methylation markers of field cancerization can be used to assess the levels of permanent methylation (i.e., methylation in stem cells) in people after *H. pylori* eradication so as to identify individuals at high risk for developing cancer despite *H. pylori* eradication. Finally, patients with conservative gastric surgery such as EMR and ESD can be evaluated to identify those at increased risk of developing metachronous tumors.

5.5 Gastric Cancer Biomarker in Gastric Juice

Proteomic analysis of gastric juice has identified a number of candidate GasCa biomarkers in this proximal fluid. Lee et al. used 2D electrophoresis to study the proteome of gastric juice samples from patients with GasCa, chronic atrophic gastritis, and other gastric conditions in comparison to gastric juice from healthy controls [3]. Alpha-1-antitrypsin was found highly elevated in gastric juice samples from 63% of GasCa patients. The potential of α-1-antitrypsin as GasCa biomarker was further investigated in independent studies [4]. Levels were measured in gastric juice samples from patients with GasCa, gastric and duodenal ulcers, as well as healthy controls. At a defined α-1-antitrypsin cutoff concentration of 717 ug/dl, the sensitivity, specificity, and AUROCC for GasCa detection were 96%, 92%, and 0.96, respectively. In another trial by the same group, a noninvasive string device was used to sample gastric juice from 93 patients with dyspepsia for a screening study [5]. The performance of gastric juice α-1-antitrypsin achieved a sensitivity, specificity, and AUROCC of 74%, 88%, and 0.84, respectively, for cancer detection. A proteomic analysis of gastric juice samples from patients with GasCa and benign gastritis uncovered 106 differential protein features [6]. Validation of the panel in independent samples achieved a sensitivity of 88% and specificity of 93% for GasCa detection. SELDI-TOF MS was used to analyze gastric juice samples from >200 patients. Five peptides showed differential levels and together achieved a diagnostic accuracy with AUROCC of 0.87 for GasCa. The overall sensitivity and specificity were 79% and 92%, respectively. 2D gel electrophoretic analysis of gastric juice samples from patients with gastritis and various stages of GasCa uncovered differential levels of α-1-antitrypsin, S100A9, and gastric intrinsic factor (GIF) between the groups [7]. Immunoblot analysis revealed potential diagnostic and prognostic utility of the three biomarkers. Early-stage GasCa was detectable with a panel of S100A9 and α-1-antitrypsin at AUROCC of 0.81, while a panel consisting of S100A9 and GIF could be used as a prognostic biomarker with AUROCC of 0.92.

A number of studies have examined the biomarker potential of noncoding RNAs in gastric juices. A review of eight studies identified LINC00153, AA17408, UCA1, RMRP, ABHD11-AS1, LINC00982, and H19 as potentially specific and reliable GasCa lncRNA biomarkers in GJ [8]. The following miRNAs, miR-9, miR-21, miR-25, miR-106a, miR-106b, miR-130b, miR-191, miR-214, miR-421, and miR-650 are upregulated, while mR-31, mir-29a, miR-148a, miR-155, miR-195, miR-218, miR-375, miR-378, and miR-429 are downregulated in GasCa. A review of four studies identified miR-21, miR-106a, miR-129, miR-133a, and miR-521 to be potential gastric juice miRNA biomarkers that demonstrate some reliability and reproducibility in GasCa detection [9]. Additionally, piR-651/823 is a potential GasCa biomarker detectable in gastric juice.

5.6 Pancreatic Cancer Biomarkers in Pancreatic Proximal Fluids

Current efforts at early detection of PanCa rely on costly and potentially invasive technologies. Endoscopic retrograde cholangiopancreatography (ERCP) is used to evaluate pancreatic ductal lesions. However, because of the possible post-procedural complication of pancreatitis, some investigators rely on magnetic resonance cholangiopancreatography (MRCP) for such evaluations. For detection of small pancreatic lesions, endoscopic ultrasound (EUS) has been a reliable approach. Of increased diagnostic value because it can detect very early lesions is ERCP with serial pancreatic juice aspiration cytologic evaluation (SPACE). This juice may be sampled through endoscopic nasopancreatic drainage (ENPD). However, PanCa is a silent disease, and these procedures are also costly and invasive and hence will not be suitable as screening tools.

Biomarker discoveries in pancreatic juice and cystic fluids have thus proven to be additional useful approach to early disease detection. PanCa protein biomarkers uncovered in pancreatic juice include IGFBP2, MMP9, S100A10, α-1-β-glycoprotein (A1BG), 14-3-3s, serine proteinase 2 (PRSS2), anterior gradient homolog 2 (AGR2), major vault protein (MVP), transthyretin (TTR), elastase 3B (ELA3B), BIG2, PSTI, and OLFM4.

Chen et al. performed the first quantitative proteomic analysis of pancreatic juice from healthy controls and patients with PanCa and pancreatitis [10, 11]. This approach enabled identification of >25 elevated proteins in patients compared to controls. Immunoblot was used to confirm the overexpression of insulin-like growth-factor binding protein 2 (IGFBP2) in pancreatic tissue and juice samples. The diagnostic performances of some of these PanCa biomarkers in pancreatic juice have been demonstrated. SELDI-TOF MS analysis of pancreatic juice samples from IPMN, PDAC, and chronic pancreatitis patients uncovered a distinct 6240 Da peak in samples from IPMN patients [12]. This peak was subsequently identified as PSTI. At a cutoff value of 25,000 ng/ml, the performance of PSTI in detecting IPMN achieved a sensitivity, specificity, PPV, and NPV of 48%, 98%, 89%, and 83%, respectively.

Chen et al. analyzed pancreatic juice samples from patients with PanIN3 and those with benign pancreatic diseases [13]. This study identified 20 proteins that were 2- to 20-fold higher in samples from patients with PanIN3 than controls. In a set of pancreatic juice samples from patients with PanIN2, PanIN3, IPMN, and PDAC, as well as patients with benign pancreatic conditions, one of the proteins, AGR2, was confirmed using ELISA to be significantly elevated in pancreatic juice from patients with premalignant pancreatic lesions. In differentiating between PanIN3 and benign disease patients, the sensitivity, specificity, and AUROCC of AGR2 were 67%, 90%, and 0.765%, respectively.

Some studies have used pancreatic juice as proximal fluid to uncover pancreatic neoplasia biomarkers that could be translated using blood as clinical samples. Park et al. used 2D electrophoresis to study pancreatic juice from PanCa patients and controls, which enabled identification of 26 abundant protein spots in cancer patient samples [14]. Immunohistochemistry was then used to confirm the overexpression of three of these proteins, peroxiredoxin 6 (PRDX6), lithostathine-1-α (REG1α), and brefeldin A-inhibited guanine nucleotide-exchange protein 2 (BIG2) in PanCa tissues. As a proximal fluid discovery biomarker that could be translated using blood, REG1α achieved a sensitivity, specificity, and AUROCC of 82.6%, 81.8%, and 0.771%, respectively, when examined in serum samples. REG1α does not appear to be specific to PanCa though, because performance decreased when samples from chronic pancreatitis patients were included as controls in the analysis. A comparative study of proteomes of six PanCa cell lines, six pancreatic juice samples from patients with PDAC, and one normal pancreatic ductal epithelial cell line uncovered seven elevated proteins associated with PDAC [15]. Five of them, OLFM4, SYNC, AGR2, PIGR, and COL6A1, were confirmed using ELISA to be significantly elevated in plasma from patients with PanCa compared to normal controls. A panel of the five biomarkers (AUROCC of 0.98) was comparable to CA19.9 (AUROCC of 0.97) in PanCa detection. However, AGR2 was able to augment the diagnostic performance of Ca19.9 to AUROCC of 1.00.

Pancreatic cystic fluid has also been used as proximal fluid for exploration of PanCa biomarkers. Pancreatic cystic fluid proteomes from patients with PDAC, IPMN, MCN, and NET were compared to those of nonmalignant patients by SELDI-TOF MS [16]. Differential protein profiles were uncovered between malignant and nonmalignant fluids, as well as between premalignant lesions (IPMN and MC). Another proteomic analysis of pancreatic cystic fluid from patients with atypia or suspicious cytological diagnosis and nonmalignant samples uncovered mucins, S100 family members, CEACAMs, and homologs of amylase as early diagnosis biomarkers [17]. The levels of these correlated with CEA levels. 2D in-gel trypsinization followed by LC-MS/MS analysis of cystic fluids from patients with IPMN, NET, serous cystadenoma, MCN, and pancreatic pseudocyst enabled identification of differential protein levels among the lesions, some of which were confirmed using immunohistochemistry on tissue samples and immunoblot on cystic fluids [18]. Of interest, one of the proteins, olfactomedin 4 (OLFM4), was associated with IPMN and MCN, while another, mucin 18 (MUC18), was associated with NET. Glycomic and glycoproteomic analysis of 21 cystic fluids from patients with various pancreatic lesions including IPMN and MCN uncovered high levels of multiple fucosylation in six of the samples [19]. Several candidate glycoproteins including pancreatic amylase and triacylglycerol lipase were found hyperfucosylated.

A systematic review of 193 studies uncovered three biomarkers that could identify malignant IPMNs with the greatest accuracy. These were pancreatic juice cytology (AUROCC of 0.84), serum CA19-9 (AUROCC of 0.81), and cystic fluid cytology (AUROCC of 0.82). The combination of pancreatic juice cytology with MUC1 and MUC2 staining of pancreatic juice improved performance with AUROCC of 0.85 [20]. A meta-analytical review of 16 studies suggests *KRAS* mutation analysis in pancreatic juice has potential as early diagnostic biomarker of PanCa [21]. In this study, the pooled sensitivity, specificity, PLR, NLR, and DOR were 59%, 87%, 4.13%, 0.42%, and 13.66%, respectively.

Should these cystic fluid biomarkers of pancreatic cancer lesion be measurable in circulation, they could be useful for disease stratification in a minimally invasive medium.

5.7 Hepatobiliary Cancer Biomarkers in Proximal Fluids

A number of hepatobiliary cancer protein biomarkers have been identified in bile. Proteomic analysis of bile from patients with malignant stenosis due to cholangiocarcinoma uncovered proteins associated with the disease [22]. Galectin-3-binding protein (Mac-2BP) was validated using ELISA in an independent study as a potential biomarker of biliary tract carcinoma [23]. The validation study included samples from patients with biliary tract carcinomas, benign biliary conditions, and primary sclerosing cholangitis. At a cutoff level of 853 ng/ml, Mac-2BP achieved a sensitivity, specificity, and AUROCC of 69%, 67%, and 0.70, respectively, in diagnosing biliary tract cancer. This performance was slightly improved by incorporating bile CA19.9 to AUROCC of 0.75. 2D electrophoretic analysis of bile identified pancreatic elastase 3B (CEL3B) as a candidate biomarker of cholangiocarcinoma [24]. The ratio of CELB3 to amylase was significantly higher in bile from patients with cholangiocarcinoma than those with gallstones. At a cutoff value of 0.065, the ratio achieved a sensitivity, specificity, and AUROCC of 82%, 89%, and 0.877, respectively, in differentiating between malignant and nonmalignant causes of biliary tract obstruction. A label-free proteomic analysis of bile from patients with pancreatobiliary cancers identified neutrophil gelatinase-associated lipocalin (NGAL) as a potential biomarker [25]. At a cutoff value of 570 ng/ml, bile NGAL could differentiate between pancreatobiliary cancer patients from those with nonmalignant conditions at a sensitivity, specificity, and AUROCC of 94%, 55%, and 0.76, respectively. The low specificity was improved to 82% (at a sensitivity of 85%) with adjusted cutoff value of 3000 ng/ml, in addition to incorporating serum CA19.9 at a cutoff value of 125 U/L. In subgroup analysis, NGAL at a cutoff value of 570 ng/ml achieved a sensitivity of 100% but at the same dismal specificity of 56% in detection of PDAC. NGAL is not specific to pancreatobiliary cancers.

Defined peptide patterns in bile were uncovered for patients with cholangiocarcinoma, primary sclerosing cholangitis (PSC), and choledocholithiasis using capillary electrophoresis MS [26]. These patterns were used to develop two diagnostic models, one for differentiating between patients with cholangiocarcinoma and PSC from choledocholithiasis, which achieved a sensitivity, specificity, and AUROCC of 93%, 86%, and 0.93%, respectively, and the other for discriminating between patients with CC and PSC that achieved a sensitivity, specificity, and AUROCC of 84%, 78%, and 0.87%, respectively. In another analysis, bile from patients with cholangiocarcinoma contained higher levels of spermatogenesis-associated protein 20 (also known as sperm-specific protein 411 (SSP411)) compared to those from patients with cholangitis [27]. The diagnostic performance of SSP411 in circulation (serum samples) achieved a sensitivity, specificity, and AUROCC of 90%, 83%, and

0.913%, respectively. Another potential malignant biliary stenosis biomarker in bile, CEA-related cell adhesion protein 6 (CEACAM6), was identified using iTRAQ proteomics [28]. The diagnostic performance of bile CEACAM6 achieved a sensitivity, specificity, PPV, NPV, AUROCC, and overall accuracy of 93.1%, 83.1%, 93.1%, 83.3%, 0.92, and 0.903%, respectively, in differentiating malignant from nonmalignant causes of biliary stenosis. These diagnostic parameters improved slightly with addition of serum CA19.9 to sensitivity, specificity, PPV, NPV, AUROCC, and overall accuracy of 96.6%, 83.3%, 93.3%, 90.9%, 0.96, and 0.927%, respectively.

5.8 Summary

- Gastric, pancreatic, and hepatobiliary cancers are among the most commonly diagnosed cancers globally. They are also associated with poor outcomes due to late presentation.
- The need for early detection so as to improve patient outcome has propelled the development and use of various imaging modalities. However, these approaches are costly and potentially invasive and may be associated with radiation exposure.
- Proximal fluids of these cancers are enriched with respective cancer-specific biomarkers that are currently being evaluated.
- Gastric cancer biomarkers in gastric juice include a-1-antitrypsin, S100A9, and several ncRNAs.
- Pancreatic cancer biomarkers in pancreatic juice include IGFBP2, MMP9, S100A10, A1BG, 14-3-3s, PRSS2, AGR2, MVP, TTR, ELA3B, BIG2, PSTI, and OLFM4.
- Hepatobiliary cancer biomarkers in bile include Mac-2BP, NGAL, CEL3B, and SSP411.
- Validated biomarkers can be used as screening tools in the at-risk population using minimally invasive sampling techniques of these fluids.

References

1. Muretto P, Ruzzo A, Pizzagalli F, et al. Endogastric capsule for E-cadherin gene (CDH1) promoter hypermethylation assessment in DNA from gastric juice of diffuse gastric cancer patients. Ann Oncol. 2008;19:516–9.
2. Muretto P, Graziano F, Staccioli MP, et al. An endogastric capsule for measuring tumor markers in gastric juice: an evaluation of the safety and efficacy of a new diagnostic tool. Ann Oncol. 2003;14:105–9.
3. Lee K, Kye M, Jang JS, et al. Proteomic analysis revealed a strong association of a high level of alpha1-antitrypsin in gastric juice with gastric cancer. Proteomics. 2004;4:3343–52.
4. Hsu PI, Chen CH, Hsieh CS, et al. Alpha1-antitrypsin precursor in gastric juice is a novel biomarker for gastric cancer and ulcer. Clin Cancer Res. 2007;13:876–83.

5. Hsu PI, Chen CH, Hsiao M, et al. Diagnosis of gastric malignancy using gastric juice alpha1-antitrypsin. Cancer Epidemiol Biomarkers Prev. 2010;19:405–11.
6. Kon OL, Yip TT, Ho MF, et al. The distinctive gastric fluid proteome in gastric cancer reveals a multi-biomarker diagnostic profile. BMC Med Genomics. 2008;1:54.
7. Wu W, Juan WC, Liang CR, et al. S100A9, GIF and AAT as potential combinatorial biomarkers in gastric cancer diagnosis and prognosis. Proteomics Clin Appl. 2012;6:152–62.
8. Virgilio E, Giarnieri E, Giovagnoli MR, et al. Long non-coding RNAs in the gastric juice of gastric cancer patients. Pathol Res Pract. 2018;214:1239–46.
9. Virgilio E, Giarnieri E, Giovagnoli MR, et al. Gastric juice microRNAs as potential biomarkers for screening gastric cancer: a systematic review. Anticancer Res. 2018;38:613–6.
10. Chen R, Pan S, Cooke K, et al. Comparison of pancreas juice proteins from cancer versus pancreatitis using quantitative proteomic analysis. Pancreas. 2007;34:70–9.
11. Chen R, Pan S, Yi EC, et al. Quantitative proteomic profiling of pancreatic cancer juice. Proteomics. 2006;6:3871–9.
12. Shirai Y, Sogawa K, Yamaguchi T, et al. Protein profiling in pancreatic juice for detection of intraductal papillary mucinous neoplasm of the pancreas. Hepatogastroenterology. 2008;55:1824–9.
13. Chen R, Pan S, Duan X, et al. Elevated level of anterior gradient-2 in pancreatic juice from patients with pre-malignant pancreatic neoplasia. Mol Cancer. 2010;9:149.
14. Park JY, Kim SA, Chung JW, et al. Proteomic analysis of pancreatic juice for the identification of biomarkers of pancreatic cancer. J Cancer Res Clin Oncol. 2011;137:1229–38.
15. Makawita S, Smith C, Batruch I, et al. Integrated proteomic profiling of cell line conditioned media and pancreatic juice for the identification of pancreatic cancer biomarkers. Mol Cell Proteomics. 2011;10(M111):008599.
16. Scarlett CJ, Samra JS, Xue A, et al. Classification of pancreatic cystic lesions using SELDI-TOF mass spectrometry. ANZ J Surg. 2007;77:648–53.
17. Ke E, Patel BB, Liu T, et al. Proteomic analyses of pancreatic cyst fluids. Pancreas. 2009;38:e33–42.
18. Cuoghi A, Farina A, Z'Graggen K, et al. Role of proteomics to differentiate between benign and potentially malignant pancreatic cysts. J Proteome Res. 2011;10:2664–70.
19. Mann BF, Goetz JA, House MG, et al. Glycomic and proteomic profiling of pancreatic cyst fluids identifies hyperfucosylated lactosamines on the N-linked glycans of overexpressed glycoproteins. Mol Cell Proteomics. 2012;11:M111 015792.
20. Tanaka M, Heckler M, Liu B et al. Cytologic analysis of pancreatic juice increases specificity of detection of malignant IPMN – a systematic review. Clin Gastroenterol Hepatol. 2019. https://doi.org/10.1016/j.cgh.2018.12.034
21. Yang J, Li S, Li J, et al. A meta-analysis of the diagnostic value of detecting K-ras mutation in pancreatic juice as a molecular marker for pancreatic cancer. Pancreatology. 2016;16:605–14.
22. Kristiansen TZ, Bunkenborg J, Gronborg M, et al. A proteomic analysis of human bile. Mol Cell Proteomics. 2004;3:715–28.
23. Koopmann J, Thuluvath PJ, Zahurak ML, et al. Mac-2-binding protein is a diagnostic marker for biliary tract carcinoma. Cancer. 2004;101:1609–15.
24. Chen CY, Tsai WL, Wu HC, et al. Diagnostic role of biliary pancreatic elastase for cholangiocarcinoma in patients with cholestasis. Clin Chim Acta. 2008;390:82–9.
25. Zabron AA, Horneffer-Van der Sluis VM, Wadsworth CA, et al. Elevated levels of neutrophil gelatinase-associated lipocalin in bile from patients with malignant pancreatobiliary disease. Am J Gastroenterol. 2011;106:1711–7.
26. Lankisch TO, Metzger J, Negm AA, et al. Bile proteomic profiles differentiate cholangiocarcinoma from primary sclerosing cholangitis and choledocholithiasis. Hepatology. 2011;53:875–84.
27. Shen J, Wang W, Wu J, et al. Comparative proteomic profiling of human bile reveals SSP411 as a novel biomarker of cholangiocarcinoma. PLoS One. 2012;7:e47476.
28. Farina A, Dumonceau JM, Antinori P, et al. Bile carcinoembryonic cell adhesion molecule 6 (CEAM6) as a biomarker of malignant biliary stenoses. Biochim Biophys Acta. 2014;1844:1018–25.

Chapter 6
Colorectal Cancer Biomarkers in Proximal Fluids

6.1 Introduction

Colorectal cancer (CRC) remains a challenge in oncology. First, they are among the most commonly diagnosed cancers, and second, they are among the leading causes of cancer-related mortality worldwide. However, tremendous efforts have been made in using the wealth of molecular genetic knowledge on this cancer in disease management. The 2018 GLOBOCAN estimated incidence, mortality, and 5-year prevalence were 1,849,518, 880,792, and 4,789,635, respectively, which places it third (after lung and breast), second (after lung), and second (after breast) in incidence, mortality, and prevalence, respectively. Whereas there are wide geographic variations in CRC incidences, the highest rate occurs in Australia and New Zealand, with the lowest in West Africa. However, the incidence is on the rise globally, and this could partly be accounted for by increased awareness and intensive screening efforts, especially in the more developed parts of the world. There are equally geographic variations in mortality rates, with the highest in Central and Eastern Europe and the lowest in West Africa.

The vast majority (up to 85%) of CRCs are sporadic with no evidence of hereditary or familial components. The risk factors for acquiring somatic gene alterations leading to the development of CRC include age (mean age at diagnosis is 66 years), consumption of diet rich in red meat and unsaturated fat, excessive alcohol use, sedentary lifestyle, and high-energy input. However, the pathophysiology may include a complex interplay between bioenergetics, inflammation, hormonal actions, and even the gut microbiome. These complex and dynamic interacting factors can cause epigenetic and genetic alterations in a vast majority of cells, creating an enlarged area of damaged mucosa consistent with the concept of field cancerization. Subsequently, clonal selection of a CRC cell to expand, grow, and form overt tumors occurs.

Improved surgical techniques coupled with adjuvant chemotherapies and novel biotherapies are making positive impacts on the 5-year survival of patients with CRC. However, this benefit is optimal mostly for patients with localized early-stage

G. D. Dakubo, *Cancer Biomarkers in Body Fluids*,
https://doi.org/10.1007/978-3-030-24725-6_6

disease (stage I disease patients have a 95%, while stage II disease patients have 82% 5-year survival). This survival rate drops to 61% in patients with regional lymph node spread (stage III) and very dismal (8%) for stage IV disease patients with distant metastasis. Yet less than 40% of all patients are diagnosed with early-stage disease. The need for improved early detection and effective therapies is urgent and is actively being pursued.

While mostly sporadic, 15–30% of CRCs have some hereditary components. Achievements made at delineating the molecular genetic alterations in hereditary CRC have helped in the elucidation of the molecular pathology of sporadic CRCs as well. Multiple genes altered in hereditary CRC and also in sporadic cancers include *APC*, *AXIN2*, *MLH1*, *MSH2*, *MSH6*, *PMS2*, *GTBP*, *LKB1*, *STK11*, *MYH*, *PTEN*, *BMPR1a*, and *DPC4*. Despite the plethora of authenticated genetic information on CRC, screening recommendations still rely on fecal occult blood test (FOBT), followed by colonoscopy to visualize and obtain biopsy samples for eventual histopathologic diagnosis. FOBT is a noninvasive assay but suffers from accuracy, while colonoscopy is invasive with possible serious complications. Therefore, validated biomarkers in body fluids should enhance CRC early detection and management. Thus, the FDA-approved *SEPT9* methylation blood test is a step in the right direction that should augment CRC screening efforts. Also easily acceptable and of additional benefit is stool DNA (sDNA) testing for CRC-specific biomarkers.

6.2 Basic Anatomy of the Colorectum

At approximately 150 cm in length, the colorectum extends from the ileocecal junction or valve to the anus (Fig. 6.1). Commonly known as the large bowel of the digestive system, the colorectum is involved with the reabsorption of water and salt so as to form a solid fecal matter that is lubricated and propelled to the anus for excretion. Anatomically, the colorectum consists of seven defined segments with relevance to cancer development, progression, and paths of invasiveness. These are the appendix, cecum, ascending colon, transverse colon, descending colon, sigmoid colon, and rectum.

A section through the colorectal wall reveals the following structural organization from the outside inwards: an outer longitudinal muscle forms separate longitudinal bands called teniae coli (absent in the rectum), an inner thick circular muscle, a submucosa with lymphoid aggregates, and a mucosa that is folded when not distended. The mucosa contains straight tubular glands that extend from the muscularis mucosa beneath. These glands contain two types of cells, the absorptive cells and mucus producing goblet cells. The goblet cells tend to aggregate at the base of the glands with the columnar absorptive cells located more on the luminal surface (hence more likely to be shed in feces). Also found in these glands are scattered basal stem cells that continuously replicate to replace the epithelium. These cells are the source of CRC stem cells. The colorectum is populated with commensal bacteria that function to help degrade food residue. Because the colorectum harbors the majority (over 90%) of the entire body microbiome, it is the subject of study of microbial dysbiosis in several cancers.

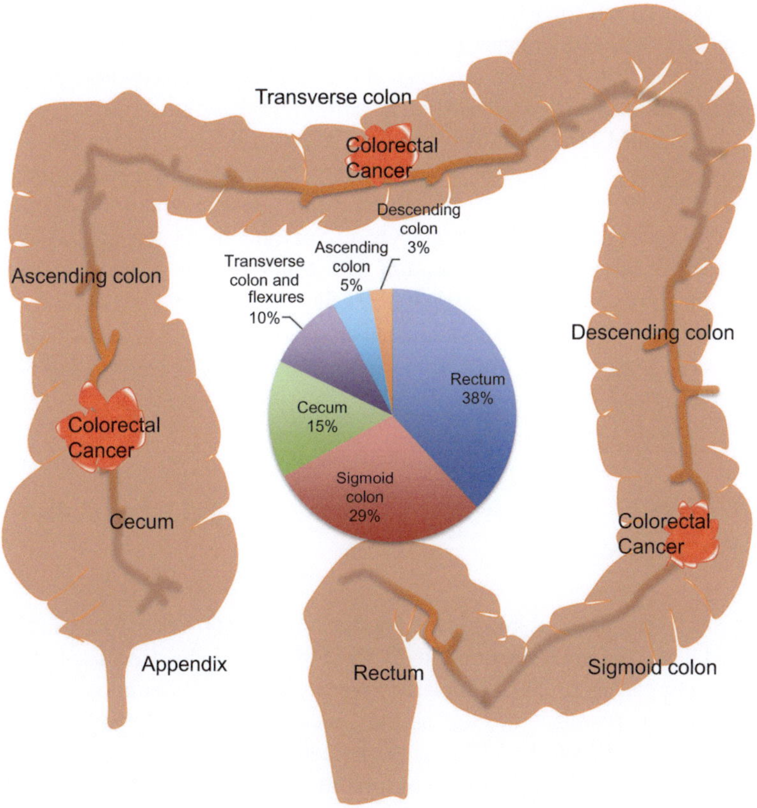

Fig. 6.1 The colorectum and anatomic distribution of colorectal cancer

6.3 Stool and Isolation of Colonocytes

Stool or human fecal matter is an excretory by-product of food digestion. It is obtained in a noninvasive manner and easily collected for CRC screening. The appearance, composition, and constitution of stool vary extensively, being influenced by diet and the health status of the individual. In addition to numerous debris and fat, human fecal matter contains several genera of microbes and shed colonic epithelial cells (colonocytes).

Fecal acquisition transportation and storage is critical to biomarker analysis. Thus, an assessment for self-fecal collection, preservation, shipment, and extraction methods at room temperature has been investigated [1]. Successful extraction of genetic material was accomplished when stored for 5 days in RNAlater and PAXgene or dried on silica gels or Whatman FTA papers. DNA with little PCR inhibition was obtained from stool stored in RNAlater and extracted using Qiagen stool methods.

In order to enrich for CRC biomarkers, some investigators isolate colonocytes for study. To isolate colonocytes, collected fecal material is immediately processed, frozen, or stored at 4 °C for less than 48 hours before processing. To process, homogenize about 2 g of stool in 50 ml of buffer (Hanks solution, 10% fetal bovine serum, and 25 mM HEPES buffer, pH 7.4) at 200 times per minute for 1–2 min. Filter homogenate solution through a nylon membrane (pore size of 512 um, which is large enough to permit passage of colonocytes while removing most debris). Add Dynabeads Epithelial Enrich (Dynal, Oslo, Norway) to the filtrate solution and incubate for 30 min at room temperature with gentle rolling. Centrifuge 15 min at room temperature and discard supernatant. Collect and store pelleted colonocytes at −80 °C until used. In a study by Onouchi et al., recovery rate of colonocytes was not reduced when samples were kept at 4 °C and colonocytes isolated within 48 hours after defecation [2].

6.4 Current Colorectal Cancer Screening and Diagnostic Procedures

CRC is commonly encountered in people over the age of 50 years. Many individuals diagnosed have no family history and do not show symptoms. Because CRC is one of the leading causes of cancer mortality worldwide, it is recommended to screen for detection of early cancerous lesions that saves lives. Screening and definite diagnosis involves noninvasive and invasive procedures. This generally involves fecal occult blood tests (FOBTs,) colonoscopy, barium enema, sigmoidoscopy, and colonography. Currently, the noninvasive FOBT is commonly used for screening, but this test is not very accurate. The sensitivity and specificity ranges for guaiac FOBT (gFOBT) are 6–83% and 65–99%, respectively, and for fecal immunochemical tests (FIT) 5–63% and 89–98%, respectively [3]. Colonoscopy, virtual colonoscopy, sigmoidoscopy, and barium enemas are invasive procedures but are very accurate at cancer detection. Hence, there is a need to identify accurate genetic markers for stratifying people for further invasive investigational procedures. Mutations in *APC, KRAS, TP53,* and BAT-26 microsatellite instability elevate the risk for colorectal adenomas and cancer. Genetic testing based on nuclear gene alterations is available for colorectal polyps, adenomas, and cancers. While approved by the FDA, stool DNA (sDNA) tests are yet to be widely available to all at average-risk individuals.

6.5 Colorectal Cancer Biomarkers in Proximal Fluid

Of the numerous biomarkers for CRC management, extensive studies have focused on FOBT and sDNA tests, with limited attention to transcript, protein, and other biomarkers.

6.5.1 Fecal Occult Blood as Colorectal Cancer Biomarkers in Proximal Fluid

CRC screening is commonly performed by detection of the widely used biomarker, occult blood in stool. These fecal blood tests are based on the tenet that neoplastic or adenomatous polyps "bleed" into stool. Guaiac-based FOBT (gFOBT) relies on detection of pseudoperoxidase activity of heme in stool samples. Confirmatory evidence for the use of gFOBT in CRC screening has been provided by a number of studies. A 30-year longitudinal study whereby participants were randomized to gFOBT or standard care revealed a 32% reduction in CRC mortality [4]. Earlier randomized controlled clinical trials in the USA, England, and Denmark had revealed significant reductions in CRC mortality with once or twice annual testing [5, 6]. Despite its usefulness, gFOBT is nonspecific because it also detects peroxidase activity of heme from other sources in stool. Thus, to prevent or reduce false-positive test results, participants must adhere to a 3-day meal regimen devoid of meat and nonsteroidal anti-inflammatory drugs (NSAIDs). Additionally, multiple testing is needed to enhance test sensitivity. The guaiac-infused Hemoccult II and its improved sensitive version, Hemoccult II Sensa (Beckman Coulter, Brea, CA), are the most commonly used gFOBTs.

An improvement to gFOBT was the development of the fecal immunochemical test (FIT). Using labeled antibodies, FIT detects the globin fraction of human hemoglobin, thus obviating other sources of heme. Because globin degrades as it passes through the gastrointestinal tract (GIT), FIT is more sensitive at detection of bleeding from the distal GIT. There are two types of FIT: quantitative (OC Sensa and Insure) and qualitative tests. Quantitative FIT is an immunoturbidimetric assay that directly measures globin levels in stool, while the qualitative assay employs lateral flow immunochromatography to determine signal positivity at a specified globin cutoff value. Many quantitative tests are however reported as positive when globin levels are above a manufacturer's recommended set threshold. Several studies have evaluated the performance of FIT in the average at-risk population. Some studies focused on the characteristics of FIT on single-time usage, while others have examined multiple testing in CRC detection. In an Italian study involving four multiple rounds of testing, 48.1% of the 2959 screening population completed all four tests [7]. Over the duration of the testing, cancer detection declined with time due to continuous detection and removal of advanced adenomas. The rate of advanced adenoma detection in this cohort was 33%. While both qualitative and quantitative FITs are similar in regard to test performance, quantitative tests have some advantages over qualitative assays. For instance, specific globin values may reflect disease stage. Additionally, the quality of quantitative FIT is higher than qualitative tests. The verdict therefore has been a preference for quantitative FIT. Quantitative FIT also permits setting of globin cutoff values that optimizes test performance. However, this must account for confounding variables such as sex and age that impact on fecal hemoglobin levels. There are studies attempting to standardize quantitative FIT to enable comparison of test performances.

Several meta-analytical studies have examined the performance of FOBTs in early CRC detection and possible cutoff values to enhance disease detection accuracy. A meta-analysis of FIT studies showed high and moderate accuracies for CRC and adenomas, respectively [8]. The diagnostic performance of FIT detecting CRC or advanced adenoma in asymptomatic patients at above-average risk for CRC (i.e., with personal or family history of CRC) was compared to colonoscopy as reference standard. Of 12 studies with 6204 participants including seven that were considered to have high or unclear bias, the pooled sensitivity, specificity, PLR, and NLR were 93%, 91%, 10.30, and 0.08, respectively, for CRC and 48%, 93%, 6.55, and 0.57 for advanced adenoma. FIT cutoff values of 15 and 25 ug/g of feces achieved the best performance with sensitivity and specificity of 93% and 94%, respectively. This indicated its usefulness for screening the at-risk population for early CRC detection. Another meta-analysis of FIT for screening CRC included 19 studies [9]. While substantial heterogeneity was uncovered between studies, the pooled sensitivity, specificity, PLR, NLR, and AUROCC were 79%, 94%, 13.10, 0.23, and 0.95, respectively. Single sample FIT achieved similar performances as several samples independent of FIT brand. Lower cutoff values increased sensitivity at the expense of specificity. Subgroup analysis revealed a sensitivity of 71% when colonoscopy was the reference standard for CRC detection. Expectedly, FIT performance for advanced adenoma was variable but overall low. For example, when qualitative tests were examined, the two top performing brands achieved sensitivity of approximately 25% in detecting advanced adenoma. However, the addition of FIT to a once-only flexible sigmoidoscopy increased sensitivity for CRC detection [10]. The overall sensitivities for cancer and advanced adenoma were, respectively, 65% and 27% for FIT alone, 65% and 67% for flexible sigmoidoscopy alone, and 89% and 75% for both. The pooled specificity for FIT was 92%. Another analysis aimed at determining optimal FOBT intervals in CRC screening focused on determining incidence of interval CRC (iCRC) following a negative FIT or gFOBT. Of 29 studies with 6,987,825 negative test result subjects, the pooled incidences of iCRC for FIT and gFOBT were 20 and 34 per 100,000 person-years, respectively [11]. This provided evidence for the superiority of FIT over gFOBT in CRC screening. Systematic reviews by Lee et al. and Katsoula et al. suggest FIT cutoff levels <20 ug/g of stool were optimal and cost-effective for CRC detection [8, 9]. A study that adjusted for confounding variables of age and sex suggests that globin level <77 ug/g of stool is an independent risk factor for the presence of advanced neoplasm with odds ratio (OR) of 3.8 (95 CI; 3.07–4.71).

While these fecal blood tests have proven useful in CRC screening in terms of reductions in mortality, there are a few noteworthy observations about them; first, GIT bleeding is not specific to CRC and not all colorectal neoplasia bleeds; second, while quantitative FIT may be superior to qualitative FIT, various studies have used different cutoff values for cancer detection making comparing studies challenging; and finally, while quantitative FIT is often reported as positive or negative, there is a need to examine the value of specific globin levels in relation to colonoscopy findings.

6.5.2 DNA Alterations as Colorectal Cancer Biomarkers in Proximal Fluid

CRC is a genetic disease characterized by mutations, microsatellite instability, and epigenetic alterations. For example, the classic tubular adenoma pathway for colorectal carcinogenesis involves loss of *APC* and activation of *KRAS* that advances adenoma growth, followed by inactivation of *TP53*. With this knowledge, as well as the numerous established genetic alterations in CRC, well-designed studies have led to the development of stool-based genetic tests for CRC screening.

Sidransky et al. first reported on detection of mutated genes (*KRAS*, *APC,* and *TP53*) in stool from CRC patients [12]. Since then several well-designed studies have confirmed these findings. Improvements in methodologies and technologies have enabled sensitive detection of gene alterations in shed neoplastic colonocytes in stool. A diagnostic proof-of-concept study involved analysis of 15-point mutations in *APC, KRAS,* and *TP53* as well as MSI detection with the marker, BAT-26. This study included 22 CRC patients, 11 patients with adenomas ≥1 cm, and 28 individuals with no evidence of CRC by colonoscopy. At a specificity of 93%, the sensitivity was 82% for adenomas and 91% for CRC [13]. Subsequent studies confirmed the rationale for sDNA investigation, because all CRC mutations detected in stool samples were present in matched primary tumor tissues and disappeared following tumor removal [14].

The first population-based screening study of sDNA for CRC detection included 2507 asymptomatic average-risk individuals aged 50 or older. The tested DNA alterations included mutations in *APC* and *KRAS*, as well as MSI (detected with BAT-26) and DNA integrity assay [15]. Performance of this first-generation sDNA panel was evaluated in comparison to Hemoccult II, while colonoscopy served as the reference standard. The overall CRC detection sensitivity of this sDNA assay was 52% compared to 13% for Hemoccult II. The sensitivities and specificities for high-grade dysplastic adenomas were 32.5% and 94.4%, respectively, for sDNA and 15% and 95.2%, respectively, for Hemoccult II test. An expanded study of sDNA panel involved 4482 average-risk individuals who were 50 years or older [16]. This study uncovered CRC detection sensitivity of 25% compared to 50% for Hemoccult II and 75% for the more sensitive Hemoccult II Sensa. The poor performance of this sDNA assay prompted the investigators to select a different panel of sDNA markers for further study. This second sDNA panel included methylation in vimentin gene (*VIM*) and mutations in *KRAS* and *APC.* CRC detection was improved with a sensitivity of 58% compared to 10% for Hemoccult II and 17% for Hemoccult II Sensa tests. These findings prompted a revision of the recommendation of CRC screening by the American College of Gastroenterology to include sDNA testing [17]. However, clinical uptake of sDNA remained unattractive due to the low sensitivity and possibly the high cost [18].

Improvements were subsequently made to the initial protocol to enhance detection of sDNA. These modifications included addition of stabilizing buffer to prevent sDNA degradation, improved DNA extraction methods, identification of new biomarker panel, and automation and enhanced analytical processes such as mutant DNA detection techniques. The second-generation panel identified included methylation of *NDRG4*, *BMP3*, *TFPI2*, and *VIM*, as well as mutations in *KRAS* and hemoglobin assay. Hybridization with oligonucleotide probes was used for target gene sequence identification, while methylated DNA was quantified using quantitative allele-specific real-time target and signal amplification (QuARTS) assay [19]. The initial pilot study using this new generation of panel biomarkers and conditions included 252 CRC patients and 133 with adenomas ≥1 cm and 293 negative colonoscopy individuals who served as control. At 90% specificity, this sDNA panel achieved a sensitivity of 54% for adenomas and 85% for CRC detection. Of interest, the sensitivity increased mirroring the increasing size of adenoma, being 54% for adenoma ≥1 cm, 63% for adenomas >1 cm, 77% for adenomas >2 cm, 86% for adenomas >3 cm, and 92% for adenomas >4 cm. These findings suggest neoplastic colonocyte shedding increases with increasing size of adenoma, which is a risk factor for progression to CRC. The encouraging findings triggered a population-based screening study that included 9899 average-risk asymptomatic individuals aged 50–84 years. The selected biomarkers for this study were methylation in *NDRG4* and *BMP3*, *KRAS* mutations, and a hemoglobin assay. The sDNA panel was compared to FIT, and colonoscopy served as reference standard for test performance in disease detection. While the specificity of 86.6% for sDNA was inferior to the 94.9% achieved for FIT, the sensitivity of this sDNA panel of 92.3% was superior to the 73.8% for FIT in CRC detection. Similarly, the sensitivity of the panel in detecting adenomas or sessile serrated polyps ≥1 cm was 42.4%, which was superior to FIT (23.8%). Whereas sDNA sensitivity was independent of tumor location, FIT sensitivity was lower for proximal tumors due to globin degradation in transit from this anatomic site. These findings led to the approval by the FDA for use of this sDNA panel in CRC screening.

Several meta-analytical studies suggest a potential for use of other stool DNA biomarkers for CRC screening. Promoter methylation of secreted frizzled-related proteins (SFRPs) has been investigated as potential fecal CRC biomarkers. A systematic review of SFRP1, 2, 4, and 5 in stool showed significantly higher pooled odds ratio (OR) in detecting CRC and benign mucosal lesions than normal mucosal samples [20]. SFRP1 and SFRP2 methylation could discriminate between CRC and benign mucosal lesions. Fecal methylated SFRP2 achieved pooled sensitivity, specificity, and AUROCC of 71%, 94%, and 0.94, respectively, in CRC detection. Analysis of 9 publications with 792 cases of SFRP promoter methylation in stool achieved pooled sensitivity, specificity, and AUROCC of 82%, 47%, and 0.70, respectively [21]. This analysis revealed low specificity. Another analysis of 38 studies involved 4867 subjects [22]. The sensitivities and specificities of different genes in detecting different stages of CRC including adenomas and hyperplastic polyps ranged from 0 to 100% and 73 to 100%. SFRP1 and SFRP2 were superior in detecting CRC with DOR of 31.67 and 35.32, respectively, for CRC and 19.72 and 13.20, respectively, for adenomas. Other potential biomarkers included methylation of *NDRG4* for CRC (DOR of 24.37) and *VIM* for adenoma (DOR of 15.21).

Other stool DNA methylation assays have demonstrated clinical utility in adenoma detection. Meta-analysis including 30 trials with 1629 cases and 1531 controls achieved pooled sensitivity, specificity, PLR, NLR, DOR, and AUROCC of 71%, 92%, 7.59, 0.33, 27.78, and 0.93, respectively [23]. Another work included 37 studies with 4484 patients [24]. Pooled sensitivity and specificity were 73% and 92%, respectively, for CRC and 51% and 92% for adenomas. Of 13 studies involving 716 CRC, 220 adenomas, and 414 healthy controls, the pooled sensitivity, specificity, PLR, NLR, DOR, and AUROCC were 78%, 90%, 9.612, 0.243, 48.21, and 0.9438, respectively, for detecting CRC, and for adenoma the pooled sensitivity, specificity, and AUROCC were 63%, 93%, and 0.9385, respectively, which suggested utility of methylation in detecting both lesions in stool [25]. A meta-analysis of 19 studies with 2356 patients achieved pooled sensitivity, specificity, PLR, NLR, and DOR of 62%, 89%, 5.66, 0.43, and 13.15 for detecting CRC or adenoma. But for adenoma alone, the sensitivity was 54% and specificity was 88% [26]. Meta-analysis of multiple stool DNA biomarkers for CRC and adenoma included 20 studies with 5876 subjects [27]. While CRC data showed no heterogeneity, risk classification and use of different markers introduced heterogeneity in advanced adenoma data. The performance was good for high-risk but not the average-risk subgroups. For the high-risk subgroup, pooled sensitivity, specificity, and AUROCC were 75.9%, 88.3%, and 0.906, respectively, for CRC and 68.3%, 91.8%, and 0.946 for adenoma. A substantially higher DOR was also uncovered for methylation than mutation biomarkers. Thus, the pooled sensitivity, specificity, and AUROCC were 75.3%, 91.3%, and 0.918 for CRC and 62.3%, 92.6%, and 0.910 for adenoma when methylation markers were used.

Conceivably, testing for multiple genes should be superior to single genes for cancer detection. However, meta-analysis of 53 studies with 7524 subjects proved otherwise. The pooled sensitivity and specificity ranged from 2 to 100% and 81 to 100%, respectively, for CRC detection [28]. Receiver operating characteristic curves and DOR suggested multiple-gene assays were not that superior to single-gene tests, with sensitivity and specificity being 48.0% and 97.02%, respectively, for single genes and 77.8% and 92.7% for multiple-gene assays. There is still some merit in multiple-gene testing.

6.5.3 Colorectal Cancer RNA Biomarkers in Proximal Fluid

Because mRNA is labile and easily degrades, it has not been an attractive target as stool-based nucleic acid target for CRC. However, the stability offered by ncRNA makes them attractive biomarkers detectable in body fluids. The use of RNA preservation buffers, however, enabled detection of *PTGS2* and *MMP7* transcripts in stool that were highly specific for CRC [29]. While several studies have examined miRNA dysregulation in colonocytes in stool, there are no validated miRNA biomarkers for CRC detection. Potential stool miRNAs for CRC detection are miR-21 and miR-106a. Further discovery, confirmatory, and validation studies are needed for deregulated ncRNA in stool neoplastic colonocytes.

6.5.4 Colorectal Cancer Protein Biomarkers in Proximal Fluid

A number of fecal proteins including calprotectin, M2 pyruvate kinase (M2-PK), CEA, DAF, haptoglobin, and S100A12 have been evaluated as potential CRC biomarkers. Of these fecal proteins, calprotectin and M2-PK are the most extensively investigated. Calprotectin is a calcium-binding protein mostly found in neutrophils and thus not cancer specific. While most widely studied, many of the studies have either not been properly powered or evaluated in the population of average-risk individuals over the age of 50 years. A study meeting these criteria included 2321 participants in the Norwegian Colorectal Cancer Prevention Screening trial. This study compared calprotectin to FIT, and its performance was lower than FIT (FlexSure OBT) in CRC detection [30]. Another meta-analysis of fecal calprotectin included 20 studies [32]. The pooled sensitivity, specificity, PLR, and NLR were 83%, 61%, 2.15, and 0.28, respectively. Overall DOR and SAUROCC for CRC detection were 7.76 and 0.81, respectively. The performance was worse for detecting adenomas with DOR and SAUROCC of 1.27 and 0.55, respectively. Calprotectin is not specific to CRC, because it has been detected in stool from patients with IBD at a high sensitivity and specificity, indicating it is more of an inflammatory than cancer-specific biomarker [31].

Studies of M2-PK have also been heterogeneous and hence been subjected to meta-analysis. A meta-analysis of six case-control and four cohort studies of stool M2-PK that had colonoscopy as reference standard was performed [33]. While the pooled sensitivity and specificity were 79% and 81%, respectively, subgroup analysis of four studies that compared M2-PK to FIT revealed inferior performance of M2-PK in CRC detection. The DOR of 67.2 for FIT was much better than the 9.5 obtained for M2-PK. While inferior to FIT, the combination of M2-PK with FIT may enhance disease detection. For example, detection of advanced adenoma was enhanced from 11 to 13 with incorporation of M2-PK [34]. Quantitative studies have used cutoff values of M2-PK to detect CRC; however, results have been variable due to set cutoff values. For example, sensitivity and specificity were 92.1% and 29.7% with a cutoff value of 1 U/ml, while at a cutoff value of 30 U/ml, a sensitivity of 11.8% was sacrificed for enhanced specificity of 97.3% [35]. With cutoff value of 4 U/ml, CRC detection sensitivity has ranged from 68 to 85%. A meta-analysis of eight studies that used 4 U/ml as cutoff value achieved pooled sensitivity, specificity, and accuracy of 79%, 80%, and 85%, respectively [36]. Another analysis of 14 trials involving 1990 subjects achieved pooled sensitivity, specificity, PLR, NLR, and AUROCC of 78%, 77%, 4.38, 0.28, and 0.86, respectively, for M2-PK in CRC detection, suggestive of it being a potential biomarker [37]. This biomarker may be useful for triaging patients for colonoscopy.

A metaproteomic approach was used to interrogate fecal proteins, and it was demonstrated that a third of them were of human origin and hence potential as CRC biomarkers [38]. Examination of six proteins in 551 stool samples coupled with Bayesian logistic regression modeling enabled identification of haptoglobin and S100A12 as candidate CRC biomarkers. These biomarkers achieved a sensitivity of

88% and specificity of 95% in detecting CRC [39]. Previously, fecal haptoglobin had been shown to perform at a sensitivity and specificity of 92% and 98% in CRC detection, and sensitivity improved to 100% when combined with fecal occult blood testing [40]. In a pilot study of 20 cases and 20 controls, Wang et al. used fecal protein biochips to assess the performance of seven proteins in CRC detection, which achieved a sensitivity of 70%, albeit at a low specificity of 40% [41].

Other stool biomarkers of potential in CRC detection are alterations in miRNA and the microbiome. A meta-analysis of stool miRNA for CRC detection revealed pooled sensitivity, specificity, and AUROCC of 76.9%, 80.6%, and 0.848, respectively, for CRC detection [42]. MiRNA panels (AUROCC of 0.918) were superior to single miRNAs (AUROCC of 0.813). But serum miRNAs were more accurate than plasma, blood, feces, and tissue samples and especially among Asians. Meta-analysis of miR-21 in multiple samples form eight studies with 986 cases and 702 controls, included stool samples [43]. Pooled sensitivity, specificity, PLR, NLR, DOR, and AUROCC were 57%, 87%, 4.4, 0.49, 9.0, and 0.83, respectively. Subgroup analysis suggested blood-based assays achieved better performances than stool-based testing. Alterations in fecal microbiome have been reported as useful CRC diagnostic biomarkers. Meta-analysis including 10 studies comprised of 13 cohorts for CRC and 7 for adenoma [44] involved 1450 CRC patients, 1421 controls, as well as 656 adenoma patients with 827 controls. Pooled sensitivity, specificity, and AUROCC were respectively 71%, 76%, and 0.80 for CRC and 36%, 73%, and 0.60 for adenoma. Extensive heterogeneity was uncovered in the analysis limiting its utility. Sources of heterogeneity were methodological (DNA extraction kits and sample sizes) as well as regional and demographic differences.

6.6 Clinical Translation of Commercial Products

Colon cancer is a genetic disease, which is either due to familial predisposition or in many cases sporadic involving somatic mutations in colonocytes. Well established is the multistep pattern described by Vogelstein's group. However, other genetic alterations are also revealed in this disease. In view of this, stool-based tests target these somatic genetic changes to alert the early signs of disease evolution. Such risk-associated biomarkers are in commercial use.

6.6.1 PreGen-Plus

PreGen-Plus is a CRC screening test recommended for people 50 years and older who are at known risk for this disease. It is a stool DNA-based test developed and commercialized by Exact Sciences Corporation using proprietary and patented technologies for mutation analysis.

Initially licensed to LabCorp®, PreGen-Plus test interrogates shed colonocytes in stool samples for CRC-associated genetic alterations. Specifically, the assay involves analysis of 21 mutations in *APC*, *KRAS*, and *TP53* known to be associated with multistep colorectal carcinogenesis. In addition, analysis of microsatellite instability at BAT-26, as well as long DNA fragments referred to as DNA Integrity Assay (DIA®), is part of data interpretation. Multiple studies have shown test sensitivity of 65% and specificity of 95%.

The test is specifically targeted at the average-risk individual whereby a positive result indicates the possibility of the presence of CRC and hence the recommendation for additional tests and examination that may include the gold standard, colonoscopy. PreGen-Plus is not recommended to replace periodic colonoscopy used for surveillance of individuals at elevated risk for CRC such as people symptomatic for CRC, or those with familial syndromes such as the hereditary CRC syndromes (e.g., HNPCC, FAP) or those with chronic inflammatory bowel disease (Crohn's disease, ulcerative colitis).

Once a prescription for a patient is sent to LabCorp®, a sample collection kit and instructions are provided to the patient. In the comfort of their own home, a stool sample (about 8 grams) is collected and mailed to LabCorp® where the test is performed. Test results are ready in 2–3 weeks for consultation with the doctor.

PreGen-Plus is not US FDA approved; however, the American Cancer Society recommends it for CRC screening.

6.6.2 ColoSure™

ColoSure™ is another stool DNA test offered by LabCorp® for CRC screening. The test has similar indications for use as PreGen-Plus. Unlike PreGen-Plus, ColoSure™ is a single marker assay that detects aberrant methylation in the vimentin gene. Licensed proprietary techniques are used to capture human DNA in stool for analysis. It is demonstrated that methylation of exon1 sequences within the non-transcribed regions of the gene is associated with CRC. The test uses methylation-specific PCR and gel electrophoresis for analysis. Multiple studies reveal a sensitivity of 72–77% and a specificity of 83–94%. The assay requires that whole stool sample of at least 36 g be collected using the proprietary ColoSure™ specimen collection kit that includes instructions and transport material. The preserved stool samples are shipped at room temperature to LabCorp® within 72 h for analysis.

6.6.3 Cologuard

Exact Sciences has developed probably the only stool-based solution to CRC screening. Because 75–85% of all CRCs are sporadic involving de novo gene methylation, mutations, and other alterations, Exact Sciences has combined methylation markers, mutation markers, and the human-specific globin fecal immunochemical test (FIT) to develop the all-encompassing multiplex assay for colorectal precancer and cancer detection. The Cologuard test, which targets *KRAS* mutation, aberrant *NDRG4* and *BMP3* methylations, and β-actin in addition to FIT, is an adjunct to colonoscopies.

6.7 Summary

- CRC remains a common diagnosis and cause of cancer-related deaths globally.
- Early detection is critical to reducing the mortalities associated with CRC.
- Screening for CRC still remains widely dependent on detection of fecal occult blood using gFOBT or FIT.
- While stool DNA tests appear superior in performance to FOBTs and have been approved by the FDA for CRC screening, they remain to be used widely in practice.
- Detection of adenoma, especially advanced adenoma, is laudable in CRC prevention. In this regard, sDNA tests have shown potential with sensitivities of 32–86% depending on panel biomarkers used and size of adenomas.
- Potential CRC biomarkers in development include gene methylation (e.g., *SFRP*) and transcripts (e.g., *PTGS2*, *MMPs*, and miRNAs), proteins (e.g., calprotectin and M2-PK), and fecal microbiome.
- While performances of some of the novel biomarkers appear better than fecal blood and current sDNA tests, they remain to be validated in randomized clinical trials.
- Commercially available stool-based CRC assays include PreGen-Plus, Cologuard, and ColoSure™.

References

1. Nechvatal JM, Ram JL, Basson MD, et al. Fecal collection, ambient preservation, and DNA extraction for PCR amplification of bacterial and human markers from human feces. J Microbiol Methods. 2008;72:124–32.
2. Onouchi S, Matsushita H, Nomura S, et al. PCR-based assessment of the recovery rate of exfoliated colonocytes or cancer cells from fecal samples depends on the storage conditions after defecation. J Gastrointestin Liver Dis. 2007;16:369–72.
3. Burch JA, Soares-Weiser K, St John DJ, et al. Diagnostic accuracy of faecal occult blood tests used in screening for colorectal cancer: a systematic review. J Med Screen. 2007;14:132–7.
4. Shaukat A, Mongin SJ, Geisser MS, et al. Long-term mortality after screening for colorectal cancer. N Engl J Med. 2013;369:1106–14.
5. Mandel JS, Bond JH, Church TR, et al. Reducing mortality from colorectal cancer by screening for fecal occult blood. Minnesota Colon Cancer control study. N Engl J Med. 1993;328:1365–71.

6. Hewitson P, Glasziou P, Watson E, et al. Cochrane systematic review of colorectal cancer screening using the fecal occult blood test (hemoccult): an update. Am J Gastroenterol. 2008;103:1541–9.
7. Crotta S, Segnan N, Paganin S, et al. High rate of advanced adenoma detection in 4 rounds of colorectal cancer screening with the fecal immunochemical test. Clin Gastroenterol Hepatol. 2012;10:633–8.
8. Katsoula A, Paschos P, Haidich AB, et al. Diagnostic accuracy of fecal immunochemical test in patients at increased risk for colorectal Cancer: a meta-analysis. JAMA Intern Med. 2017;177:1110–8.
9. Lee JK, Liles EG, Bent S, et al. Accuracy of fecal immunochemical tests for colorectal cancer: systematic review and meta-analysis. Ann Intern Med. 2014;160:171.
10. Niedermaier T, Weigl K, Hoffmeister M, Brenner H. Diagnostic performance of flexible sigmoidoscopy combined with fecal immunochemical test in colorectal cancer screening: meta-analysis and modeling. Eur J Epidemiol. 2017;32:481–93.
11. Wieten E, Schreuders EH, Grobbee EJ, et al. Incidence of faecal occult blood test interval cancers in population-based colorectal cancer screening: a systematic review and meta-analysis. Gut. 2018;68(5):873–81.
12. Sidransky D, Tokino T, Hamilton SR, et al. Identification of ras oncogene mutations in the stool of patients with curable colorectal tumors. Science. 1992;256:102–5.
13. Ahlquist DA, Skoletsky JE, Boynton KA, et al. Colorectal cancer screening by detection of altered human DNA in stool: feasibility of a multitarget assay panel. Gastroenterology. 2000;119:1219–27.
14. Syngal S, Stoffel E, Chung D, et al. Detection of stool DNA mutations before and after treatment of colorectal neoplasia. Cancer. 2006;106:277–83.
15. Imperiale TF, Ransohoff DF, Itzkowitz SH, et al. Fecal DNA versus fecal occult blood for colorectal-cancer screening in an average-risk population. N Engl J Med. 2004;351:2704–14.
16. Ahlquist DA, Sargent DJ, Loprinzi CL, et al. Stool DNA and occult blood testing for screen detection of colorectal neoplasia. Ann Intern Med. 2008;149:441–450, W481.
17. Rex DK, Johnson DA, Anderson JC, et al. American College of Gastroenterology guidelines for colorectal cancer screening 2009 [corrected]. Am J Gastroenterol. 2009;104:739–50.
18. Levin B, Brooks D, Smith RA, Stone A. Emerging technologies in screening for colorectal cancer: CT colonography, immunochemical fecal occult blood tests, and stool screening using molecular markers. CA Cancer J Clin. 2003;53:44–55.
19. Imperiale TF, Ransohoff DF, Itzkowitz SH, et al. Multitarget stool DNA testing for colorectal-cancer screening. N Engl J Med. 2014;370:1287–97.
20. Yang Q, Huang T, Ye G, et al. Methylation of SFRP2 gene as a promising noninvasive biomarker using feces in colorectal cancer diagnosis: a systematic meta-analysis. Sci Rep. 2016;6:33339.
21. Zhou Z, Zhang H, Lei Y. Diagnostic value of secreted frizzled-related protein 2 gene promoter hypermethylation in stool for colorectal cancer: a meta-analysis. J Cancer Res Ther. 2016;12:30–3.
22. Mojtabanezhad Shariatpanahi A, Yassi M, Nouraie M, et al. The importance of stool DNA methylation in colorectal cancer diagnosis: a meta-analysis. PLoS One. 2018;13:e0200735.
23. Qian LY, Zhang W. The diagnostic value of DNA hypermethylation in stool for colorectal cancer: a meta-analysis. J Cancer Res Ther. 2014;10 Suppl:287–91.
24. Zhang H, Qi J, Wu YQ, et al. Accuracy of early detection of colorectal tumours by stool methylation markers: a meta-analysis. World J Gastroenterol. 2014;20:14040–50.
25. Yuan Y, Qu B, Yan J, et al. Diagnostic value of aberrant gene methylation in stool samples for colorectal cancer or adenomas: a meta-analysis. Panminerva Med. 2015;57:55–64.
26. Luo YX, Chen DK, Song SX, et al. Aberrant methylation of genes in stool samples as diagnostic biomarkers for colorectal cancer or adenomas: a meta-analysis. Int J Clin Pract. 2011;65:1313–20.

27. Yang H, Xia BQ, Jiang B, et al. Diagnostic value of stool DNA testing for multiple markers of colorectal cancer and advanced adenoma: a meta-analysis. Can J Gastroenterol. 2013;27:467–75.
28. Zhai RL, Xu F, Zhang P, et al. The diagnostic performance of stool DNA testing for colorectal Cancer: a systematic review and meta-analysis. Medicine (Baltimore). 2016;95:e2129.
29. Takai T, Kanaoka S, Yoshida K, et al. Fecal cyclooxygenase 2 plus matrix metalloproteinase 7 mRNA assays as a marker for colorectal cancer screening. Cancer Epidemiol Biomark Prev. 2009;18:1888–93.
30. Hoff G, Grotmol T, Thiis-Evensen E, et al. Testing for faecal calprotectin (PhiCal) in the Norwegian colorectal Cancer prevention trial on flexible sigmoidoscopy screening: comparison with an immunochemical test for occult blood (FlexSure OBT). Gut. 2004;53:1329–33.
31. von Roon AC, Karamountzos L, Purkayastha S, et al. Diagnostic precision of fecal calprotectin for inflammatory bowel disease and colorectal malignancy. Am J Gastroenterol. 2007;102:803–13.
32. Ye X, Huai J, Ding J. Diagnostic accuracy of fecal calprotectin for screening patients with colorectal cancer: a meta-analysis. Turk J Gastroenterol. 2018;29:397–405.
33. Li R, Liu J, Xue H, Huang G. Diagnostic value of fecal tumor M2-pyruvate kinase for CRC screening: a systematic review and meta-analysis. Int J Cancer. 2012;131:1837–45.
34. Leen R, Seng-Lee C, Holleran G, et al. Comparison of faecal M2-PK and FIT in a population-based bowel cancer screening cohort. Eur J Gastroenterol Hepatol. 2014;26:514–8.
35. Shastri YM, Loitsch S, Hoepffner N, et al. Comparison of an established simple office-based immunological FOBT with fecal tumor pyruvate kinase type M2 (M2-PK) for colorectal cancer screening: prospective multicenter study. Am J Gastroenterol. 2008;103:1496–504.
36. Uppara M, Adaba F, Askari A, et al. A systematic review and meta-analysis of the diagnostic accuracy of pyruvate kinase M2 isoenzymatic assay in diagnosing colorectal cancer. World J Surg Oncol. 2015;13:48.
37. Huang JX, Zhou Y, Wang CH, et al. Tumor M2-pyruvate kinase in stool as a biomarker for diagnosis of colorectal cancer: a meta-analysis. J Cancer Res Ther. 2014;10(Suppl):C225–8.
38. Verberkmoes NC, Russell AL, Shah M, et al. Shotgun metaproteomics of the human distal gut microbiota. ISME J. 2009;3:179–89.
39. Karl J, Wild N, Tacke M, et al. Improved diagnosis of colorectal cancer using a combination of fecal occult blood and novel fecal protein markers. Clin Gastroenterol Hepatol. 2008;6:1122–8.
40. Xing PX, Young GP, Ho D, et al. A new approach to fecal occult blood testing based on the detection of haptoglobin. Cancer. 1996;78:48–56.
41. Wang HP, Wang YY, Pan J, et al. Evaluation of specific fecal protein biochips for the diagnosis of colorectal cancer. World J Gastroenterol. 2014;20:1332–9.
42. Yan L, Zhao W, Yu H, et al. A comprehensive meta-analysis of MicroRNAs for predicting colorectal Cancer. Medicine (Baltimore). 2016;95:e2738.
43. Jiang JX, Zhang N, Liu ZM, Wang YY. Detection of microRNA-21 expression as a potential screening biomarker for colorectal cancer: a meta-analysis. Asian Pac J Cancer Prev. 2014;15:7583–8.
44. Zhang X, Zhu X, Cao Y, et al. Fecal fusobacterium nucleatum for the diagnosis of colorectal tumor: a systematic review and meta-analysis. Cancer Med. 2019;8:480–91.

Chapter 7
Renal Cell Carcinoma Biomarkers in Proximal Fluids

7.1 Introduction

Renal cell carcinoma (RCC), the commonest variant of renal cancers, still poses a challenge to oncologists, because metastatic RCC (mRCC) is inevitably a fatal disease. Globally, RCC is about the 14th most commonly diagnosed cancer, matching that of pancreatic cancer. The 2018 global estimated incidence, mortality, and 5-year prevalence were 403,262, 175,098, and 1,025,730, respectively. There are geographic and regional variations in the epidemiology of RCC. Age-standardized ratio puts the Czech Republic, Lithuania, Slovakia, and the USA among the countries with the highest incidences, while the Netherlands and Iceland have the lowest rates. In the USA, 65,340 new cases and 14,970 deaths were estimated for 2018, with the vast majority occurring in men (American Cancer Society). While these statistics may not seem alarming, the problem is that RCC incidence has been on the rise since the early 1990s, probably due to enhanced detection by imaging. More worrisome is the fact that the incidence some of the known risk factors are on the rise as well, suggesting the incidence of RCC may mirror these rising risk factors in the future. While the incidence tends to be low in the resource-poor parts of the world, mortality is very high in these regions due to late presentation and ineffective management from lack of resources.

There are myriads of risk factors for RCC. Age is an unmodifiable risk factor for RCC, because it is most commonly diagnosed in people over the age of 64 years. It is also racially associated, at least in the USA, being more common in African-Americans and American Indians than the general US population. Dialysis, high blood pressure, and associated administration of diuretics elevate the risk for RCC. Modifiable risks are smoking, obesity, and occupational exposure to substances such as cadmium, herbicides, and organic solvents, especially trichloroethylene. Some genetic diseases elevate the risks for RCC as well. These genetic factors include von Hippel-Lindau (VHL) disease (with *VHL* mutations), hereditary papil-

G. D. Dakubo, *Cancer Biomarkers in Body Fluids*,
https://doi.org/10.1007/978-3-030-24725-6_7

lary renal cell carcinoma (HPRCC, with mutations in *MET*), and hereditary leiomyomatosis and renal cell cancer (HLRCC, with mutations in fumarate hydratase and *SDHB*).

The dismal outcome of RCC is due to late diagnosis. There are currently no screening recommendations for RCC, and early lesions cannot be detected by palpation. While imaging can detect small tumors, they are inaccurate at differentiating between benign and malignant lesions. Thus, biomarkers representative of renal tumor biology and hence specific to RCC behavior are needed for accurate early detection, classification, staging, prognosis, and treatment predictions. There are such biomarkers available awaiting validation and translation. However, obtaining tumor tissue for biomarker analyses is invasive and nonrepresentative of tumor heterogeneity. Thus, assaying such biomarkers in body fluids offers a much better alternative and should advance renal oncology.

7.2 Basic Anatomy of the Urinary System

The kidneys, ureters, bladder, and urethra constitute the urinary system. The system functions to produce and excrete urine. Additionally, the kidneys secrete rennin and erythropoietin that control blood pressure and hematopoiesis, respectively. Acid-base balance and maintenance of fluid volume are other functions of the system.

Bean-shaped in structure, the kidneys are located outside the peritoneum in the posterior abdominal wall. On the superior aspect, in the renal fat are the adrenal glands. Located on the concave or medial side is the hilum that is surrounded by loose connective tissue-filled space and the renal sinus and houses the renal artery, renal vein, and renal pelvis.

A section through the kidney reveals a thick connective tissue capsule, a lighter-appearing cortex, and a darker-looking and deep-seated medulla (Fig. 7.1). The medulla is cone-shaped and composed of numerous renal pyramids. In between these conical structures are extensions of the renal cortical tissue referred to as renal columns. The apexes of the renal pyramids extend into the renal pelvis to form the renal papilla. Urine empties at the renal papilla into minor calyces that coalesce to form a major calyx. Several major calyces join to form the large funnel-shaped renal pelvis that exits the kidney as the ureters into the urinary bladder.

The renal corpuscles and renal tubules constitute the nephron, the functional unit of the kidney. The renal corpuscles contain rich capillaries organized into the glomeruli. Each of these capillary beds is encapsulated by a bilayer of epithelial cells called Bowman's or glomerular capsule. This capsule has an inner (visceral) layer of specialized epithelial cells called podocytes that surround the glomerular capillaries and an outer (parietal) layer of simple squamous epithelial cells.

Arterial blood enters and leaves the renal corpuscle at the arterial pole. Upon filtration in the glomerular capillaries, the filtrate enters the urinary space between the visceral and parietal layers of the glomerular capsule and leaves at the urinary

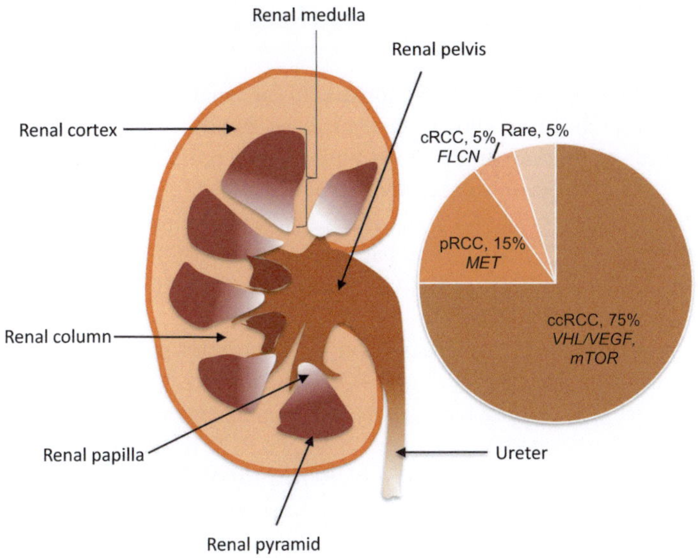

Fig. 7.1 Structure of the kidney and proportions of the histopathologic types of renal tumors in association with the most common genetic alterations. *pRCC* papillary RCC, *ccRCC* clear cell RCC, *cRCC* chromophobe RCC

pole into convoluted renal tubule. Urine then enters the collecting tubules, collecting ducts, papillary ducts, and the minor calyces. The process of blood filtration, reabsorption of substances and nutrients, and secretion of waste products produces urine. About 99% of the urinary filtrate is indeed reabsorbed. Given its function of filtering blood from the entire body, urine should essentially contain disease biomarkers from extrarenal sources.

7.3 Collection and Processing of Urine

The collection and processing of urine will usually follow a standard operating procedure. However, in general, urine will be voided into a larger container, with the appropriate or required amount transferred into a smaller container (this container may contain preservatives) using a pipette. The remaining urine and other suppliers are then discarded appropriately. The container is sealed, labeled, and shipped to the laboratory or returned to the requesting physician. Note that additional instructions may be provided depending on the specific indicated analysis. Urine stored at room temperature can be safely preserved in EDTA for up to a week without loss of DNA integrity. Storage at −20 °C or −80 °C for up to 4 weeks (28 days) preserved DNA well irrespective of addition of preserving agent. In order to prevent possible bacterial overgrowth, Pen-Strep can be added without it negatively affecting DNA preservation [1].

7.4 Renal Cell Carcinoma Biomarkers in Urine

There is paucity of data on urinary biomarkers for renal cancer. Only recently has the number of publications shown some increase, but this is still dismal compared to other cancer biomarkers in proximal fluids. Some protein biomarkers including aquaporin 1 (AQP1), perilipin 2 (PLIN2), NMP22, NGAL, KIM1, and MMPs have been investigated, but only AQP1 and PLIN2 have shown promise as sensitive and specific clear cell RCC (ccRCC) and papillary RCC (pRCC) biomarkers. Emerging biomarkers include urinary miRNAs, metabolites, volatile organic compounds (VOCs), and gene methylations.

There has been extensive investigation of the urinary proteome for RCC biomarkers with some promise. Urinary AQP1 and PLIN2 levels were assessed as ccRCC and pRCC screening biomarkers in a clinical setting [2]. Both biomarkers were significantly elevated in patients with known RCC than healthy controls and a prospectively screened population. The AUROCC for AQP1 and PLIN2 as single or panel biomarkers was 0.990 or greater, with sensitivity and specificity of 95% and 91% or higher, respectively, when compared to the healthy and screening populations. Three of the 720 screened population with biomarker levels suggestive of RCC had renal masses by computed tomography scan, of which 2 had confirmed RCC on subsequent evaluation. These biomarkers have thus proven to serve as useful screening and diagnostic biomarkers for RCC, as well as differential diagnosis of renal masses. The specificity of AQP1 and PLIN2 for RCC was further uncovered when levels were compared to other urothelial tumors and benign renal masses [3]. The concentrations of AQP1 and PLIN2 were, respectively, 29 and 36 relative absorbance units/mg urinary creatinine (UCr), which were significantly higher than the <10 absorbance units/mg UCr found in urine from patients with bladder, prostate, and chromophobe renal tumors, as well as benign oncocytomas and angiomyolipomas, which were comparable to healthy controls. The AUROCC ranged from 0.99 to 1.0 for both biomarkers in detecting RCC. Urinary AQP1 and PLIN2 appear highly sensitive and specific for ccRCC and pRCC [4]. In a clinical study, their utility could have prevented surgical interventions in 23% of patients with benign renal masses. Moreover, the mandatory required biopsy of small renal masses for confirmatory diagnosis could have been avoided in 74% of patients with elevated AQP1 and PLIN2 levels as evidence of ccRCC and pRCC. Urinary AQP1 and PLIN2 concentration in relation to tumor size, grade, and stage was assessed [5]. Median levels of AQP1 and PLIN2 concentration were 35-fold and 9-fold higher, respectively, in RCC patients than controls. Sensitivity and specificity were perfect for AQP1 and 92% and 100%, respectively, for PLIN2. Both urinary biomarker concentrations correlated with tumor size and stage (T1 and T2, but not T3). No association was found for tumor grade. The urinary levels of AQP1 and PLIN2 in RCC patients were, respectively, 11–23-fold and 17–25-fold greater than patients with common renal diseases such as urinary tract infection, diabetic nephropathy, and glomerulonephritis. This further confirms the specific associations of these biomarkers with ccRCC and pRCC. The elevated urine AQP1 and PLIN2 levels decreased by 83% and 84%, respectively, after tumor removal [6]. Sreedharan et al.

confirmed the diagnostic potential of AQP1 for RCC [7]. However, their assay needed to be performed on freshly collected urine samples because archival specimens showed an absence of detectable AQP1.

Urinary KIM1 and NGAL levels have been associated with RCC. Preoperative urinary levels of KIM1 correlated with tissue levels and pathological features of ccRCC in surgical specimens [8]. Preoperative KIM1 levels were significantly higher in ccRCC than controls, and the levels declined to control levels postoperative. Urinary KIM1 levels were significantly associated with tumor KIM1 levels and pathological features such as tumor size, Fuhrman grade, pathologic stage (pT), TNM stage, lymphovascular invasion, and type of surgery (radical or partial nephrectomy). While urinary levels of NGAl and KIM1 are suggested as biomarkers for RCC, their sensitivity and specificity have been called into question [9]. The median urinary levels of these biomarkers were significantly elevated in RCC than control samples; however, there was substantial overlap of NGAL levels between RCC patients and controls, thus limiting its sensitivity and specificity. While KIM1 concentration did not show such overlap between cases and controls, KIM1 is not specific to RCC either, as levels are also associated with many types of renal injuries and pathologies.

Other proteins that might be of relevance in RCC are cathepsin D, survivin, NMP22, and brain-type fatty acid-binding protein (B-FABP). Analysis of conditioned RCC cell medium enabled identification of cathepsin D as potential RCC biomarker that was validated in urinary samples from RCC patients, healthy controls, and patients with benign renal diseases [10]. The elevated levels were significantly associated with overall survival (OS; hazard ratio, HR = 1.33) and cancer-specific survival (HR = 1.36). Multivariate analysis showed some aspect of it being of an independent prognostic value for OS. Urinary survivin levels achieved a diagnostic accuracy with AUROCC of 0.763 for RCC [11]. This was improved to 0.920 when combined with urinary LAPTM4B that alone had an AUROCC of 0.704. Urinary NMP22 levels were significantly higher in RCC patients than controls. Values ≥10 U/ml were uncovered in 60.5% of cancer patient samples [12]. A nonsignificant trend of increasing levels with pT stage was observed. Another study found NMP22 levels to be significantly increased in cancer patients (13.69 U/ml) than controls (3.03 U/ml) [13], but levels ≥10 U/ml were detected in 40% of RCC samples. Urinary B-FABP levels were associated with RCC because it could be detected in urinary samples from cancer patients but not healthy controls or post-nephrectomy urinary samples [14].

Proteomic analysis of proximal cyst fluid associated with RCC identified elevated 14-3-3 protein beta/alpha levels in cancer patients [15]. The increased levels were confirmed in urinary and other samples (tissue and serum) from cancer patients. In this pilot study, this urinary biomarker achieved an AUROCC of 0.8813 in detecting RCC. Another study confirmed the elevated urinary levels of 14-3-3 protein beta/alpha in samples from ccRCC patients compared to healthy controls and patients with angiomyolipoma [16]. The elevated levels were associated with advanced tumor stage as determined by pT, lymph node status, and distant metastasis, and this conferred poor OS outcomes. The levels remained significant even in patients with small-sized carcinomas compared to angiomyolipoma patients, suggesting its additional value in discriminating between the two conditions.

The use of multiple proteomic approaches enabled identification of 354 proteins in 3 groups of samples: (i) Fuhrman good, (ii) poor prognosis, and (iii) healthy control groups [17]. Quantitative proteomics found 49 elevated and 40 decreased proteins in urine from ccRCC patients that were related to good prognosis. Decreased and associated with Fuhrman good prognosis and healthy control groups were kininogen 1, uromodulin, apolipoprotein D, polyubiquitin, and CD59 glycoprotein. Elevated in patient samples were apolipoprotein A, fibrinogen, and haptoglobin. The levels of kininogen, apolipoprotein D, fibrinogen, and haptoglobin were also confirmed by 2DE LC-MS/MS or 2DE MALDI-TOF quantitative analysis. Chinello et al. evaluated the clinicopathologic correlation of urinary peptidome biomarkers for ccRCC [18]. Five, 15, and 26 peptides demonstrated significant alterations in concentrations associated with tumor grade, size, and pT, respectively. Fifteen and nine urinary peptides also showed significant alterations in patients at different pT stages or grades, even at very early stages. C1RL, A1AGx, ZAG2G, PGBM, MMP23, G162, ADA19, G3P, RSPH3, DREB, NOTC2, SAB2, and CC168 were identified as urinary proteins. MS analysis identified Raf kinase inhibitor protein (RKIP) to be modulated (reduced) in ccRCC tissue samples [19]. Using ELISA, immunoblot, and microarray assays, RKIP and its phosphorylated form, pRKIP, were modulated in urinary samples from ccRCC patients. Independent analysis confirmed the ability of using RKIP and pRKIP to differentiate ccRCC patients from healthy controls, and prediction of cancer-specific and progression-free survival was accurate at a cutoff value of 10 ng/ml/g Pr/UCr. Phosphorylated RKIP was undetectable in urine and tissue samples of cancer patients. Frantzi et al. applied CE-MS to identify 86 urinary peptides associated with RCC, of which sequences were obtained for 40 [20]. In an independent set of samples, this peptide panel achieved a sensitivity and specificity of 80% and 87%, respectively. The specificity for RCC was further confirmed by comparing urinary levels to age-matched controls, patients with related cancer and renal diseases. In silico predictions suggested cleavage and modified activities of some of these peptides including cathepsins, ADAMTS, and kallikreins.

SELDI-TOF MS of urine uncovered potential RCC biomarkers of molecular weights 4020, 4637, 5070, and 5500 Da that achieved a sensitivity and specificity of 67.8% and 81.4% in blind validation sample set [21]. ClinProt proteomic analysis of urine from ccRCC patients and controls identified a cluster of 3 signals at m/z 1827, 1914, and 1968 that could discriminate between cases and controls [22]. The combined diagnostic performance achieved a sensitivity of 100% and specificity of 85% in the test set of samples. One of these biomarkers was identified as Tamm-Horsfall protein. Another SELDI-TOF MS in a Brazilian cohort of RCC patients and controls uncovered downregulation of urinary secreted and membrane 1 precursor (protein K12) and mannan-binding lectin-associated serine protease-2 (MASP-2) in urine from RCC patients compared to controls [23]. Urinary proteome identification of biomarkers for VHLD patients uncovered α-1-antitrypsin (A1AT) and β-2-glycoprotein 1 (APOH) to be overabundant only in the urine from VHLD patients with history of ccRCC [24].

Urinary miRNA dysregulation has been associated with RCC. miR-15a was upregulated in ccRCC compared to benign renal oncocytoma patients, and the elevated levels were measurable in urinary samples [25]. Indeed, urinary miR-15a was undetectable in patients with oncocytomas, chromophobe carcinomas, and urinary tract inflammation, suggesting its specificity for ccRCC. Mean urinary miR-15a levels were substantially different between preoperative RCC (2.50E-01 RFU), benign renal masses (1.32E-03 RFU), and healthy controls (3.36E-05 RFU), and the levels correlated with sizes of RCC [26]. Levels decreased by 99.53% on the eighth day post-nephrectomy. At a cutoff value of 5.00E-06 RFU, the sensitivity and specificity were 98.1% and 100%, respectively, in differentiating patients with RCC from those with benign renal masses. Petrozza et al. examined whether tissue-associated miRNAs (miR-21-5p, miR-210-3p, and miR-22-3p) were elevated in urine from ccRCC patients [27]. This analysis identified miR-210-3p to be significantly increased in urine from preoperative ccRCC patients, and levels significantly decreased postoperative. Thus, urinary miR-210-3p could serve as noninvasive diagnostic biomarker and is also useful for monitoring completeness of surgical resection of ccRCC. Global urinary miRNA profiling and independent validation studies identified sets of miRNAs as useful noninvasive biomarkers for ccRCC [28]. Combination of miR-126-3p and miR-449a (AUROCC of 0.84) and miR-126-3p and miR-34b-5p (AUROCC of 0.79) significantly differentiated ccRCC from controls. miR-126-3p and miR-34b-5p could differentiate small renal masses (AUROCC of 0.79) from controls. Useful in differentiating ccRCC from benign renal lesions were combined miR-126-3p and miR-486-5p (AUROCC of 0.85). Elevated urinary ccRCC miRNAs returned to healthy control levels after surgery. Urinary let-7 miRNAs including let-7a, let-7b, let-7c, let-7d, let-7e, and let-7 g were significantly higher in ccRCC than control samples [29]. The best in diagnostic accuracy was urinary let-7a, with sensitivity, specificity, and AUROCC of 71%, 81%, and 0.8307, respectively. Urinary cell-free miR-210 was significantly higher in ccRCC than control samples, and the levels decreased a week after surgery [30]. The sensitivity, specificity, and AUROCC were 57.8%, 80.0%, and 0.76, respectively. Although decreased in RCC tissue samples, the levels of PIWI-interacting RNA (piR823) was elevated in serum and urine samples from cancer patients compared to controls [31]. As a biomarker, the diagnostic performance achieved AUROCC of 0.6264 for serum and 0.7433 for urinary samples, which demonstrate a potential for urinary piR823 in RCC detection.

Genome-scale metabolic modeling to elucidate metabolic reprogramming in ccRCC led to discovery of coordinated regulation of glycosaminoglycans (GAGs) biosynthesis at both the message and protein levels [32]. Derivation of three GAG scores based on alterations detected in urine and plasma samples could distinguish metastatic ccRCC at 93.1–100% accuracy. A systems biology approach also identified measurements of GAGs aggregated into diagnostic score biomarkers. Patients with "high vs. low" urinary GAG scores had significantly different survival outcomes [33]. The 2-year PFS rate was 53.3% vs. 100%, and OS rate was 73.3% vs. 100% for patients with high vs. low urinary GAG scores. As a continuous variable, this urinary systems biology biomarker was an independent predictor of progression-free survival (PFS; HR = 4.62) and OS (HR = 10.13) of ccRCC patients. Another study found an increase in urinary GAG excretion in RCC patients that correlated with tumor size, multifocality, but not tumor stage [34].

Metabolomic analyses have uncovered elevated levels of hydroxybutyryl carnitine, decanoylcarnitine, propanoylcarnitine, carnitine, dodecanoylcarnitine, and norepinephrine sulfate in urine and tissue samples from ccRCC patients compared to controls [35]. A pilot study of urinary and serum metabolomics identified alterations in glycolytic and tricarboxylic acid (TCA) cycle intermediates as RCC biomarkers [36]. In discriminating between stages, urinary metabolites achieved AUROCC of 0.83 for benign vs. pT1 tumors and 0.98 for benign vs. pT3 tumors. GC-MS coupled with principal component analysis (PCA) and orthogonal partial least squares discriminant analysis (PLS-DA) enabled the identification of urinary metabolites for differential diagnosis of RCC [37]. Pentamic acid, malonic acid, glutamic acid, adipic acid, aminoquinoline, quinoline, indole acetic acid, and tryptophan were significantly elevated in urine from RCC patients compared to controls. Significantly elevated in urine from RCC compared to other urologic cancers were pentanoic acid, phenylalanine, and 6-methoxy-nitro quinolone. Another metabolomic analysis uncovered differential levels of quinolate, 4-hydroxybenzoate, and gentisate between RCC patients and controls, and these metabolites reflect amino acid metabolism and the Warburg effect [38]. Their biomarker potential requires further investigation.

Potential discriminatory urinary volatile organic compounds (VOCs) for RCC have been discovered. A panel of 21 urinary VOCs could discriminate RCC patients from controls [39]. Among these, consistently and significantly altered were 2-oxopropanal and 2,5,8-trimethyl-1,2,3,4-tetrahydronaphthalene-1-ol. As biomarkers of RCC, 11 VOC biomarkers (phenol; decanal; 1,6-dioxacyclododecane-7,12-dione; 1-bromo-1-(3-methyl-1-pentenylidene)-2,2,3,3-tetramethyl-cyclopropane; nonanal; 3-ethyl-3-methylheptane; isolongifolene-5-ol; 2,5-cyclohexadiene-1,4-dione, 2,6-bis(1,1-dimethylethyl); tetradecane; aniline; and 2,6,10,14-tetramethylpentadecane) were elevated, while 3 (styrene, 4-heptanone, and dimethylsilanediol) were decreased in RCC patients compared to healthy control samples [40]. This unique VOC profile could potentially aid in RCC detection.

Less attractive and thus less focused on are urinary genetic biomarkers. However, some attempts have been made in this aspect in RCC detection. Quantitative methylation-specific PCR (MSP) analysis of methylated *RASSF1A* in urinary samples was positive at 84.6% of samples from RCC patients [41]. In this pilot study, the sensitivity, specificity, and AUROCC were 84.6%, 100%, and 0.923, respectively, for RCC detection. The robust performance of methylation biomarkers in body fluids should lend impetus to further study of their clinical utility in RCC urinary samples. Extracellular vesicle (EV) content may prove useful for RCC detection. Urinary EV three-gene signature including *GSTA1*, *CEBPA*, and *PCBD1* were decreased in ccRCC patient samples and increased to normal control levels after surgery [42]. RCC urinary exosomal protein content differs substantially from those of control subjects by comparative proteomic analysis [43].

Research efforts at discovery of novel urinary biomarkers for RCC need to be encouraged, as the potential exists.

7.5 Non-urogenital Cancer Biomarkers in Urine

The urge to search for noninvasive body fluid biomarkers has led to investigation of non-urogenital tract cancer biomarkers in urine. Illustrated here are urinary biomarkers for breast, lung, pancreatic, and ovarian cancers.

7.5.1 Urinary Biomarkers for Breast Cancer

Biomarkers in urine have been discovered for their potential utility in BrCa management. These mostly include miRNAs and proteins. The differential levels of four breast cancer miRNAs in urine have been demonstrated [44]. Compared to healthy controls, breast cancer patients harbored significantly elevated levels of mR-155 (median urinary miRNA levels of 1.49 vs. 0.25), but reduced levels of miR-21 (2.27 vs. 5.07), miR-125b (0.71 vs. 1.62), and miR-451 (0.02 vs. 0.59).

Levels of urinary MMP9 and ADAM12 were associated with 5 times elevated risk for developing atypical hyperplasia and 13 times risk for lobar carcinoma in situ [45]. However, the elevated ADAM12 levels could not be confirmed by an independent study [46]. A complex of MMP6 and NGAL was demonstrated to be significantly elevated in urine from women with metastatic breast cancers compared to controls [47]. The elevated levels of NGAL were confirmed by immunohistochemistry and in vitro assays and were also associated with increased breast cancer cell proliferation and poor patient prognosis. However, increased NGAL expression is not specific to breast cancer as levels are increased in cancers such as colorectal, bladder, liver, pancreatic, and ovarian cancer, as well as in renal failure.

7.5.2 Urinary Biomarkers for Lung Cancer

Potential lung cancer biomarkers have been sought in many body fluids to help with early detection to improve the poor prognosis associated with the numerous late-stage diagnoses. Thus, urinary biomarkers of lung cancer have been pursued. Mainly explored are mutations and alterations in protein and metabolite levels.

Urinary cfDNA prior to and following treatment was monitored for *EGFR* mutations as predictive outcome in NSCLC patients [48]. Mean concentration of *EGFR* mutations in 130 *EGFR* mutation-positive patients was 220 ± 237copies/ml. Posttreatment, *EGFR* mutations were undetectable in a significant number of patients, while others had significant decline. Six months posttreatment, 91% of patients with high levels of urinary *EGFR* mutations relapsed, indicative of the presence of minimal residual disease. Urinary *KRAS* mutation detection could predict survival outcomes in NSCLC patients [49]. Detection of T790M and *EGFR* mutations in urine could improve compliance in this mutation testing for lung cancer management. Urinary *EGFR* mutations, including detection of acquired T790M mutations, demonstrated clinical utility in management of NSCLC patients [50]. Moreover, detection of urinary *EGFR* mutations had clinical utility for treatment monitoring with TKI [51]. Urinary testing for T790M mutation detection as a strategy for patient selection to receive third-generation TKI had increased detection rate of 7% compared to tissue testing [52]. Of clinical relevance, urinary testing was positive in some patients who could not be biopsied or whereby tissue results were indeterminate. Because of enhanced TKI therapy, urinary testing increased PFS and OS by 0.44 and 0.35 months, respectively. Cost savings from avoidance of biopsy, potential biopsy-related complications, and tissue testing was US $1243–$1680 per patient.

Urinary proteomic profiling identified five biomarkers including ferritin light chain, MAPK1-interacting protein 1 like (MAPK1IP1L), fibrinogen beta chain (FGB), RAB33B, and RAB15 that could discriminate lung cancer patients from healthy controls and those with other common solid tumors with AUROCC of 0.8747–0.9853 [53]. Other urinary peptides for lung adenocarcinoma validated to be upregulated using immunohistochemical analysis are IGKC, AAT, SH3BGRL3, osteopontin, and gelsolin [54]. A urinary three-biomarker panel consisting of IGFBP1, SIL-1Ra, and CEACAM1 could discriminate between NSCLC patients and controls at a sensitivity of 72% and specificity of 100%. Of note, the performance decreased when controls were patients with benign lung conditions, and specificity was limited when considering several cancers and tuberculosis [55].

A number of urinary lung cancer metabolite biomarkers were examined in subjects prior to diagnosis. Elevated creatine riboside was associated with lung cancer risk with an odds ratio (OR) of 2.0, while N-acetylneuraminic acid achieved an OR of 5.3 among European-Americans, although race was insignificant in modifying the association (haznadar m, cai q 2016). Both metabolite levels increased with increasing tumor size. Urinary N(1),N(12)-diacetylspermine (DiAcSpm) levels were determined and used to establish a ratio (DiAcSpm/cutoff) for predicting prognosis of lung cancer patients [56]. The median ratio was higher in NSCLC (especially squamous cell carcinoma) patients than controls, and the elevated levels were associated with pT, histologic invasive factors, and unfavorable outcome in patients with complete cancer resection. This ratio was an independent indicator in multivariate Cox regression analysis with HR of 4.652. A review of urinary metabolites for lung, breast, bladder, prostate, and ovarian cancer identified pteridines, modified nucleosides, and acylcarnitines to be associated with cancer development and progression [57].

7.5.3 Urinary Biomarkers for Pancreatic Cancer

The challenging early detection of pancreatic cancer has propelled the search for noninvasive diagnostic biomarkers in several body fluids including urine. This urinary search for pancreatic cancer biomarkers has mostly involved proteomic and metabolomic approaches in addition to miRNA alterations. Urinary biomarkers for pancreatic cancer risk prediction, diagnosis, and differential diagnosis from chronic pancreatitis have been uncovered in a number of pilot studies.

Urinary PGE2 metabolite measurement as an indicator of PGE2 overproduction and pancreatic cancer risk was examined in a case-control study ([58]. Compared to the lowest levels (first quartile), the odds for pancreatic cancer risk demonstrated a positive trend from second to fourth quartile. The OR was 1.63 (second quartile), 1.55 (third quartile), and 1.94 (fourth quartile), and this dose-associated risk was more pronounced in people with body mass index of <25 kg/m^2 compared to those overweight.

Potential differential pancreatic cancer diagnostic urinary biomarkers have also been demonstrated. Of 127 differential levels of proteins between pancreatic cancer and chronic pancreatitis patients, 101 were identified using MALDI-TOF MS. These urinary proteins included annexin A2, gelsolin, and CD59 that proved difficult to be validated using immunoblot [59]. Using ELISA and multivariate logistic regression analyses and controlling for age and sex, urinary MMP2 and TIMP1 were identified as independent predictors of pancreatic cancer [60]. While urinary MMP2 was an independent predictor of pancreatic neuroendocrine tumors (PNETs), TIM1 could differentiate between the two, suggesting their usefulness in differential diagnosis of pancreatic cancer. Analysis of urine using CE-MS analysis of urine enabled identification of statistically differential peptides that were included in a peptide multimarker model for differential diagnosis of pancreatic cancer from chronic pancreatitis [61]. Validation of this model achieved a sensitivity, specificity, and AUROCC of 87%, 85%, and 0.93, respectively. Identified and validated using immunoassays and immunohistochemistry was fetuin-A. By in silico analysis, increased meprin A activity in pancreatic cancer was identified and demonstrated using IHC to be associated with neoangiogenesis. Urinary metabolomics have also been used to identify pancreatic cancer metabolites (1). H-NMR spectroscopic analysis of urine found significant metabolite concentration differences between patients with pancreatic cancer and controls consisting of healthy individuals and those with benign pancreatic conditions [62]. Multivariate orthogonal partial least squares discriminant analysis achieved AUROCC of 0.988 for differentiating between pancreatic cancer and healthy controls and 0.958 from those with benign pancreatic diseases. Given their resilience in body fluids, urinary miRNAs have been associated with pancreatic cancer. Differential urinary miRNA between patients with pancreatic cancer and controls consisting of patients with chronic pancreatitis and healthy subjects was identified using Affymetrix microarrays and validated in an independent sample set using RT-PCR [63]. Significantly elevated levels were observed for miR-143, miR-221, and miR-30e between stage I cancer patients and healthy controls; miR-143, miR-223, and miR-204 between stage I and stage II–IV patients; and miR-223 and miR-204 between early-stage cancer and chronic pancreatitis patients. The diagnostic performance between stage I disease and healthy control in terms of sensitivity, specificity, and AUROCC was 83%, 88.5%, and 0.862 for miR-143, which increased to 83.3%, 96.2%, and 0.923 when combined with miR-30e. This pilot study suggests the potential of urinary miRNAs in early detection of pancreatic cancer.

7.5.4 Urinary Biomarkers for Ovarian Cancer

A number of urinary miRNAs are associated with ovarian cancer. In prospectively collected urinary samples from women scheduled for gynecological surgery, miR-92a and miR-200b were upregulated, while miR-100 and miR-106b were decreased in ovarian cancer patients compared to women with benign gynecological conditions [64]. A microarray analysis of urinary samples from ovarian cancer patients compared to control group of healthy women and those with benign gynecological conditions uncovered increased levels of miR-30a-5p and decreased levels of 37 miRNAs in ovarian serous adenocarcinoma samples [65]. The elevated levels of miR-30a-5p reduced following surgery and were devoid in samples from patients with gastric and colorectal cancers, suggestive of some specificity of this miRNA for ovarian serous adenocarcinoma.

7.6 Summary

- RCC is a common urogenital tract cancer.
- Known risk factors of RCC include age, uncontrolled hypertensive patients on diuretics, race, smoking, obesity, occupational carcinogen exposure, and genetics.
- Late diagnosis is the primary reason for the dismal survival outcomes associated with RCC.
- Of the numerous urinary biomarkers uncovered, AQP1 and PLIN2 show promise as sensitive and specific biomarkers for ccRCC and pRCC.
- Emerging urinary biomarkers for RCC include alterations in VOCs, mutations, miRNAs, and metabolites.
- Biomarkers of non-urogenital cancers including breast, lung, pancreatic, and ovarian cancers have been explored in urine with some promising findings.

References

1. Bosschieter J, Bach S, Bijnsdorp IV, et al. A protocol for urine collection and storage prior to DNA methylation analysis. PLoS One. 2018;13:e0200906.
2. Morrissey JJ, Mellnick VM, Luo J, et al. Evaluation of urine aquaporin-1 and perilipin-2 concentrations as biomarkers to screen for renal cell carcinoma: a prospective cohort study. JAMA Oncol. 2015;1:204–12.
3. Morrissey JJ, Mobley J, Figenshau RS, et al. Urine aquaporin 1 and perilipin 2 differentiate renal carcinomas from other imaged renal masses and bladder and prostate cancer. Mayo Clin Proc. 2015;90:35–42.
4. Song JB, Morrissey JJ, Mobley JM, et al. Urinary aquaporin 1 and perilipin 2: can these novel markers accurately characterize small renal masses and help guide patient management? Int J Urol. 2019;26:260–5.
5. Morrissey JJ, Mobley J, Song J, et al. Urinary concentrations of aquaporin-1 and perilipin-2 in patients with renal cell carcinoma correlate with tumor size and stage but not grade. Urology. 2014;83:256 e259–14.
6. Morrissey JJ, Kharasch ED. The specificity of urinary aquaporin 1 and perilipin 2 to screen for renal cell carcinoma. J Urol. 2013;189:1913–20.
7. Sreedharan S, Petros JA, Master VA, et al. Aquaporin-1 protein levels elevated in fresh urine of renal cell carcinoma patients: potential use for screening and classification of incidental renal lesions. Dis Markers. 2014;2014:135649.
8. Mijuskovic M, Stanojevic I, Milovic N, et al. Tissue and urinary KIM-1 relate to tumor characteristics in patients with clear renal cell carcinoma. Int Urol Nephrol. 2018;50:63–70.
9. Morrissey JJ, London AN, Lambert MC, Kharasch ED. Sensitivity and specificity of urinary neutrophil gelatinase-associated lipocalin and kidney injury molecule-1 for the diagnosis of renal cell carcinoma. Am J Nephrol. 2011;34:391–8.
10. Vasudev NS, Sim S, Cairns DA, et al. Pre-operative urinary cathepsin D is associated with survival in patients with renal cell carcinoma. Br J Cancer. 2009;101:1175–82.
11. Yang Y, Xu J, Zhang Q. Detection of urinary survivin using a magnetic particles-based chemiluminescence immunoassay for the preliminary diagnosis of bladder cancer and renal cell carcinoma combined with LAPTM4B. Oncol Lett. 2018;15:7923–33.
12. Kaya K, Ayan S, Gokce G, et al. Urinary nuclear matrix protein 22 for diagnosis of renal cell carcinoma. Scand J Urol Nephrol. 2005;39:25–9.
13. Huang S, Rhee E, Patel H, et al. Urinary NMP22 and renal cell carcinoma. Urology. 2000;55:227–30.
14. Teratani T, Domoto T, Kuriki K, et al. Detection of transcript for brain-type fatty acid-binding protein in tumor and urine of patients with renal cell carcinoma. Urology. 2007;69:236–40.
15. Minamida S, Iwamura M, Kodera Y, et al. 14-3-3 protein beta/alpha as a urinary biomarker for renal cell carcinoma: proteomic analysis of cyst fluid. Anal Bioanal Chem. 2011;401:245–52.
16. Kaneko S, Matsumoto K, Minamida S, et al. Incremental expression of 14-3-3 protein beta/alpha in urine correlates with advanced stage and poor survival in patients with clear cell renal cell carcinoma. Asian Pac J Cancer Prev. 2016;17:1399–404.
17. Sandim V, Pereira Dde A, Kalume DE, et al. Proteomic analysis reveals differentially secreted proteins in the urine from patients with clear cell renal cell carcinoma. Urol Oncol. 2016;34(5):e11–25.
18. Chinello C, Cazzaniga M, De Sio G, et al. Tumor size, stage and grade alterations of urinary peptidome in RCC. J Transl Med. 2015;13:332.
19. Papale M, Vocino G, Lucarelli G, et al. Urinary RKIP/p-RKIP is a potential diagnostic and prognostic marker of clear cell renal cell carcinoma. Oncotarget. 2017;8:40412–24.
20. Frantzi M, Metzger J, Banks RE, et al. Discovery and validation of urinary biomarkers for detection of renal cell carcinoma. J Proteome. 2014;98:44–58.

21. Wu DL, Zhang WH, Wang WJ, et al. Proteomic evaluation of urine from renal cell carcinoma using SELDI-TOF-MS and tree analysis pattern. Technol Cancer Res Treat. 2008;7:155–60.
22. Bosso N, Chinello C, Picozzi SC, et al. Human urine biomarkers of renal cell carcinoma evaluated by ClinProt. Proteomics Clin Appl. 2008;2:1036–46.
23. Alves G, Pereira DA, Sandim V, et al. Urine screening by Seldi-Tof, followed by biomarker identification, in a Brazilian cohort of patients with renal cell carcinoma (RCC). Int Braz J Urol. 2013;39:228–39.
24. Mandili G, Notarpietro A, Khadjavi A, et al. Beta-2-glycoprotein-1 and alpha-1-antitrypsin as urinary markers of renal cancer in von Hippel-Lindau patients. Biomarkers. 2018;23:123–30.
25. von Brandenstein M, Pandarakalam JJ, Kroon L, et al. MicroRNA 15a, inversely correlated to PKCalpha, is a potential marker to differentiate between benign and malignant renal tumors in biopsy and urine samples. Am J Pathol. 2012;180:1787–97.
26. Mytsyk Y, Dosenko V, Borys Y, et al. MicroRNA-15a expression measured in urine samples as a potential biomarker of renal cell carcinoma. Int Urol Nephrol. 2018;50:851–9.
27. Petrozza V, Pastore AL, Palleschi G, et al. Secreted miR-210-3p as non-invasive biomarker in clear cell renal cell carcinoma. Oncotarget. 2017;8:69551–8.
28. Butz H, Nofech-Mozes R, Ding Q, et al. Exosomal MicroRNAs are diagnostic biomarkers and can mediate cell-cell communication in renal cell carcinoma. Eur Urol Focus. 2016;2:210–8.
29. Fedorko M, Juracek J, Stanik M, et al. Detection of let-7 miRNAs in urine supernatant as potential diagnostic approach in non-metastatic clear-cell renal cell carcinoma. Biochem Med (Zagreb). 2017;27:411–7.
30. Li G, Zhao A, Peoch M, et al. Detection of urinary cell-free miR-210 as a potential tool of liquid biopsy for clear cell renal cell carcinoma. Urol Oncol. 2017;35:294–9.
31. Iliev R, Fedorko M, Machackova T, et al. Expression levels of PIWI-interacting RNA, piR-823, are deregulated in tumor tissue, blood serum and urine of patients with renal cell carcinoma. Anticancer Res. 2016;36:6419–23.
32. Gatto F, Volpi N, Nilsson H, et al. Glycosaminoglycan profiling in patients' plasma and urine predicts the occurrence of metastatic clear cell renal cell carcinoma. Cell Rep. 2016;15:1822–36.
33. Gatto F, Maruzzo M, Magro C, et al. Prognostic value of plasma and urine glycosaminoglycan scores in clear cell renal cell carcinoma. Front Oncol. 2016;6:253.
34. Sarica K, Turkolmez K, Soygur T, et al. Evaluation of urinary glycosaminoglycan excretion in patients with renal cell carcinoma. Eur Urol. 1997;31:54–7.
35. Niziol J, Bonifay V, Ossolinski K, et al. Metabolomic study of human tissue and urine in clear cell renal carcinoma by LC-HRMS and PLS-DA. Anal Bioanal Chem. 2018;410:3859–69.
36. Falegan OS, Ball MW, Shaykhutdinov RA, et al. Urine and serum metabolomics analyses may distinguish between stages of renal cell carcinoma. Metabolites. 2017;7:E6.
37. Zhang L, Li L, Kong H, Zeng F. Urinary metabolomics study of renal cell carcinoma based on gas chromatography-mass spectrometry. Nan Fang Yi Ke Da Xue Xue Bao. 2015;35:763–6.
38. Kim K, Taylor SL, Ganti S, et al. Urine metabolomic analysis identifies potential biomarkers and pathogenic pathways in kidney cancer. OMICS. 2011;15:293–303.
39. Monteiro M, Moreira N, Pinto J, et al. GC-MS metabolomics-based approach for the identification of a potential VOC-biomarker panel in the urine of renal cell carcinoma patients. J Cell Mol Med. 2017;21:2092–105.
40. Wang D, Wang C, Pi X, et al. Urinary volatile organic compounds as potential biomarkers for renal cell carcinoma. Biomed Rep. 2016;5:68–72.
41. Minciu R, Tudor A, Pupca G, et al. Renal cancer diagnosed by noninvasive methods from body fluids by quantitative methylation-specific PCR(qMSP). Clin Lab. 2016;62:1563–8.
42. De Palma G, Sallustio F, Curci C, et al. The three-gene signature in urinary extracellular vesicles from patients with clear cell renal cell carcinoma. J Cancer. 2016;7:1960–7.
43. Raimondo F, Morosi L, Corbetta S, et al. Differential protein profiling of renal cell carcinoma urinary exosomes. Mol BioSyst. 2013;9:1220–33.

44. Erbes T, Hirschfeld M, Rucker G, et al. Feasibility of urinary microRNA detection in breast cancer patients and its potential as an innovative non-invasive biomarker. BMC Cancer. 2015;15:193.
45. Pories SE, Zurakowski D, Roy R, et al. Urinary metalloproteinases: noninvasive biomarkers for breast cancer risk assessment. Cancer Epidemiol Biomark Prev. 2008;17:1034–42.
46. Nyren-Erickson EK, Bouton M, Raval M, et al. Urinary concentrations of ADAM 12 from breast cancer patients pre- and post-surgery vs. cancer-free controls: a clinical study for biomarker validation. J Negat Results Biomed. 2014;13:5.
47. Yang J, Bielenberg DR, Rodig SJ, et al. Lipocalin 2 promotes breast cancer progression. Proc Natl Acad Sci U S A. 2009;106:3913–8.
48. Hu T, Shen H, Huang H, et al. Urinary circulating DNA profiling in non-small cell lung cancer patients following treatment shows prognostic potential. J Thorac Dis. 2018;10:4137–46.
49. Xie F, Li P, Gong J, et al. Urinary cell-free DNA as a prognostic marker for KRAS-positive advanced-stage NSCLC. Clin Transl Oncol. 2018;20:591–8.
50. Li F, Huang J, Ji D, et al. Utility of urinary circulating tumor DNA for EGFR mutation detection in different stages of non-small cell lung cancer patients. Clin Transl Oncol. 2017;19:1283–91.
51. Chen S, Zhao J, Cui L, Liu Y. Urinary circulating DNA detection for dynamic tracking of EGFR mutations for NSCLC patients treated with EGFR-TKIs. Clin Transl Oncol. 2017;19:332–40.
52. Sands J, Li Q, Hornberger J. Urine circulating-tumor DNA (ctDNA) detection of acquired EGFR T790M mutation in non-small-cell lung cancer: an outcomes and total cost-of-care analysis. Lung Cancer. 2017;110:19–25.
53. Zhang C, Leng W, Sun C, et al. Urine proteome profiling predicts lung Cancer from control cases and other tumors. EBioMedicine. 2018;30:120–8.
54. Wang W, Wang S, Zhang M. Identification of urine biomarkers associated with lung adenocarcinoma. Oncotarget. 2017;8:38517–29.
55. Nolen BM, Lomakin A, Marrangoni A, et al. Urinary protein biomarkers in the early detection of lung cancer. Cancer Prev Res (Phila). 2015;8:111–9.
56. Takahashi Y, Sakaguchi K, Horio H, et al. Urinary N1, N12-diacetylspermine is a non-invasive marker for the diagnosis and prognosis of non-small-cell lung cancer. Br J Cancer. 2015;113:1493–501.
57. Burton C, Ma Y. Current trends in cancer biomarker discovery using urinary metabolomics: achievements and new challenges. Curr Med Chem. 2019;26:5–28.
58. Cui Y, Shu XO, Li HL, et al. Prospective study of urinary prostaglandin E2 metabolite and pancreatic cancer risk. Int J Cancer. 2017;141:2423–9.
59. Weeks ME, Hariharan D, Petronijevic L, et al. Analysis of the urine proteome in patients with pancreatic ductal adenocarcinoma. Proteomics Clin Appl. 2008;2:1047–57.
60. Roy R, Zurakowski D, Wischhusen J, et al. Urinary TIMP-1 and MMP-2 levels detect the presence of pancreatic malignancies. Br J Cancer. 2014;111:1772–9.
61. Schonemeier B, Metzger J, Klein J, et al. Urinary peptide analysis differentiates pancreatic cancer from chronic pancreatitis. Pancreas. 2016;45:1018–26.
62. Davis VW, Schiller DE, Eurich D, et al. Pancreatic ductal adenocarcinoma is associated with a distinct urinary metabolomic signature. Ann Surg Oncol. 2013;20(Suppl 3):S415–23.
63. Debernardi S, Massat NJ, Radon TP, et al. Noninvasive urinary miRNA biomarkers for early detection of pancreatic adenocarcinoma. Am J Cancer Res. 2015;5:3455–66.
64. Zavesky L, Jandakova E, Turyna R, et al. Evaluation of cell-free urine microRNAs expression for the use in diagnosis of ovarian and endometrial cancers. A pilot study. Pathol Oncol Res. 2015;21:1027–35.
65. Zhou J, Gong G, Tan H, et al. Urinary microRNA-30a-5p is a potential biomarker for ovarian serous adenocarcinoma. Oncol Rep. 2015;33:2915–23.

Chapter 8
Urinary Bladder Cancer Biomarkers in Proximal Fluids

8.1 Introduction

Being the most commonly diagnosed cancer of the urinary tract, the 2018 global estimated cases of bladder cancer (BlCa) were 424,082 for men and 125,311 for women. For both sexes, however, BlCa was 10th in incidence (549,393 for 2018) and 13th cause of cancer-related mortality (199,922 for 2018). But for men, it was the 9th (compared to 17th for women) cause of cancer-related deaths (148,270 for 2018 in men). In the USA, the projected estimates for BlCa were 62,380 and 18,810 for men and women, respectively, while mortality figures stood at 12,520 for men and 4,720 for women. Although the incidence of BlCa has remained quite stable over the past few years, it is among the top ten most commonly diagnosed cancers globally.

BlCa is a disease mostly caused by environmental carcinogenic effects on the genome. Tobacco smoke carcinogens cause a substantial number (~50%) of BlCa. Additionally, occupational chemical exposures such as working in the rubber industry are established risk factors. Because of these risk associations, the prevalence of BlCa is five times higher in men than women. Additionally, this is a disease of the aged, having a median diagnostic age of 65 years.

Over 90% of BlCa is of urothelial cell origin. Many (about 75%) of these are diagnosed early when the lesion is confined to the mucosa and submucosa. These tumors are referred to as non-muscle-invasive BlCa (NMIBC). The remaining 25% of BlCa are muscle-invasive BlCa (MIBC), whereby cancer cells will have already infiltrated the muscle wall of the urinary bladder. However, about 70% of these NMIBC patients will develop recurrences within 2 years after treatment as a consequence of "field cancerization," whereby almost the entire urothelium is exposed to the same carcinogen and hence at elevated risk of developing cancers in the future. BlCa is also dichotomized into low-grade and high-grade tumors based on tumor biology. Low-grade tumors are superficial papillary multifocal tumors that may progress to advanced-stage disease. These tend to be associated with good prognosis.

G. D. Dakubo, *Cancer Biomarkers in Body Fluids*,
https://doi.org/10.1007/978-3-030-24725-6_8

High-grade tumors are nodular, and tend to invade early, and hence are associated with adverse outcomes. In general, early-stage in situ BlCa or low-grade tumors have a favorable outcome with a 5-year survival rate of about 94–96%. But this survival rate is markedly reduced to about 6% in advanced-stage disease.

Early-stage BlCa is usually asymptomatic. Clinical suspicion is made in patients presenting with blood in the urine (hematuria), increased frequency (polyuria) and urgency of urination, or discomfort/pain on urination. But these symptoms are non-specific to BlCa and could occur in other bladder conditions such as bladder infection. Thus, a diagnostic workup including urine cytology, cystoscopy, and possible biopsy of suspicious lesions for histopathologic evaluation is needed. But early BlCa may not shed cancer cells into the urine, thus making urine cytology insensitive (apart from also being dependent on pathologist experience). Cystoscopy is invasive and may not detect early lesions (without overt histopathologic appearance). Thus, the need for authenticated early detection noninvasive biomarkers should improve the outlook, at least for patients with elevated risk factors. This has primarily been explored in urinary samples for BlCa screening and management, but circulating biomarkers have also been examined and could be useful in disease prognosis and treatment decision-making.

8.2 Need for "Body Fluid Biopsy" Biomarkers

The presence of hematuria from BlCa is often associated with late presentation. Many people who present with hematuria do not have BlCa. Although specific, the gold standard for BlCa detection, cytology, falls short in sensitivity. Cystoscopy enables visualization and biopsy of suspicious lesions. However, this is invasive and costly and not amenable to screening for BlCa. The sensitivity of cystoscopy for BlCa detection is 80% for white light cystoscopy, but much higher (96%) for fluorescence-guided cystoscopy using 5-aminolevulinic acid or 5-ALA or its hexyl ester, hexaminolevulinate 5-ALA (Hexvix®, Photocure, Oslo, Norway). These sensitivities are much lower with regard to detection of early-stage disease such as dysplasia and carcinoma in situ (CIS). The sensitivity for white light cystoscopy is 48% for dysplasia and 68% for CIS, while hexaminolevulinate cystoscopy is 93% for dysplasia and 95% for CIS. Therefore, for early detection of curable cancers, noninvasiveness and cost-effective approaches to targeting biomarkers are needed. Surveillance and prognostication of BlCa also benefit from urinary biomarker tests.

8.3 The Urinary Bladder

The urinary bladder receives urine from the ureters and stores it temporarily before voiding or micturition (Fig. 8.1). Its structure and design are hence reflected on these functions. A section through the wall of the bladder reveals an outer serosa

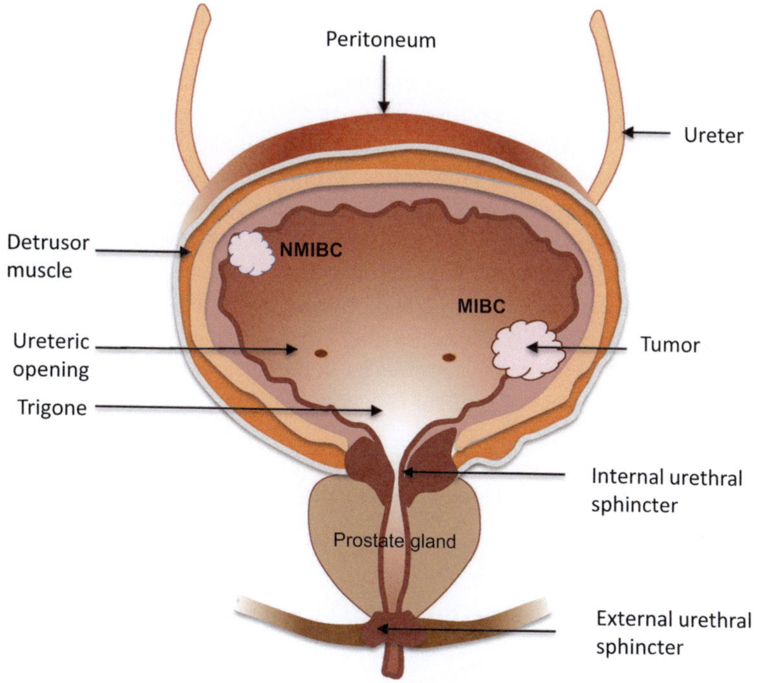

Fig. 8.1 Anatomy of the urinary bladder

covering, a middle muscularis, and an inner mucosa. The serosa is a simple squamous epithelium found only in the upper surface of the bladder. Fibrous adventitia covers the rest of the bladder. The muscularis consists of a layer of loosely arranged smooth muscle and elastic tissues, which contract to expel urine. The smooth muscle cells are arranged into inner longitudinal, middle circular, and outer longitudinal layers. This relationship is less evident when sectioned longitudinally, but clearly discernible on oblique section. The mucosa consists of the transitional epithelium (urothelium) and its supporting connective tissue. The cells vary in thickness depending on whether the bladder is distended or relaxed. It varies from about three-cell layers in the stretched bladder to about five-cell layers in the empty bladder.

8.3.1 Field Cancerization of the Urinary Bladder

Urothelial BlCa is uniquely characterized by simultaneous or metachronous development of multifocal tumors with identical or variable histological features in the urinary bladder or tract of a single patient. Urothelial BlCa is commonly accompanied by surrounding abnormal urothelium, with histopathologic features ranging from dysplasia to carcinoma in situ. Two distinct concepts have been proposed to help explain this phenomenon. First is the "field cancerization" hypothesis, which postulates that multiple cells become initiated or partially transformed as a result of carcinogenic insults and acquire independent genetic alterations. Therefore, multifocal tumors would arise synchronously or metachronously from distinct transformed cells. The second hypothesis proposes that multifocal tumors are descendants of a single transformed cell that proliferates and spreads through the urothelium via intraluminal or intraepithelial seeding. Intraepithelial spread may occur through the continuous proliferation and migration of transformed cells throughout the urothelium. Intraluminal seeding could occur through the release of cancer cells from the primary lesion followed by the spread and implantation of the tumor cells at different sites of the urothelium. It should be noted that clonal expansion of the spread cancerous or precancerous cells might cause field cancerization. Therefore, there are two possible mechanisms of field cancerization in urothelium, one involving multiclonal neoplastic alterations in response to carcinogenic insults and the other, a clonal expansion and spread from a single transformed progenitor cell. These transformed cells are a rich source of early detection and surveillance biomarkers.

8.4 Approaches to Detection and Diagnosis of Bladder Cancer

Symptomatic hematuria triggers the following investigations for BlCa diagnosis:

- Urinary cytology for detection of abnormal cells
- Urine culture to rule out infectious cause of hematuria
- Flow cytometry for DNA ploidy detection as biomarker of BlCa
- Cystoscopy and biopsy of suspicious lesions for definite diagnosis
- Intravenous pyelogram to detect growths from filling defects in the bladder

Cystoscopy is the gold standard for BlCa diagnosis that is often coupled with void urinary cytology. Cystoscopy is the direct visualization of the bladder epithelium via an instrument (a cystoscope) that is inserted into the urethra and directed into the bladder. It allows biopsy of suspicious lesions for histopathologic evaluation. However, it is expensive, invasive, and uncomfortable and may require anesthesia. Cytology relies on visual identification of cells from the bladder. Upon sample preparation, a cytologist or pathologist examines the slides and classifies the cells as either normal, atypical/indeterminate, suspicious, or cancerous. Although this method is the gold standard for BlCa detection, cytology is insensitive being affected by confounding factors such as benign bladder conditions (e.g., infection and inflammation), which may produce false-positive results. It is also operator-dependent and thus suffers from both inter- and intraobserver errors. Worse still, urinary cytology is insensitive in detecting early-stage disease (non-muscle-invasive pTa-pT1 cancer), for which the sensitivity is 20–40% for low-stage and low-grade (I and II) cancers. High-grade cancers are detected at a much better rate of over

80%. Overall though, cytology has a sensitivity of 44% but a high specificity of 96%. This explains why it is often combined with cystoscopy for BlCa management.

The numerous advantages of cytology are it being noninvasive; being comfortable for patients; having high specificity; being not confounded by hematuria or chemicals such as pH and salt; being inexpensive (inexpensive equipment and reasonable operating cost); not being subjected to artifacts such as amplification, normalization, and other errors of molecular assays; and not requiring special patient preparation. The drawbacks for urinary cytology are it being subjective and some urinary samples being devoid of cells for analysis. Additionally, it suffers from poor compliance with the best approach of requiring three serial first-morning void specimens to reduce sampling error.

8.5 Urinary Bladder Cancer Biomarkers in Proximal Fluid

Sidransky et al. pioneered the successful use of a molecular genetic approach to assay tumor-associated *TP53* mutations in urine from BlCa patients [1]. They used multiple techniques including the polymerase chain reaction, mutant-specific oligonucleotide hybridization, and sequencing techniques to screen for mutations in clinical samples as a diagnostic possibility. Since then the field of detecting cancer biomarkers in urine and other body fluids has tremendously been advanced.

8.5.1 DNA Methylation as Urothelial Bladder Cancer Biomarkers in Proximal Fluid

Epigenetic changes in tumor suppressor genes are frequent events in BlCa. Some established tumor suppressor genes are methylated at very high frequencies (e.g., *APC* is methylated in about 69% of BlCa). Importantly, these changes occur early in bladder carcinogenesis, being observed in curable stage Ta and Tis lesions. Methylation-specific PCR (MSP) analysis of *APC*, *RASSF1A*, and *p14/ARF* in urine specifically detects BlCa at a sensitivity of 87%. Obviously a sensitivity of 91% from gene methylation is much superior in BlCa detection compared to urine cytology of 50%. Genes commonly methylated in urine from BlCa patients include *CDH1*, *CDH13*, *CDKN2A*, *RARβ*, *APC*, *DAPK*, and *RASSF1A*. Of clinical relevance, *CDH1* methylation is an independent prognostic factor, and *DAPK* methylation is an indicator of recurrence. Moreover, compared to cytology with detection sensitivity of 45.5%, methylation of *CDH1*, *RARβ*, *DAPK,* and *CDKN2A* performs much better at BlCa detection (sensitivity of 90.9%). Urinary methylation assays therefore hold promise for BlCa early detection, chemoprevention, surveillance, and disease monitoring for recurrence. Myriads of studies have been performed, mostly using quantitative and non-quantitative MSP. Similar to other urothelial cancer biomarkers, the use of methylation biomarkers for BlCa requires that methylation markers in urine must not be in other cells of the urinary tract or associated with benign bladder conditions such as infections or benign hematuria. Many studies have controlled for these factors. Methylation in tissue should also match urinary methylation to confirm their cancer cell origin. Methylation markers must also be age-matched to control for aging-associated methylation.

Pathetically, many methylation markers for early detection mostly lack validation in independent experiments. However, a prospective multicenter study with both training and validation sets achieved promising cancer detection accuracy. Because of the increased sensitivity with some reported promising specificities closer to cytology (the gold standard), methylation biomarkers appear superior to cytology. Methylation markers for surveillance have not been widely studied, albeit a few studies show promise in detection of recurrent tumors, especially in patients with tumors that harbor similar gene methylation.

However, a number of studies provide evidence for urinary methylation as BlCa biomarkers. Analysis of epigenomic alterations, especially DNA methylation, in body fluids holds promise for management of cancer. In BlCa, analysis of DNA methylation in urinary exfoliated cells has been successfully demonstrated using various methodologies. Diagnostic performances have been encouraging with sensitivities of 80–90% and high specificities of up to 100% in some series. Several genes including *DAPK*, *RARβ*, *CDH*, *CDKN2A*, *BCL2*, *TERT*, *APC*, *RASSF1A*, *p14/ARF*, *NID2*, *TWIST1*, *MGMT*, *GSTP1*, *TCF21*, *PCDH17*, *PENK*, *SOX11*, *DBC1*, *NKX6-2*, *CA10*, and *MYO3* have shown altered methylation statuses in urine from BlCa patients. Summarized here are some studies attesting to the diagnostic performances of these methylation biomarkers. Chan et al. examined a panel consisting of *DAPK*, *RARβ*, *CDH*, and *CDKN2A* in urine and demonstrated a sensitivity of 91% and specificity of 76% for BlCa detection [2]. *DAPK*, *BCL2*, and *TERT* were methylated in as many as 78% of urine from BlCa patients [3]. Methylation of *APC*, *RASSF1A*, and *p14/ARF* in urine achieved a sensitivity and specificity of 87% and 100%, respectively, for BlCa detection [4]. Hoque et al. analyzed methylation of 9 genes in urine, and methylation was demonstrated in at least 1 of *CDKN2A*, *p14/ARF*, *MGMT*, and *GSTP1* in 175 samples from BlCa patients [5]. This methylation pattern in urine matched those in primary tumors. A logistic regression analysis uncovered a sensitivity of 82% and specificity of 96% for BlCa detection. In a large cohort of 500 urine samples analyzed using quantitative MSP, methylation of *TWIST* and *NID2* achieved a sensitivity and specificity of 90% and 93%, respectively, in detecting BlCa. This performance was superior to cytology in this cohort [6]. A multigene predictive model consisting of *MYO3A*, *CA10*, *NKX6-2*, *DBC1*, and either *SOX11* or *PENK* methylation in urine achieved a sensitivity of 85% and specificity of 95% in BlCa detection [7]. In a pilot study using small volumes of urine, methylation of *CDKN2A*, *NID2*, and *BCL2* achieved a sensitivity of 81% and specificity of 86% in BlCa detection [8]. Hypermethylation of *KCNV1*, *TAL1*, *VAX1*, *CFTR*, and *PROX1* in urine is associated with BlCa. The performance of this panel achieved a sensitivity and specificity of 88.9% and 87.3%, respectively [9]. Meta-analytical review of urinary *CDH13* promoter methylation uncovered its association with BlCa risk (OR = 7.71) [10]. The association with high-grade tumors (OR = 2.22), multifocal tumors (OR = 1.45), and MIBC (OR = 3.42) was also realized. Moreover, the association was higher in Asian (OR = 35.18) than Caucasian (OR = 8.86) populations.

8.5.2 Genomic Alterations as Urothelial Bladder Cancer Biomarkers in Proximal Fluid

DNA alterations, including chromosomal, microsatellite, and mutations underlie urothelial carcinogenesis. Expectedly, some of these genomic alterations have been successfully demonstrated in urinary samples from BlCa patients. In void urine from patients, analysis using 17–20 microsatellite markers across several chromosomes uncovered the most frequent alterations to be on chromosomes 8p and 9p [11]. In patients with recurrent BlCa, of nine microsatellite markers, six achieved an overall accuracy of 86% in BlCa detection [12]. In a large cohort of 300 patients, multiple mutations in five genes were uncommon in individual genes, including *FGFR3*. However, mutations in one or more genes were found in 88% of primary tumors and at the same frequency in recurrent tumors [13]. These mutations were demonstrable in urine from BlCa patients.

8.5.3 Gene Transcript Alterations as Urothelial Bladder Cancer Biomarkers in Proximal Fluid

Both coding and noncoding gene transcript alterations in urine have been evaluated as possible BlCa biomarkers.

8.5.3.1 Coding Transcripts

Understandably, transcriptomic studies of BlCa have mostly focused on primary cancer tissue samples. These analyses have uncovered a number of altered transcripts associated with BlCa and have shown utility in disease detection, staging, recurrence, and outcome predictions, as well as subtype stratification. Some validated altered tissue transcripts have been demonstrated in urinary samples as well. Probing of BlCa tissues at various stages (Ta, T1, and > T1) enabled identification of *IGFBP5*, *HOXA13*, *CDC2*, and *MDK* as BlCa biomarkers. Urinary assay of this panel achieved a sensitivity and specificity of 85% and 80%, respectively, for BlCa detection. The best performance was however achieved with stage >T1 and > 1-cm-diameter tumors [14]. A commercial assay of this panel, called uRNA assay (Pacific

Edge Ltd., Dunedin, New Zealand), was developed and evaluated in comparison to cytology and the established NMP22 ELISA assay. Among 485 patients presenting with hematuria, at a predetermined specificity of 85%, the sensitivity of uRNA (62%) was superior to cytology and the NMP22 assay. A modification to this assay enhanced BlCa detection to 82% among this cohort [15]. Hanke et al. used whole urine, clarified urine, and urothelial cell pellets to profile expression of a selected panel of genes in 98 subjects [16]. The ratio of expressed virus E26 oncogene homolog 2 (ETS2) to urokinase plasminogen activator (uPA) in whole urine was sensitive and specific at 75% and 100%, respectively, for BlCa detection. Other genes assayed in urine for BlCa detection include *KRT20*, *BIRC5*, *HYAL1*, and *MUC7*. These genes have shown enhanced BlCa detection using 2–3 panel assays with sensitivities ranging from 62% to 90% [17]. Survivin (*BIRC5*) mRNA as a single biomarker in urine has been investigated for BlCa diagnosis and has achieved sensitivities and specificities of 64–83% and 88–93%, respectively. However, sensitivity is low for low-grade tumors.

Whole transcriptome analysis of exfoliated urothelial cells is promissory for identification of altered expressed gene profile for BlCa. Rosser et al. subjected transcriptome profiles of 90 urothelial cell samples to feature selection algorithm to uncover the optimal gene signature for BlCa [18]. RT-PCR analysis of the 14-gene signature panel achieved a sensitivity and specificity of 90% and 100%, respectively, for BlCa detection in independent urothelial samples [19]. This performance was much superior to cytology that detected only 35% of tumors in this cohort. A similar strategy was previously used to select an optimal 12-gene signature from 384 altered genes identified in primary tissue samples. Similarly, RT-PCR analysis of this gene panel achieved a sensitivity of 89% and specificity of 95% for BlCa detection among a cohort of 211 subjects [20].

8.5.3.2 Noncoding Transcripts

The stability of miRNA in body fluids due in part to being in complexes with macromolecules or enclosure in exosomes makes them attractive disease biomarkers that can be deployed in a noninvasive fashion. Profiling of BlCa tissue samples has uncovered miRNA deregulation in BlCa, and some of these are demonstrable in urinary samples. BlCa miRNAs have utility in disease detection, complementary cancer diagnosis by cytology, tumor stratification, and possible prognosis because some are associated with advanced tumor grade and stage.

Hanke et al. profiled 157 miRNAs in urinary samples [21]. The ratio of miR-126 to miR-182 could discriminate BlCa at a sensitivity of 72% and specificity of 82%. In another panel of 15 miRNAs, the combined utility of miR-15b, miR-135b, and miR-1224-3b achieved a sensitivity of 94.1% in BlCa detection, albeit at a low specificity of 51% [22]. Urinary miR-96 and miR-183 could complement cytology in BlCa detection and also correlated with advanced tumor grade and stage [23]. Puerta-Gil et al. could detect and stratify BlCa using the combination of miR-222 and miR-452 [24].

The numerous studies of urinary miRNA involved in BlCa have been subjected to meta-analytical reviews. The diagnostic role of urinary miRNA in blood and urine for BlCa detection inclusive of 22 studies with 4558 cases and 4456 controls achieved pooled sensitivity, specificity, and AUROCC of 74%, 78%, and 0.83, respectively. Blood-based and panel miRNA assays performed better, and diagnostic performance was also better in Asian than Caucasian populations [25]. Of 14 studies involving 1128 BlCa and 1057 matched controls, the pooled sensitivity, specificity, PLR, NLR, DOR, and AUROCC of urinary miRNA biomarkers were 71%, 75%, 2.8, 0.39, 7.0, and 0.79, respectively [26]. Subgroup analysis uncovered the influence of ethnicity and miRNA profiling on the diagnostic accuracy. Cheng et al. assessed the diagnostic accuracy of urinary miRNA by meta-analysis of 23 studies from 9 articles involving 719 cases and 494 controls [27]. Pooled sensitivity, specificity, PLR, NLR, DOR, and AUROCC were 75%, 75%, 3.03, 0.33, 9.07, and 0.81, respectively. Accuracy improved with urine supernatant assays and use of panel miRNAs. Finally, another urinary miRNA BlCa diagnostic performance meta-analyzed achieved the highest sensitivity and specificity of 86.6% (in urine sediments) and 85.3% (in voided urine), respectively, when multiple miRNAs were used [28]. The performance was independent of sample type (voided, supernatant, or sediment). The potential of urinary miRNA has been demonstrated by these studies. However, improvements are still needed and coordinated clinical validation is awaited.

8.5.4 Proteomic Alterations as Urothelial Bladder Cancer Biomarkers in Proximal Fluid

Urinary proteomic biomarker discovery, validation, and clinical utility in BlCa management have been approached in two ways: analyses of established altered proteins in BlCa as single or panel biomarkers and discovery of novel BlCa biomarkers in primary tumor samples using various advanced high-throughput proteomic technologies, with subsequent development of urinary assays.

Abogunrin et al. evaluated 23 BlCa-associated proteins in urinary samples from 80 BlCa patients and 77 healthy controls [29]. Univariate analysis uncovered nine of these proteins to show significant differential levels in urine between the two groups. The performance of these biomarkers in BlCa detection was significantly enhanced by incorporating age and smoking history. Out of the nine informative biomarkers, a panel consisting of BTA, NMP22, EGF, thrombomodulin, and serum CEA achieved a sensitivity of 91% and specificity of 80% in cancer detection. Examination of immune mediators including cytokines and 15 HSPs in urine uncovered HSP60 and IL-13 to significantly enhance BlCa detection compared to single biomarkers [30].

Proteomic studies have identified altered signature proteins for BlCa detection, characterization, and prognosis. Novel BlCa proteins and peptides have also been uncovered in urinary samples from BlCa patients. Vlahou et al. examined urinary protein profiles between patients with transitional cell carcinoma (TCC) and healthy controls by SELDI-TOF MS [31]. This approach enabled identification of five novel biomarkers and many protein clusters for BlCa. As BlCa classification biomarkers, the combination of the altered proteins and clusters significantly enhanced BlCa classification. One of the biomarkers, α-defensin, was confirmed in BlCa cells, and cross-validation in independent urinary samples achieved an accuracy superior to commercially available BlCa screening tests. A well-designed study whereby urinary protein biomarkers were detected by CE-MS in a training set and further improved in a separate cohort of patients and controls consisting of healthy individuals and patients with nonmalignant urogenital diseases enabled the identification of 22-signature diagnostic urinary biomarkers for BlCa. In a validation study, these urinary biomarkers could accurately classify all cancer patients [32]. Application of iTRAQ technique to pooled urine from patients and controls enabled identification of 55 differentially expressed candidate proteins. Significantly elevated in urine from BlCa patients was APOA1, which was confirmed using ELISA to have high diagnostic potential [33]. Profiling of urinary samples by glycoprotein enrichment technique enabled identification of BlCa glycoproteins, of which α-1-antitrypsin (SERPINA1/A1AT) achieved a sensitivity and specificity of 74% and 80%, respectively, for BlCa detection in an independent assessment using ELISA [34]. The MD Anderson group led by Goodison used an integrated proteomic and genomic profiling of urine to uncover BlCa diagnostic biomarkers. Urinary concentrations of 14 of the biomarkers (IL-8, MMP-9, MMP-10, SDC1, CCL18, PAI-1, CD44, VEGF, ANG, CA9, A1AT, OPN, PTX3, and APOE) were assessed by ELISA. Panels of 2–3 of these biomarkers have been also analyzed using ELISA [35–37]. A multivariate analysis enabled identification of eight biomarkers that could detect BlCa at a sensitivity and specificity of 92% and 97%, respectively, but the combination of three of the eight biomarkers (IL-8, VEGF, and APOE) was equally highly accurate at sensitivity of 90% and specificity of 97%. These performances were superior to current urine tests including cytology for BlCa detection [38].

Immunoassays targeting fragments of KTR 8 and 18 in urine have been developed for BlCa detection. The various test kits demonstrate sensitivities of 50–61% and specificities of 63–97%. These assays have relatively high false-positive rates and low sensitivity for low-grade tumors. Two transcription factors, BLCA-1 and BLCA-4, show potential as early BlCa detection biomarkers because they are both elevated early in BlCa development. BLCA-4 is elevated in urothelial cancer and adjacent benign cells, but not in normal bladder cells. ELISA assays for BLCA-4 have achieved sensitivities and specificities of 89–96% and 90–100%, respectively [39]. Similarly, BLCA-1 assay achieved sensitivity and specificity of 80% and 87%, respectively.

Several urinary proteins studied as BlCa biomarkers have been subjected to meta-analytical reviews. The diagnostic accuracy of urinary BLCA-4 for BlCa detection was analyzed using nine studies with 1119 subjects [40]. The performance according to pooled sensitivity, specificity, PLR, NLR, DOR, and AUROCC were

93%, 97%, 48.16, 0.08, 534.03, and 0.9607, respectively, which suggest BLCA-4 is a promising BlCa diagnostic biomarker. A couple of meta-analyses have been performed on urinary CYFRA21-1. Meta-analysis of urinary and serum CYFRA21-1 for BlCa inclusive of only three case-control studies suggests its accuracy for metastatic rather than localized disease [41]. Thus, as a diagnostic biomarker, it might be useful for differentiating early stage localized from metastatic disease. Another meta-analysis of urinary CYFRA21-1 included 16 studies with 1262 cases and 1223 controls [42]. The pooled sensitivity, specificity, and AUROCC were 82%, 80%, and 0.87, respectively. Participant selection and verification biases were uncovered. The potential value of urinary CYFRA21-1 for BlCa needs clarification. Urinary KTR 20 for BlCa detection was meta-analyzed using 27 studies [43]. The pooled sensitivity, specificity, PLR, NLR, DOR, and AUROCC were 79%, 90%, 8.17, 0.23, 35.29, and 0.90, respectively. Performance was higher for higher-grade and higher-stage tumors. Moreover, test accuracy was better for RT-PCR or PCR assays than immunoassays. Urinary fibronectin in BlCa detection included eight studies involving 744 cancer patients [44]. Pooled sensitivity, specificity, DOR, and AUROCC were 80%, 79%, 15.18, and 0.83, respectively. The performance was augmented when used with cystoscopy, which achieved a sensitivity and specificity of 86% and 89%, respectively. Urinary UCA1 for BlCa detection was analyzed in six studies of 578 cases and 562 controls [45]. The pooled sensitivity, specificity, PLR, NLR, DOR, and AUROCC were 81%, 86%, 5.85, 0.22, 27.01, and 0.88, respectively. While there was evidence of publication bias, ethnicity contributed to heterogeneity in sensitivity.

A urinary ten-plex biomarker in comparison to single biomarkers for BlCa detection was meta-analyzed in 1173 patients [46]. The ten-plex urinary protein biomarkers included interleukin-8, matrix metalloproteinases 9 and 10, angiogenin, apolipoprotein E, syndecan 1, α-1-antitrypsin, plasminogen activator inhibitor-1, carbonic anhydrase 9, and vascular endothelial growth factor A. There was a higher OR (3.46) for the ten-plex than any single biomarker independent of tumor stage or grade.

8.5.5 Metabolomic Alterations as Urothelial Bladder Cancer Biomarkers in Proximal Fluid

Although preliminary, metabolomic analyses have been successfully applied to urinary samples from BlCa patients. Issaq et al. analyzed urine from 41 cancer and 48 healthy controls by HPLC [47]. Analysis of metabolite differences between the groups enabled at least 40 of the 41 cancer patients to be identified. Similar urinary metabolomic analysis uncovered 15-metabolite signature that achieved perfect BlCa detection rate in a cohort of 24 patients [48]. In another pilot study of 58 specimens, a 35-metabolite signature could distinguish normal and benign bladder from BlCa. Moreover, this signature could potentially identify tumor stages and grades [49].

8.5.6 Extracellular Vesicle Alterations as Urothelial Bladder Cancer Biomarkers in Proximal Fluid

Extracellular vesicles (EVs), especially exosomes, can preferentially be enriched with cancer-derived cargo including nucleic acids and proteins. With the development of technologies for EV isolation from body fluids, EVs and their cargo are becoming important potential noninvasive cancer biomarkers. EVs have been successfully isolated from urine. Using a microfluidic chip-based system, EVs were isolated from patients with and without BlCa. The levels of urinary EVs were significantly higher in cancer patients than controls and could be used for BlCa detection, but this is not specific to BlCa. Apart from EV enumeration, alterations of their content have been demonstrated in urine from BlCa patients. Indeed, several genetic and protein biomarkers of potential interest in BlCa have been uncovered in urinary EVs. Urinary exosomal lncRNA levels were elevated in BlCa patients compared to controls, and the lncRNA, HOTAIR, was associated with epithelial-mesenchymal transition and poor prognosis [50]. Also elevated in urinary EVs are HOX-AS-2 and MALAT1 [51]. A microarray platform (with >850 different tumor miRNAs) was used to analyze urinary exosomal miRNAs from BlCa patients and healthy controls. This enabled identification of 26 significantly dysregulated miRNAs (23 down and 3 up) between patients with high-grade tumors and controls. However, among this cohort, miR-375 appeared to predict patients with high-grade BlCa, while low-grade tumors were associated with miR-146a [52]. Transcripts of urinary *SLC2A1*, *GPRC5A*, and *KRT17* in EVs were elevated in pT1 and higher-stage BlCa and could be used to detect NMIBC with AUROCC of 0.56–0.64 for pTa, 0.62–0.80 for pTis, and 0.82–0.86 for pT1, as well as pT2 and higher MIBC with AUROCC of 0.72–0.90 [53]. Proteomic approaches have also been successfully used to characterize proteins in EVs from urine and BlCa cell lines. This proteomic approach enabled identification of α-1-antitrypsin and histone cluster 1 H2B family member K (H2B1K) in urine from BlCa patients. Threefold elevation of H2B1K levels could accurately predict disease recurrence.

8.5.7 Urinary Cytology for Urinary Bladder Cancer Detection

The gold standard noninvasive test for BlCa detection is voided urine cytology (VuC). As such, newer molecular BlCa biomarkers and assays are measured against urinary cytology. Because low-grade and early-stage tumors shed few cancer cells, cytology is insensitive in detecting these tumors. Hence, the overall sensitivity of VuC is low for BlCa detection. Because molecular assays often involve some aspects of target amplification, their sensitivities for early-stage tumors are high and hence often outperform VuC. Urinary enrichment techniques, coupled with cystoscopy, help offset the low performance of cytology for BlCa detection. VuC has variable sensitivities (25–95%). High sensitivities are demonstrable in high-grade tumors (80–90%) and carcinoma in situ (98–100%). Moreover, VuC has a false-positive rate of up to 12% due to morphological cellular changes caused by inflammation. VuC however has a number of advantages including high specificity, low equipment cost, and refractory from amplification artifacts and chemical confounders such as salt concentration and pH changes that can affect molecular assays. The main disadvantages of VuC are low sensitivity, sampling errors, cost associated with requirement of a pathologist, and interobserver variation. The indecisiveness of atypical and suspicious lesions could result in psychological trauma to patients and possible costly invasive procedures on follow-up.

8.5.8 Meta-analytical Review of Commercial Biomarkers in Proximal Fluid

A systematic review and meta-analysis of urinary BlCa biomarkers included 57 studies [54]. Evaluated biomarkers included NMP22, BTA, FISH, ImmunoCyt/Scimedx, and Cxbladder. Cystoscopy and histopathology were reference standards. The ranges of sensitivity, specificity, PLR, and NLR were 57–82%, 74–88%, 2.52–5.53, and 0.21–0.48, respectively. Sensitivity increased with advanced-stage tumors by grade and stage. Qualitative NMP22 and quantitative BTA had no differences in diagnostic accuracies. While sensitivity was better for biomarkers and cytological evaluation than biomarkers alone, about 10% of BlCas were still missed. The accuracy of these biomarkers is dismal as substantial proportions of BlCa are still being missed and others have false-positive rates. Accuracy is especially poor for early-stage low-grade and low-stage tumors. Another systematic review and meta-analysis of commercially available urinary BlCa biomarkers was conducted to determine their performances in evaluating primary hematuria [55]. The included biomarkers were AssureMDx, BTA, Cxbladder, NMP22, UroVysion, and uCyt+. The ranges in sensitivity and specificity were 67–95% and 68–93%, respectively. There was significant heterogeneity between studies, and the quality of evidence was moderate due to inadequate blinding. While the biomarkers may have superior sensitivity, their specificities are lower than cystoscopy in evaluating hematuria. It was concluded that they were inadequate to replace cystoscopy in the evaluation of primary hematuria, but AssureMDx could be used to triage patients for cystoscopy.

8.6 Clinical Translation of Commercial Products

Bladder cancer is probably the only cancer that has advanced tremendously with regard to noninvasive screening and monitoring. Commercial tests are developed that can even be done at the point-of-care with rapid results for interpretations or at the comfort of the patient's home. The uptake of such tests is high given the facile mode of performance (easy instructions to follow) and painless noninvasive nature of the tests. Not surprisingly therefore, such tests, although not all are necessarily excellent in performances, have received US FDA clearances for use. Additionally, many of these tests are marketed globally. The leading commercial products include UroVysion and the Ikoniscope technology, NMP22, BTA, and ImmunoCyt/uCyt+, with AssureMDx™ and Cxbladder being newer commercial tests yet to be FDA approved (Table 8.1).

8.6.1 *UroVysion™*

UroVysion™ is the first DNA probe test approved by the FDA for diagnosis and monitoring of BlCa. It is a FISH assay that interrogates the copy numbers of chromosomes 3, 7, and 17, as well as loss of the short arm of chromosome 9 (9p21). Loss of 9p21 results in the loss of the tumor suppressor functions of *CDKN2A*, and this is a known associated BlCa biomarker. The test involves a multiplex of four fluorescent probes for each chromosomal locus and hence produces four distinct colors. The probes are designated as chromosome enumeration probe (CEP) and locus-specific identifier (LSI). The spectral colors associated with each chromosome are CEP3 (red), CEP7 (green), CEP17 (aqua), and LSI9p21 (gold). The test is easy to perform. Urine is collected and centrifuged to pellet cells, and these are smeared and dried on a microscope slide. The DNA of the cells and the probes together with blocking probes are denatured and hybridized. Following washes and DAPI nuclei counterstain, the slides are examined and analyzed under a microscope. UroVysion™ test has several advantages over other BlCa urine tests. It demonstrates such a high sensitivity, especially when combined with cytology. The combined sensitivity with cytology of 97% is higher than cytology and cystoscopy combined (88%). Of even much clinical relevance is its high detection rate (96%, compared to cytology rate of 71%) of high-grade urothelial carcinomas (carcinoma in situ) with flat appearance that can evade even cystoscopy scrutiny. Additionally, being a FISH assay, UroVysion™ is unaffected by infection, hematuria, cytology, or even bacillus Calmette-Guérin immunotherapy commonly used to treat BlCa.

8.6.2 *Ikoniscope® Robotic Digital Microscopy Platform*

Ikonisys has developed a digital microscopy system that enables easy, economical, and unbiased analysis of FISH of clinical samples. The Ikoniscope is a digital robotic and fully automated walk-away microscopy. The instrument is a proprietary epifluorescence microscopy designed to automatically load and handle slides, stains, captures images in real time, analyzes the images, and generates a report on possible diagnosis. Up to 175 slides can be handled simultaneously, thus making the throughput really high. The workstation includes the ikonisoft explorer, which is an

Table 8.1 Commercially available urinary bladder cancer tests

Test	Target	Assay	Sensitivity (%)	Specificity (%)	FDA approval status/ uses
UroVysion™	Aneuploidy of chromosomes 3, 7, and 17. Loss of 9p21 locus	FISH	63 (30–86)	87 (63–95)	Yes/diagnosis and monitoring
NMP22®BC test	NMP22	Sandwich immunoassay	69 (26–100)	77 (41–92)	Yes/monitoring
NMP22®BladderChek®	NMP22	Sandwich immunoassay	58 (51–85)	88 (77–96)	Yes
BTA stat®	Complement factor H-related protein	Colorimetric immunoassay	64 (29–83)	77 (56–86)	Yes/diagnosis and monitoring
BTA TRAK®	Complement factor H-related protein	Sandwich immunoassay	65 (53–91)	74 (28–83)	Yes/diagnosis and monitoring
ImmunoCyt™	CEA and mucins (2)	Immunofluorescence cytology	78 (52–100)	78 (63–79)	Yes/monitoring
AssureMDx™	Gene methylation and mutations	Methylation and mutation detection	93	85	No
Cxbladder	Expression of five genes	RT-PCR	82	85	No

automated cell suspension staining software that enables user-established scanning and analytical parameters. The IkoniLAN® server is a network connectivity that links up with other ikoniscopes internally and externally and enables interlaboratory data sharing and interpretation, thus improving the level of accuracy and hence care. An Internet-based viewing of data can be accomplished via the IkoniWAN™.

8.6.3 NMP22® Bladder Cancer Test

Altered cellular states in cancer are associated with nuclear matrix protein (NMP) changes. There is ample evidence of NMP-specific signatures for various cancers including breast, renal, prostate, and colorectal cancers. NMPs are released into the circulation and other body fluids. The NMP technology license was obtained by Matritech from the Massachusetts Institute of Technology and is being currently used to develop a battery of tests for cancer management. The NMP22® test kit is an FDA-approved quantitative microplate immunoassay developed for the management of BlCa. Not only is this test good for monitoring cancer patients; it is accurate at early detection of BlCa as the levels of NMP22 are elevated in urine even at the early stages of cancer. The NMP® BladderChek® test is an FDA-approved test for point-of-care analysis of urine samples. A study published in JAMA showed that early-stage BlCa could be missed with cystoscopy alone, but when cystoscopy is combined with NMP22® BladderChek® test, sensitivity could be as high as 99% [56]. The NMP22® BladderChek® test helps in the diagnosis and monitoring of BlCa. The test is CLIA waived for in-office use, economical, and widely reimbursed. Results are available in 30 min, and the assay uses only four drops of urine.

8.6.4 BTA Test

Bladder tumor-associated antigen (BTA) is a complement factor H-related protein (CFHrp), which is a variant of complement factor H involved in control of the complement system. Apparently, tumor cells highly express CFHrp, and this is to protect them from destruction by the immune system. These antigens are made and shed into the urine of cancer patients and hence can be detected as biomarkers of the disease. The BTA stat® test is a qualitative immunoassay designed for the detection of BlCa antigens in urine of cancer patients. It can be performed at the point-of-care and is used mainly for monitoring of tumor recurrence. It is a quick assay with a turnaround time of just 5 min. It is prescribed for home use, and the results are interpreted in conjunction with urine cytology. BTA TRAK® quantitative is a quantitative ELISA assay that also measures CFHrp levels in urine. Both assays are US FDA-approved tests for BlCa management.

8.6.5 *ImmunoCyt™/uCyt™*

This assay is a fluorescent microscopic method for detection of BlCa using a cocktail of three monoclonal antibodies targeted at the expression levels of sulfated mucin-glycoproteins and glycosylated forms of the carcinoembryonic antigen in urine. The test improves the sensitivity of cytology for BlCa detection and is cleared by the FDA for BlCa monitoring. In high-risk individuals, uCyt+™ is used as a research assay to screen for BlCa occurrence.

8.6.6 *AssureMDx™*

Developed by MDxHealth, AssureMDx™ is a noninvasive urine-based test for BlCa detection in patients presenting with hematuria. The test is composed of gene methylation (*TWIST1, ONECUT2*, and *OTX1*) and mutation (*HRAS, FGFR3,* and *TERT*) panel that helps rule out the presence of BlCa risk due to its validated high negative predictive value of 99%. Conceivably, the high NPV suggests AssureMDx™ could help prevent or spare 77% of symptomatic patients with hematuria from invasive cystoscopy evaluation. Additionally, validated sensitivity of 93% and specificity of 85% could identify individuals with elevated risk for BlCa who will therefore be candidates for cystoscopy. The test is available as a laboratory-developed test performed in the company's College of American Pathologists and CLIA-accredited facility in Irvine, California.

8.6.7 *Cxbladder*

Pacific Edge Ltd. is a cancer diagnostic company that developed and launched Cxbladder urine-based test for BlCa. The Cxbladder assay measures the expression levels of five genes (*MDK, HOXA13, CDC/CDK1, IGFBP5*, and *CXCR2*) in urine. Similar to AssureMDx™, Cxbladder could help rule out BlCa in 60% of patients presenting with hematuria and hence spare them from further invasive procedures. There are three Cxbladder assays, each with a specific intended use. For the low-risk patient presenting with hematuria, Cxbladder Triage test helps rule out the presence of BlCa. Cxbladder Detect test is intended for enhanced detection of BlCa in the high-risk patient. Used in combination with cystoscopy, Cxbladder Detect could identify 97% of high-grade tumors. Finally, Cxbladder Monitor is used to monitor for early detection of recurrence and thus help reduce the number of invasive procedures needed for detection of disease relapse.

8.7 Summary

- BlCa is the most commonly diagnosed urinary tract cancer, especially in men.
- About 75% of BlCa is diagnosed at the NMIBC stage that is associated with good prognosis.
- The urothelium is exposed to carcinogens (e.g., from tobacco) that create widespread genetic imprints of preconditioned cancer fields.
- Early detection biomarkers in preconditioned cancer fields should enable translation into precancer detection for active surveillance and chemoprevention.
- There are numerous validated urinary biomarkers for BlCa that have been developed into commercial products.
- Current US FDA-approved BlCa urinary biomarker tests include UroVysion™, NMP22® Bladder Cancer Test, BTA test, and ImmunoCyt™/uCyt™.

References

1. Sidransky D, Von Eschenbach A, Tsai YC, et al. Identification of p53 gene mutations in bladder cancers and urine samples. Science. 1991;252:706–9.
2. Chan MW, Chan LW, Tang NL, et al. Hypermethylation of multiple genes in tumor tissues and voided urine in urinary bladder cancer patients. Clin Cancer Res. 2002;8:464–70.
3. Friedrich MG, Weisenberger DJ, Cheng JC, et al. Detection of methylated apoptosis-associated genes in urine sediments of bladder cancer patients. Clin Cancer Res. 2004;10:7457–65.
4. Dulaimi E, Uzzo RG, Greenberg RE, et al. Detection of bladder cancer in urine by a tumor suppressor gene hypermethylation panel. Clin Cancer Res. 2004;10:1887–93.
5. Hoque MO, Begum S, Topaloglu O, et al. Quantitation of promoter methylation of multiple genes in urine DNA and bladder cancer detection. J Natl Cancer Inst. 2006;98:996–1004.
6. Renard I, Joniau S, van Cleynenbreugel B, et al. Identification and validation of the methylated TWIST1 and NID2 genes through real-time methylation-specific polymerase chain reaction assays for the noninvasive detection of primary bladder cancer in urine samples. Eur Urol. 2010;58:96–104.
7. Chung W, Bondaruk J, Jelinek J, et al. Detection of bladder cancer using novel DNA methylation biomarkers in urine sediments. Cancer Epidemiol Biomark Prev. 2011;20:1483–91.
8. Scher MB, Elbaum MB, Mogilevkin Y, et al. Detecting DNA methylation of the BCL2, CDKN2A and NID2 genes in urine using a nested methylation specific polymerase chain reaction assay to predict bladder cancer. J Urol. 2012;188:2101–7.
9. Zhao Y, Guo S, Sun J, et al. Methylcap-seq reveals novel DNA methylation markers for the diagnosis and recurrence prediction of bladder cancer in a Chinese population. PLoS One. 2012;7:e35175.
10. Chen F, Huang T, Ren Y, et al. Clinical significance of CDH13 promoter methylation as a biomarker for bladder cancer: a meta-analysis. BMC Urol. 2016;16:52.
11. von Knobloch R, Hegele A, Brandt H, et al. Serum DNA and urine DNA alterations of urinary transitional cell bladder carcinoma detected by fluorescent microsatellite analysis. Int J Cancer. 2001;94:67–72.
12. Roupret M, Hupertan V, Yates DR, et al. A comparison of the performance of microsatellite and methylation urine analysis for predicting the recurrence of urothelial cell carcinoma, and definition of a set of markers by Bayesian network analysis. BJU Int. 2008;101:1448–53.

13. Kompier LC, Lurkin I, van der Aa MN, et al. FGFR3, HRAS, KRAS, NRAS and PIK3CA mutations in bladder cancer and their potential as biomarkers for surveillance and therapy. PLoS One. 2010;5:e13821.
14. Holyoake A, O'Sullivan P, Pollock R, et al. Development of a multiplex RNA urine test for the detection and stratification of transitional cell carcinoma of the bladder. Clin Cancer Res. 2008;14:742–9.
15. O'Sullivan P, Sharples K, Dalphin M, et al. A multigene urine test for the detection and stratification of bladder cancer in patients presenting with hematuria. J Urol. 2012;188:741–7.
16. Hanke M, Kausch I, Dahmen G, et al. Detailed technical analysis of urine RNA-based tumor diagnostics reveals ETS2/urokinase plasminogen activator to be a novel marker for bladder cancer. Clin Chem. 2007;53:2070–7.
17. Christoph F, Weikert S, Wolff I, et al. Urinary cytokeratin 20 mRNA expression has the potential to predict recurrence in superficial transitional cell carcinoma of the bladder. Cancer Lett. 2007;245:121–6.
18. Rosser CJ, Liu L, Sun Y, et al. Bladder cancer-associated gene expression signatures identified by profiling of exfoliated urothelia. Cancer Epidemiol Biomark Prev. 2009;18:444–53.
19. Urquidi V, Goodison S, Cai Y, et al. A candidate molecular biomarker panel for the detection of bladder cancer. Cancer Epidemiol Biomark Prev. 2012;21:2149–58.
20. Mengual L, Burset M, Ribal MJ, et al. Gene expression signature in urine for diagnosing and assessing aggressiveness of bladder urothelial carcinoma. Clin Cancer Res. 2010;16:2624–33.
21. Hanke M, Hoefig K, Merz H, et al. A robust methodology to study urine microRNA as tumor marker: microRNA-126 and microRNA-182 are related to urinary bladder cancer. Urol Oncol. 2010;28:655–61.
22. Miah S, Dudziec E, Drayton RM, et al. An evaluation of urinary microRNA reveals a high sensitivity for bladder cancer. Br J Cancer. 2012;107:123–8.
23. Yamada Y, Enokida H, Kojima S, et al. MiR-96 and miR-183 detection in urine serve as potential tumor markers of urothelial carcinoma: correlation with stage and grade, and comparison with urinary cytology. Cancer Sci. 2011;102:522–9.
24. Puerta-Gil P, Garcia-Baquero R, Jia AY, et al. miR-143, miR-222, and miR-452 are useful as tumor stratification and noninvasive diagnostic biomarkers for bladder cancer. Am J Pathol. 2012;180:1808–15.
25. Xiao S, Wang J, Xiao N. MicroRNAs as noninvasive biomarkers in bladder cancer detection: a diagnostic meta-analysis based on qRT-PCR data. Int J Biol Markers. 2016;31:e276–85.
26. Ding M, Li Y, Wang H, et al. Diagnostic value of urinary microRNAs as non-invasive biomarkers for bladder cancer: a meta-analysis. Int J Clin Exp Med. 2015;8:15432–40.
27. Cheng Y, Deng X, Yang X, et al. Urine microRNAs as biomarkers for bladder cancer: a diagnostic meta-analysis. Onco Targets Ther. 2015;8:2089–96.
28. Kutwin P, Konecki T, Borkowska EM, et al. Urine miRNA as a potential biomarker for bladder cancer detection – a meta-analysis. Cent Eur J Urol. 2018;71:177–85.
29. Abogunrin F, O'Kane HF, Ruddock MW, et al. The impact of biomarkers in multivariate algorithms for bladder cancer diagnosis in patients with hematuria. Cancer. 2012;118:2641–50.
30. Margel D, Pevsner-Fischer M, Baniel J, et al. Stress proteins and cytokines are urinary biomarkers for diagnosis and staging of bladder cancer. Eur Urol. 2011;59:113–9.
31. Vlahou A, Schellhammer PF, Mendrinos S, et al. Development of a novel proteomic approach for the detection of transitional cell carcinoma of the bladder in urine. Am J Pathol. 2001;158:1491–502.
32. Theodorescu D, Wittke S, Ross MM, et al. Discovery and validation of new protein biomarkers for urothelial cancer: a prospective analysis. Lancet Oncol. 2006;7:230–40.
33. Chen YT, Chen CL, Chen HW, et al. Discovery of novel bladder cancer biomarkers by comparative urine proteomics using iTRAQ technology. J Proteome Res. 2010;9:5803–15.
34. Yang N, Feng S, Shedden K, et al. Urinary glycoprotein biomarker discovery for bladder cancer detection using LC/MS-MS and label-free quantification. Clin Cancer Res. 2011;17:3349–59.

35. Urquidi V, Goodison S, Kim J, et al. Vascular endothelial growth factor, carbonic anhydrase 9, and angiogenin as urinary biomarkers for bladder cancer detection. Urology. 2012;79:1185 e1181–6.
36. Urquidi V, Goodison S, Ross S, et al. Diagnostic potential of urinary alpha1-antitrypsin and apolipoprotein E in the detection of bladder cancer. J Urol. 2012;188:2377–83.
37. Urquidi V, Kim J, Chang M, et al. CCL18 in a multiplex urine-based assay for the detection of bladder cancer. PLoS One. 2012;7:e37797.
38. Goodison S, Chang M, Dai Y, et al. A multi-analyte assay for the non-invasive detection of bladder cancer. PLoS One. 2012;7:e47469.
39. Myers-Irvin JM, Landsittel D, Getzenberg RH. Use of the novel marker BLCA-1 for the detection of bladder cancer. J Urol. 2005;174:64–8.
40. Cai Q, Wu Y, Guo Z, et al. Urine BLCA-4 exerts potential role in detecting patients with bladder cancers: a pooled analysis of individual studies. Oncotarget. 2015;6:37500–10.
41. Kuang LI, Song WJ, Qing HM, et al. CYFRA21-1 levels could be a biomarker for bladder cancer: a meta-analysis. Genet Mol Res. 2015;14:3921–31.
42. Huang YL, Chen J, Yan W, et al. Diagnostic accuracy of cytokeratin-19 fragment (CYFRA 21-1) for bladder cancer: a systematic review and meta-analysis. Tumour Biol. 2015;36:3137–45.
43. Mi Y, Zhao Y, Shi F, et al. Diagnostic accuracy of urine cytokeratin 20 for bladder cancer: a meta-analysis. Asia Pac J Clin Oncol. 2018;4(4):353–63.
44. Dong F, Shen Y, Xu T, et al. Effectiveness of urine fibronectin as a non-invasive diagnostic biomarker in bladder cancer patients: a systematic review and meta-analysis. World J Surg Oncol. 2018;16:61.
45. Cui X, Jing X, Long C, et al. Accuracy of the urine UCA1 for diagnosis of bladder cancer: a meta-analysis. Oncotarget. 2017;8:35222–33.
46. Masuda N, Ogawa O, Park M, et al. Meta-analysis of a 10-plex urine-based biomarker assay for the detection of bladder cancer. Oncotarget. 2018;9:7101–11.
47. Issaq HJ, Nativ O, Waybright T, et al. Detection of bladder cancer in human urine by metabolomic profiling using high performance liquid chromatography/mass spectrometry. J Urol. 2008;179:2422–6.
48. Pasikanti KK, Esuvaranathan K, Ho PC, et al. Noninvasive urinary metabonomic diagnosis of human bladder cancer. J Proteome Res. 2010;9:2988–95.
49. Putluri N, Shojaie A, Vasu VT, et al. Metabolomic profiling reveals potential markers and bioprocesses altered in bladder cancer progression. Cancer Res. 2011;71:7376–86.
50. Yan TH, Lu SW, Huang YQ, et al. Upregulation of the long noncoding RNA HOTAIR predicts recurrence in stage Ta/T1 bladder cancer. Tumour Biol. 2014;35:10249–57.
51. Berrondo C, Flax J, Kucherov V, et al. Expression of the long non-coding RNA HOTAIR correlates with disease progression in bladder cancer and is contained in bladder cancer patient urinary exosomes. PLoS One. 2016;11:e0147236.
52. Andreu Z, Otta Oshiro R, Redruello A, et al. Extracellular vesicles as a source for non-invasive biomarkers in bladder cancer progression. Eur J Pharm Sci. 2017;98:70–9.
53. Murakami T, Yamamoto CM, Akino T, et al. Bladder cancer detection by urinary extracellular vesicle mRNA analysis. Oncotarget. 2018;9:32810–21.
54. Chou R, Buckley D, Fu R, et al. Emerging approaches to diagnosis and treatment of non-muscle-invasive bladder cancer. Rockville: Agency for Healthcare Research and Quality; 2015.
55. Sathianathen NJ, Butaney M, Weight CJ, et al. Urinary biomarkers in the evaluation of primary hematuria: a systematic review and meta-analysis. Bladder Cancer. 2018;4:353–63.
56. Grossman HB, Soloway M, Messing E, et al. Surveillance for recurrent bladder cancer using a point-of-care proteomic assay. JAMA. 2006;295:299–305.

Chapter 9
Prostate Cancer Biomarkers in Proximal Fluids

9.1 Introduction

Globally, prostate cancer (PrCa) is the most commonly diagnosed non-cutaneous malignancy and a major cause of cancer-related deaths in men. In 2018, the estimated incidence was 1,276,106 with 358,989 case fatalities and 5-year prevalence of 3,724,658 worldwide. The mortality rate falls significantly below the incidence rate, while the prevalence is high, being third (after breast and colorectal cancers). These observations are partly due to intense screening detection of mostly indolent tumors, especially in the more developed world. Consistent with this possibility, most cases of PrCa (about 70%) are diagnosed in the more developed parts of the world such as Australia, New Zealand, North America, and Europe. The geographic regions second to the aforementioned with increased PrCa diagnosis include the Caribbean, South America, and South Africa, with the lowest incidence rate in Asia.

Prostate cancer is screened for by the prostate-specific antigen (PSA) test and digital rectal examination (DRE), whereby an abnormal finding in either of these leads to prostate biopsy for evident histopathologic diagnosis. But because of biopsy sampling errors (because it randomly samples small volume of the gland), false-negative outcomes are concerns to the urologic community. Similarly, clinical trials have shown that the finding and treatment of clinically insignificant tumors is even of a major concern not only from an economic perspective but also the physical and psychological harm it brings to the patient. This heightened evaluation of men over 50 years leads to overdiagnosis and overtreatment.

Similar to breast and other cancers, PrCa is very heterogeneous, with unpredictable disease course. Some tumors may grow slowly (indolent cancers), and yet others can be very aggressive and extremely lethal. Due to the obvious limitations of PSA, and that DRE detected tumors are not early cancers, the need for accurate early detection biomarkers is being actively sort after. Of even much importance are biomarkers that can accurately differentiate between indolent and aggressive can-

G. D. Dakubo, *Cancer Biomarkers in Body Fluids*,
https://doi.org/10.1007/978-3-030-24725-6_9

cers (the Holy Grail PrCa biomarker). Thus, companion diagnostic biomarkers that can be assayed noninvasively, preferably at the community level or at home (point-of-care technologies), will be an extremely helpful armamentarium.

Castrate-resistant PrCa (CRPC) poses a major challenge in PrCa management. Prostate cancers are addicted to androgen signaling for survival. Androgen deprivation is therefore a mainstay therapeutic strategy; however, the PrCa cell eventually becomes resistant to these treatments, which is a major issue with PrCa management. While advances are being made to develop alternate and more effective pharmacologic agents, docetaxel remains the first-line chemotherapeutic agent. Although this treatment has major toxicity issues, only ~50% of men will demonstrate some response. Noninvasive companion diagnostic and predictive biomarkers are needed, and these should be included in drug development protocols.

Because it is obtained following a noninvasive or minimally invasive procedure, urinary biomarkers in proximal fluids for PrCa management are being vehemently explored for clinical utility. A large number of targets, either singly or in combination as panels, have been studied, and some validated and developed into commercial products for PrCa detection and management. Noteworthy, many of the studies are mainly academic, which often involve either small sample sizes or have not been replicated or validated. Therefore, this chapter only examines those markers that are either in use or have shown promise in multiple validation studies.

9.2 Anatomy of the Prostate Gland

The size of the prostate gland varies from a walnut to a small apple. It is located at the bladder neck and the most proximal urethra, the prostatic urethra, into which opens the ejaculatory ducts from the testes. The base abuts the bladder neck and the apex is distal to the bladder. The urethra emerges at the apex of the gland as the membranous urethra. The prostate is composed of tubuloacinar glands embedded in a fibromuscular stroma. A partial capsule surrounds the posterior and lateral aspects, while the apex and anterior are made of glandless fibromuscular stroma. There are three main zones of the prostate gland: the transition zone, made up of only 5% of the gland, surrounds the prostatic urethra, surrounding the ejaculatory ducts is the central zone (20% of the gland), and the remainder of the gland is called the peripheral zone from where most prostate cancer arises (Fig. 9.1). The gland secrets prostatic fluid into semen and also helps urinary flow by its muscular contractions that squeeze the urethra.

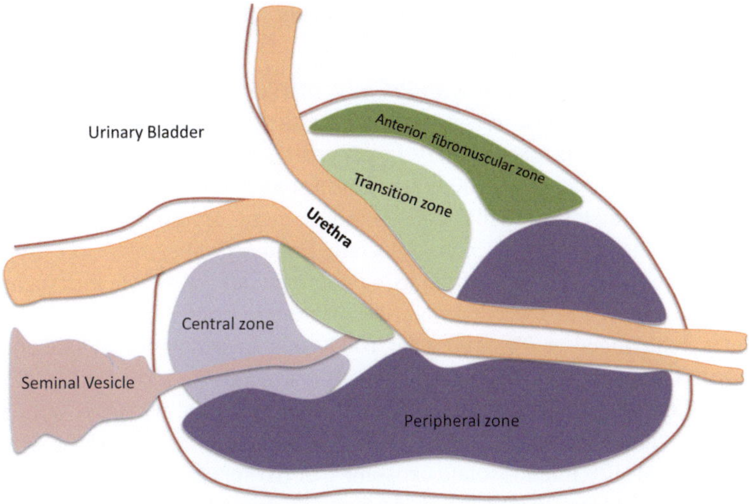

Fig. 9.1 Zones of the prostate gland. PrCa rarely occurs in the anterior zone; however, the few that arise from this zone are difficult to sample by biopsy

9.3 Proximal Fluids for Prostate Cancer Detection

PrCa biomarkers have been explored using different proximal fluid urinary samples. These include midstream urine, first morning catch urine, 12- and 24-h urine collection, catheterized urine, pre- and post-biopsy urine, urine collected after digital rectal examination and prostatic massage (post-DRE urine), and expressed prostatic secretion, which is urine collected by urethral milking following prostate massage. Mostly used for PrCa biomarker assays is post-DRE urine, which simply represents the first-catch urine following an attentive digital examination and massage of the prostate by an expert. The procedure is carried out with the aim of dislodging exfoliated epithelial cells and other prostatic secretions into the urethra such that they will be enriched for in the first-catch urine for PrCa biomarkers. Again, biomarkers explored in this medium should have minimal overlap with other biomarkers of structures of the urinary system. Thus, this fluid is often used to validate PrCa-specific biomarkers.

Post-DRE urine procedure and collection involve attentive digital rectal examination with massage performed by applying at least three strokes per lobe. The patient is then instructed to void the first 20–30 ml of urine into a larger container. The remaining urine is voided. Placing a mark on the container facilitates volumetric accuracy. A pipette is used to transfer the desired amount of urine into a tube to be sent for processing. The volume of required urine depends on test parameters, and the container may contain preservatives. The remaining urine and other materials are discarded appropriately. The container is capped, labeled, and shipped to the processing facility.

9.3.1 Purification of Urinary Exosomes

Urinary exosomes are enriched with PrCa biomarkers. Hence, exosomes purification is used to isolate these for analysis. Prostatic secretions contain at least two types of extracellular vesicles, namely, larger prostasomes (150–500 nm in size) and smaller-sized exosomes (30–100 nm). Prostasomes are normal component of semen. Prostate ductal epithelial cells produce them. Exosomes are cup-shaped structures actively secreted by cells, especially PrCa cells.

Urinary exosomes can be purified using commercially available kits such as the one from Norgen Biotek Corporation or by differential centrifugation. About 30 ml of urine is centrifuged at 300–500 g for 10–20 min to remove cells. The collected supernatant is subjected to further centrifugation at 2000–16,000 g for 15–20 min to remove cellular debris. Exosomes in filtrate can be purified by either (i) filtration through 0.45 um pore-sized filter, followed by ultracentrifugation of filtrate at 100,000 g for 90–120 min to isolate exosomes, or (ii) supernatant that can be underlayed with 30% sucrose/D2O cushion prior to ultracentrifugation. Exosomes in the cushion are then washed with filtered PBS. Purified exosomes can then be stored at −80 °C for later use or used immediately for downstream analysis.

9.4 Issues with Current Prostate Cancer Screening

Uncertainty still lingers on screening for early detection of PrCa, which still relies on PSA testing coupled with digital rectal examination (DRE) for detectable abnormalities in the gland. While not recommended by most medical organizations and institutions, PSA screening is suggested for men 50 years and older and younger men (age 45) who have known PrCa risk factors. For definite diagnosis, a biopsy is obtained for histopathologic examination. Detected cancer is then histologically graded to determine degree of aggression and staged using various imaging modalities to determine management strategies. Prostate biopsies are done under transrectal ultrasound (TRUS) guidance, or MRI-TRUS fusion, which is expected to enhance the accuracy of cancer detection on biopsy. MRI-TRUS fusion technology blends images from MRI and TRUS to provide a 360-degree prostate map to help improve biopsy accuracy.

There are a number of drawbacks in all these screening and diagnostic interventions. The PSA test has limited accuracy as evident from the PCPT trial data whereby out of 9050 men who were biopsied due to abnormal PSA, only 2050 were positive for cancer (22.6% detection rate) [1]. In fact, there is no rational cutoff value of PSA for accurate cancer detection. PSA is a continuous variable, such that even levels <1 ng/ml are associated with 7% risk of PrCa. Thus, urologists use PSA in conjunction with nomograms to improve accuracy; however, primary care physicians do not use nomograms. There is actually no consensus on intervals for PSA testing. Another issue is that PSA kinetics is affected by subclinical prostatitis, which is the commonest cause of variations in PSA levels, especially short-term increases. Moreover, PSA levels are affected by prostatic stimulation from any source (DRE, bike riding), ethnicity, BMI (obesity), sun exposure (levels are low in summer from effects of vitamin D), and age (benign prostatic hyperplasia – BPH). PSA is androgen-dependent, being inhibited by androgen depletion such that men with low testosterone can present with false low PSA. A common and frequently unrecognized cause of androgen depletion is hypogonadism. While an annual PSA rise of 0.75 ng/ml is suggestive of PrCa, normal men do demonstrate such rise and decline in PSA levels.

Thus, any uncertainty triggers a biopsy, such that the biggest utility of PSA is driving urologists to perform biopsies. But elevated PSA with negative biopsy presents a dilemma because of the difficulty with risk estimation. Cancer detection on first biopsy is operator-dependent (average rate is 35%). Anatomically, the anterior part of the gland is not easily accessible to biopsy (many men in active surveillance harbor anterior tumors). Also, the anterolateral horn is not easy to sample using conventional procedures. However, anterior tumors are rearer than posterior tumors. False-negative rate is also high because 25–30% of initial negative biopsies are positive on second biopsy.

Prostate biopsy procedure is also associated with a number of complications. These include hematuria and hematospermia that can last for months and are worrisome to patients. Urosepsis is another concern. The push to increase the number of biopsy cores, in association with emerging drug (e.g., quinolones)-resistant strains, increases the incidence of sepsis post-biopsy. Many urosepsis cases (about 10%) are treated as outpatients, but significant cases requiring hospitalization are on the rise. Biopsy of the prostate gland can also cause voiding symptoms such as frequency, urgency, nocturia, and dysuria, and multiple biopsies (three or more) can cause erectile dysfunction. Many men refuse a second biopsy because of the pain and possible complications associated with the initial procedure. Local anesthesia is not always effective, and the skill set of the urologist is paramount to efficacious anesthesia.

Finally, diagnosing PrCa in biopsy encounters a number of challenges, especially when the tumor foci are small. There is interobserver variability. Diagnosing atypical small acinar proliferation requires expertise that not all pathologists possess. Also, mimickers of PrCa including atrophy, post-atrophic hyperplasia, granulomatous and xanthogranulomatous prostatitis, and malakoplakia may confound diagnosis. Thus, uncertainty case rates are probably high (6–14%). Sample mix-up could potentially lead to unnecessary treatment.

All these issues with PrCa screening and diagnosis call for better biomarkers for PrCa detection. Of even much relevance will be noninvasive biomarkers (the Holy Grail biomarker) that could inform at diagnosis as to the future indolence vs. aggressive behavior of the tumor.

9.5 Prostate Cancer Biomarkers in Proximal Fluids

There is a plethora of identified PrCa biomarkers. However, as with biomarker translation in general, only a few appear promising as many fail during validation. Promising urinary PrCa biomarkers include prostate cancer antigen 3 (PCA3), transmembrane protease, serine 2 (TMPRSS2), ETS-related gene (ERG), SAM pointed domain ETS transcription factor (SPDEF), second chromosome locus associated with prostate-1 (SChLAP1), homeobox C6 (HOXC6), and distal-less homeobox 1 (DLX1). Developed into commercially available PrCa assays are PCA3 as a single biomarker (Progensa PCA3 or uPM3™), exosomal PCA3, ERG, and SPDEF as a panel biomarker (ExoDx), and HOXC6 and DLX1 as panel biomarker (SelectMDx). In development are PCA3, TMPRSS2-ERG, and PSA panel assay (Mi-Prostate Score or MiPS) and SChLAP1 and TMPRSS2-ERG as single biomarker assays. While all these assays have diagnostic utility, only ExoDx (due to SPDEF) and SChLAP1 have associated prognostic potential.

9.5.1 DNA Methylation as Prostate Cancer Biomarkers in Proximal Fluids

There have been extensive investigations on gene promoter methylation biomarkers in PrCa. Of the numerous potential genes, GSTP1 has been the most extensively studied with potential noninvasive utility. GSTP1 is a detoxification enzyme involved in catalyzing the conjugation of hydrophobic and electrophilic molecules that contain reduced glutathione. The four isoforms of GSTP1 are alpha (α), mu (μ), pi (π), and theta (θ). GSTP1 is involved in xenobiotic (substances foreign to the body) metabolism, which may explain why its loss of function is associated with cancer.

As a PrCa biomarker, promoter methylation of GSTP1 (mGSTP1) is absent in over 90% of PrCa. Moreover, as a possible early detection biomarker, mGSTP1 is detectable in 70% of prostatic intraepithelial neoplasia (PIN) and 6% of proliferative inflammatory atrophy (PIA). Methylated GSTP1 has been detected in ejaculates and urine from PrCa patients [2–5]. As a urinary biomarker for PrCa, mGSTP1 has been studied with various clinical potential. Goessl et al. demonstrated mGSTP1 in urinary sediments from 2% of BPH, 29% of PIN, 68% of early intracapsular PrCa, and as many as 78% of locally advanced or systemic PrCa [4]. The diagnostic performance yielded a sensitivity and specificity of 73% and 98%, respectively. In 100 men referred for core needle biopsy for suspicion of PrCa, the sensitivity and specificity of urinary mGSTP1 were 75% and 98%, respectively, which contrasted with a sensitivity of 88% and specificity of 91% using biopsy samples [6]. A significant difference of mGSTP1 was uncovered between stage III (100%) and II (20%) disease patients ($p = 0.05$). Large-scale multicenter study is needed to establish the clinical utility of urinary mGSTP1 in PrCa.

Meta-analyses have been performed to evaluate the performances of some urinary methylated biomarkers. *GSTP1* promoter methylation was analyzed in six body fluids (plasma, serum, blood, urine, ejaculate, and prostatic secretions) as PrCa screening biomarker [7]. Pooled specificity in plasma, serum, and urine was 89% at a sensitivity of 52%. While sensitivity was comparable to PSA, the high specificity of *GSTP1* methylation in plasma, serum, and urine could complement PSA testing. The association of *RASSF1A* promoter methylation and PrCa was reviewed and meta-analyzed using 19 studies [8]. Promoter methylation was associated with PrCa risk (OR = 9.58) and Gleason score (OR = 2.58). Subgroup analysis indicated tissue rather than urinary *RASSF1A* methylation was associated with Gleason score (OR = 3.09), PSA (OR = 2.75), and tumor stage (OR = 1.74). Thus, tissue *RASSF1A* methylation could augment PrCa diagnosis and possible prognostication. Should this demonstrate PrCa "field cancerization," it could be useful for determining and guiding rebiopsy decisions.

9.5.2 Genetic Alterations as Prostate Cancer Biomarkers in Proximal Fluids

A number of fusion genes have been discovered to mediate PrCa biology and have served as useful biomarkers in PrCa detection. The transmembrane protease, serine 2 (TMPRSS2) and ETS-related gene (ERG) map to chromosome 21q22 and are separated by less than 3 megabase of DNA. In a large percentage of PrCa (40–78%), and some PIN lesions (21%), intergenic deletion of segments between these two genes leads to the TMPRSS-ERG fusion rearrangement. Other rearrangements of these genes account for the remaining fusion products in PrCa. While the most common fusion gene in PrCa, the prevalence appears to be dependent on ethnicity.

The ETS gene family is differentially expressed in PrCa. Using a novel bioinformatic tool referred to as "cancer outlier profile analysis (COPA)," a strong outlier profile of ERG and ETS variant gene 1 (ETV1) were uncovered in 57% of PrCa samples [9]. Indeed, overexpression of ERG was demonstrated in 72% of PrCa. Further investigation found that the 5' untranslated region of the androgen-regulated TMPRSS2 gene was fused to ERG or ETV1 in a majority (>90%) of PrCa that overexpressed these ETS genes. Other ETS family members, including ETV4 and ETV5, are also fused to TMPRSS2; however, the overexpression frequencies of these genes in PrCa are lower than ERG. A noninvasive detection of TMPRSS-ERG in urine has been developed. In a pilot study, this fusion gene was absent in urinary samples from healthy young men, females, and post-radical prostatectomy patients. However, it was present in 34.8% of samples from PrCa patients and 18.2% of men with negative biopsy outcomes [10]. A systematic review of 18 studies on urinary TMPRSS2-ERG fusion for PrCa detection was conducted [11]. Meta-analysis was performed on 15 of the 18 studies, of which 9 showed unclear risk of bias. The odds ratio (OR) was 2.24 for the association of the PrCa with TMPRSS2-ERG fusion. In regard to samples, urine had the best OR of 2.79, and this increased to 3.55 when detecting DNA template. Thus, urinary TMPRSS2-ERG DNA molecular assay had diagnostic value for PrCa.

The prognostic relevance of TMPRSS-ERG in PrCa remains unclear. TMPRSS-ERG levels in post-DRE urine have been positively correlated with elevated serum PSA, Gleason score, and pathological stage and also associated with Gleason score $\geq$ 7 (indicative of clinically significant PrCa) and PrCa mortality. The increased urinary levels were associated with Epstein criteria for significant PrCa, which include tumor volume, Gleason score, percentage of cancer per core biopsy, and number of positive cores. Thus, cancer-specific mortality has been associated with TMPRSS-ERG expression [12]. TMPRSS-ERG biomarker levels improved the predictive accuracy of Gleason score and stage of the European Randomized Study of Screening for Prostate Cancer risk calculator (ERSPCrc) [13]. Other studies could associate TMPRSS2-ERG and PCA3 in increased detection of PrCa, but failed to uncover a correlation of TMPRSS2-ERG with Gleason score [14, 15].

Notably, the value of TMPRSS-ERG and PCA3 in PrCa detection may differ among ethnic or racial groups, because African-American men appear not to benefit from PrCa detection using these biomarkers [16]. Also, while TMPRSS-ERG fusion is less frequent (at 11%) in China, a different fusion gene product, TTTY15-USP9Y was identified in post-DRE urine from 226 Chinese men with PrCa. In preliminary diagnostic evaluation, elevated urinary TTTY15-USP9Y fusion product achieved a high AUROCC of 0.828 [17]. In addition, incorporating TTTY15-USP9Y score in models involving patient age, PSA levels, and prostate volume could have prevented unnecessary prostate biopsies. Combining TTTY15-USP9Y score and PSA levels significantly ($p = 0.001$) improved PrCa detection.

9.5.3 Gene Transcript Alterations as Prostate Cancer Biomarkers in Proximal Fluids

9.5.3.1 Coding Transcripts

Microarray analysis enabled discovery of dysregulated transcripts in PrCa. Of the 39 potential PrCa biomarkers discovered, 8 (*HOXC4*, *HOXC6*, *DLX1*, *TDRD1*, *ONECUT2*, *NKAIN1*, *MS4A8B,* and *PPFIA2*) were elevated in urinary precipitate from PrCa patients compared to non-cancer controls [18]. HOXC6 on chromosome 12 and DLX1 on chromosome 2 are two homeobox genes that demonstrated upregulated expression in PrCa [19]. HOXC6 plays a role in epithelial proliferation. Tudor domain containing 1 (TDRD1) is a target of ERG and is upregulated in concert with ERG in PrCa. Differential transcript levels of *HOXC6*, *DLX1*, and *TDRD1* in urine for PrCa detection, monitoring of progression, and response have been validated in a multicenter study [18]. The performance of the three-gene panel for predicting aggressive PrCa (AUROCC of 0.77) was much superior to PSA (AUROCC of 0.72) and PCA3 (AUROCC of 0.68). The predictive accuracy was further enhanced to AUROCC of 0.81 by incorporating PSA levels. Urinary HOXC6 levels were significantly higher in men with PrCa than those with negative biopsies. The potential clinical utility of urinary HOXC6 mRNA led to the development of HOXC6 assay for PrCa detection and monitoring [19].

9.5.3.2 Noncoding Transcripts

Both long and short noncoding RNAs are found dysregulated in PrCa. Promising lncRNA for noninvasive PrCa management are PCA3 and *SChLAP1*. Prostate cancer gene 3 (PCA3), also known as "differential display code 3" (DD3), is a PrCa biomarker established to aid in PrCa management. Given the issues encountered in current prostate cancer diagnosis, PCA3 performance will help urologists stratify patients for invasive procedures, thus reducing patient anxiety, pain, and waste of healthcare resources. Bussemaker et al. identified PCA3 in 1999 using differential display, and its overexpression in PrCa was demonstrated using northern blot analysis [20]. PCA3 is a PrCa-specific biomarker because of its exclusive overexpression in PrCa. Analysis of tissue samples revealed overexpression in over 90% of localized and metastatic PrCa samples. Located on chromosome 9q21.1, PCA3 encodes a long nonprotein transcript. This realization came from analysis of the open reading frame (ORF), which revealed many exonic stop codons. The lack of protein expression prompted methodological developments to measure the noncoding PCA3 transcript in clinical samples.

Urinary PCA3 has been extensively investigated and validated to establish its clinical utility or intended use. An initial sensitive PCR assay was developed to enable detection and measurement of low-level expression on the background of numerous normal cells. A median 66-fold overexpression in PrCa compared to normal prostatic tissues was uncovered using fluorescent-based qRT-PCR assay. Indeed, in prostatic tissue samples with less than 10% cancer cells, an 11-fold overexpression was demonstrated, indicating the feasibility of translating this platform technology using body fluid samples with diluted targets. Expectedly, PCA3 was measurable in post-DRE void urinary sediments from men suspected of having PrCa based on elevated PSA (> 3.0 ng/ml). In comparison to biopsy diagnosis in this cohort of 108 men at risk, the sensitivity and specificity were 67% and 83%, respectively. The NPV was 90%, indicating its utility could reduce the number of repeat biopsy procedures. Gen-Probe Inc., the then exclusive global license holder, transferred and optimized the assay using its transcript-mediated amplification (TMA) APTIMA technology. The PCA3 assay, also known as Progensa® PCA3 in Europe, has a predictive score, which is a ratio of PCA3 to PSA transcripts (PCA3/PSA × 1000). A score of >35 achieved a sensitivity and specificity of 66% and 76%, respectively. PSA sensitivity was 65% in this cohort, but with a dismal specificity of 47%. Thus, various scores (20, 35, and 50) have been examined with different accuracies. The urinary PCA3 test has been developed into US FDA-approved product indicated for men with negative biopsy outcomes despite elevated PSA levels. In a multicenter study, both PCA3 and TMPRSS-ERG added significant predictive value to the ERSPC risk calculator [15]. The AUROCC increased from 0.799 to 0.833, when PCA3 was added to the calculator, and to 0.842 when both PCA3 and TMPRSS-ERG were included. However, only TMPRSS-ERG added value to the ERSPC calculator in predicting Gleason score and clinical tumor stage. PCA3 has also been incorporated in nomograms for PrCa detection on initial biopsy. In a nomogram with age, serum PSA, prostate volume, and PCA3, PrCa detection improved by 4.5–7.1% [21, 22]. In the REDUCE trial, PCA3 scores were significantly associated with positive rebiopsy and correlated with Gleason scores [23].

The performance of urinary PCA3 has been subjected to numerous meta-analyses, with consistent proven results. Performance of urinary PCA3 scores for accurate detection of PrCa was analyzed in 9 studies with 1721 suspected PrCa individuals [24]. The pooled sensitivity, specificity, AUROCC, and Q-value were 83%, 40%, 3.11, 0.6842, and 0.6404 for PCA3 score of 20. A score of 35 sacrificed sensitivity (66%), DOR (2.84), and SAUROCC (0.6715) for specificity (63%). Thus, the diagnostic accuracy was high for PCA3 score of 20. Systematic review and meta-analysis of PCA3 scores for making repeat biopsy decision included 11 studies of moderate to high quality, although study heterogeneity was uncovered [25]. The SAUROCC for a PCA3 score of 20 for PrCa inclusive of was 0.81–0.85.

Multiple reviews have demonstrated the clinical utility of PCA3 in making accurate rebiopsy decisions. Systematic review and meta-analysis of urinary PCA3 in PrCa detection included 46 clinical trials with 12,295 subjects [26]. Pooled sensitivity, specificity, PLR, NLR, DOR, and AUROCC were 65%, 73%, 2.23, 0.48, 5.31, and 0.75, respectively, indicating moderate potential as a diagnostic biomarker. Another meta-analysis of urinary PCA3 for PrCa diagnosis included 13 trials with 3245 study subjects [27]. Pooled sensitivity, specificity, PLR, NLR, DOR, and AUROCC were 62%, 75%, 6.16, 0.50, 5.49, and 0.75, respectively. Systematic review and meta-analysis of urinary PCA3 for making prostate rebiopsy decision achieved pooled sensitivity, specificity, PLR, NLR, DOR, and AUROCC of 82%, 96.2%, 2.36, 0.51, 4.89, and 0.7441 [25], indicating its diagnostic potential in avoiding unnecessary biopsies. Another systematic review and meta-analysis of urinary PCA3 included 14 studies of moderate to high quality [28]. Pooled sensitivity, specificity, PLR, and NLR were 85%, 96%, 22.21, and 0.15, respectively. This was acceptably accurate for PrCa detection. Thus, this biomarker was subjected to extensive scrutiny before clinical translation.

SChLAP1, also called LINC00913, is associated with PrCa biology. Prensner et al. first characterized this lncRNA and showed it to promote development of PrCa by inhibiting the tumor suppressor complex, SWI/SNF [29]. Of clinical relevance, SChLAP1 expression is associated with more aggressive PrCa. High levels of SChLAP1 expression were significantly correlated with increasing Gleason score and tumor stage ($P < 0.005$) and increased time to development of lethal PrCa [30]. Moreover, SChLAP1 expression levels could significantly predict PrCa metastasis within 10 years [31]. A commercial assay of SChLAP1 for PrCa screening is yet to become available.

Several miRNAs demonstrate differential levels in various media between PrCa and healthy men. Consistently evaluated and found to have clinical utility are circulating miRNA-141 and miR-375. Levels of these two miRNAs in circulation have been associated with Gleason scores, metastasis, and lymph node status. Circulating miRNA-141 was 46-fold elevated in circulation of metastatic PrCa patients compared to healthy controls. Evidence also suggest these miRNAs are microvesicular or exosomal because levels of both miRNAs are increased in these microparticles of cancer patients.

miRNAs have also been explored in urinary samples from PrCa patients. miR-107, miR-141, miR-200b, miR-375, and miR-574-3b have showed differential levels in urinary samples from PrCa patients and healthy control men. While urinary miR-141 and miR-375 were not discriminatory as their circulating levels did, levels of miR-107 and miR-574-3p were significantly higher in patients than controls. Due to protocol and methodological differences, consensus data on urinary miRNA for PrCa are missing. Consistently evaluated to exhibit differential levels are miR-21, miR-141, miR-200b, miR-221, and miR-375. However, demonstrating their clinical utility has been problematic. For example, levels of miR-21 and miR-375 were decreased in urine from PrCa patients [32], while elevated miR-375 was associated with stages of PrCa [33]. Further studies are needed to establish their role in PrCa.

9.5.4 Alpha-Methylacyl-CoA Racemase as Prostate Cancer Biomarker

Alpha-methylacyl-CoA racemase (AMACR) is an enzyme involved in peroxisomal β-oxidation of branched-chain fatty acids from dietary meat and dairy products. The mRNA of this gene is overexpressed up to ninefold in PrCa compared to normal prostatic tissues. Consistently, elevated levels of AMACR protein has been demonstrated in PrCa. A diagnostic performance study of needle biopsy samples by immunohistochemistry achieved a sensitivity of 97% at a perfect specificity of 100%. Basal cell hyperplasia, atrophic glands, urothelial cells, or metaplasia is devoid of AMACR overexpression, which enhances its specificity for PrCa detection.

Technologies have been developed to assay AMACR in various body fluid samples for PrCa detection and management. Immunoassays were developed for assaying AMACR in tissue and serum samples. An AMACR activity assay using extracts from PrCa needle biopsies performed at detecting PrCa with sensitivity and specificity of 92.3% and 89.2%, respectively. A serum immunoreactivity assay also achieved good performance in differentiating PrCa patients from healthy controls at a sensitivity of 61.6% and specificity of 71.8%. Urinary assays include protein and transcript detection by Western blot and RT-PCR analysis, respectively. A Western blot analysis of post-DRE urine was successful at PrCa detection achieving a sensitivity and specificity, PPV, and NPV of 100%, 58%, 72%, and 88%, respectively. Detection of AMACR transcripts in post-DRE urine has been demonstrated with possible utility in identifying men with significant disease. A multiplex assay of AMACR transcript detection and PCA3 scores could successfully detect PrCa at a sensitivity and specificity of 81% and 84%, respectively, which is an immense improvement of using only urinary PCA3 score.

9.5.5 Prostate-Specific Membrane Antigen as Prostate Cancer Biomarker

Prostate epithelial cells express the transmembrane glycoprotein, prostate-specific membrane antigen (PSMA), and the levels are much higher in PrCa than benign prostatic tissues. PSMA can therefore be considered a PrCa biomarker. Elevated levels correlate with some clinicopathologic features including pathological stage, tumor grade, aneuploidy, and biochemical recurrence. However, the lack of sensitive immunoassay has hampered its clinical translation. Because PSMA mRNA levels also correlate with protein levels, a combination of ProteinChip arrays and SELDI-TOF MS technologies enabled quantification of PSMA in serum samples. Preliminary analysis revealed higher mean PSMA levels in men with PrCa than BPH. Prostate epithelial cells also express a spliced variant of PSMA, PSM. Because expression of PSM is much higher than PSMA in normal prostatic tissues, while PSMA levels are higher than PSM in PrCa tissues, a ratio of PSMA to PSM indicates disease progression, which suggest a prognostic role for this ratio. In post-DRE urinary sediments, PSMA was superior to PCA3 and PSGR in disease prediction. At a defined specificity of 70%, PSMA, PCA3, and PSGR achieved sensitivities of 64%, 46%, and 61%, respectively, in PrCa detection. A multiplex assay of the three genes enhanced the sensitivity to 68% at the same specificity of 70%. PSMA has also been targeted therapeutically with development of immunotherapeutic agents, radionucleotides, and targeted toxins.

9.5.6 Urinary Exosomes as Prostate Cancer Biomarkers

Exosomes are shed into urine, and their levels are much higher in PrCa patients than healthy men. The biomarker potential of urinary exosomes stems from their stability in urine as well as being enriched with tissue-specific biomolecules. Urinary exosomes collected after prostatic massage is enriched for coding and noncoding transcripts. TMPRSS-ERG gene fusion, PSA, and PCA3 are among transcripts that have been detected in exosomes from PrCa patients. Exosomal TMPRSS-ERG fusion gene biomolecules correlate with higher Gleason scores. Androgen deprivation therapy (ADT) appears to have a negative effect on the abundance of urinary exosomes, because ADT was associated with loss of expression of androgen-regulated molecules including TMPRSS-ERG, PCA3, and PSA. The loss of expression of these biomolecules correlated with response to ADT and disease regression. Methodological refinements should enhance recovery and analysis of urinary exosomes for clinical translation.

9.6 Clinical Translation of Commercial Products

9.6.1 PRoGensa

The Progensa® PCA3 assay is a urine-based in vitro nucleic acid amplification test for predicting PrCa on rebiopsy. The assay measures the concentration of PCA3 and PSA transcripts and calculates the ratio of PCA3 RNA molecules to PSA RNA molecules (PCA3 Score) in post-digital rectal exam (DRE) first-catch male urine specimens. The test result is indicated for use in conjunction with other patient information to aid in the decision for repeat biopsy in men 50 years of age or older who have had one or more previous negative prostate biopsies and for whom a repeat biopsy would be recommended by a urologist based on current standard of care. The PCA3 score cutoff is 25, meaning a reduced likelihood of cancer detection upon rebiopsy if the score is <25. Collected urine is chilled at 2–8 °C and transferred to urine specimen transport tube within 4 h of collection. Freezing of unprocessed specimen is unacceptable.

9.6.2 ExoDx Assay

The ExoDx assay is a urine test based on exosomal cargo. The assay targets expression of ERG, PCA3, and SPDEF. Elevated levels of SPDEF correlate with increased PrCa aggressiveness and metastatic potential [34]. Combination of the ExoDx panel with PSA, age, race, and family history could better predict significant PrCa (GS ≥ 7) than these parameters alone. Additionally, this panel could help prevent 27% of biopsies. At a sensitivity of 92%, only 8% of GS ≥ 7 cancers could have been missed [35]. A commercial launch was in September 2016, and the test is currently only available from the manufacturer and performed in a certified Clinical Laboratory Improvement Amendments (CLIA) laboratory. It has yet to be approved by the FDA.

9.6.3 SelectMDx Assay

SelectMDx is a commercially available PrCa assay targeting urinary expression levels of *HOXC6* and *DLX1,* which are normalized to *PSA* mRNA. HOXC6 and DLX1 could accurately predict clinically significant PrCa with an overall AUROCC of 0.76 [36]. The performance improved to AUROCC of 0.90 when combined with PSA density, DRE results, previous biopsy, PSA, family history, and age [37]. Although available, this is still an investigational assay yet to be approved by the FDA.

9.6.4 Michigan Prostate Score

The Michigan Prostate Score (MiPS) is currently in development and not yet commercially available due to the need to perform cost-benefit analyses. It is a panel assay targeting expression of PCA3, TMPRSS2-ERG, and PSA in urine. The assay is based on a score generated after transcription-mediated amplification of the target genes. The TMPRSS2-ERG and PCA3 levels are normalized to PSA levels, and the score is generated using a multivariable regression model. Studies have demonstrated the clinical utility of the MiPS. First, the MiPS could better predict the presence of both PrCa and significant PrCa (AUROCC of 0.751) than PSA alone (AUROCC of 0.585), PCA3 and PSA (AUROCC of 0.726), and TMPRSS2-ERG and PSA (AUROCC of 0.693) [38]. Second, incorporating the MiPS into PCPT nomogram could lead to avoidance of 35–47% of biopsies while missing the diagnosis of 1–2.3% of clinically significant PrCa.

9.7 Summary

- Cancer of the prostate gland is an age-associated affliction that is the most commonly diagnosed male malignancy globally.
- While not generally recommended, PSA testing remains the screening tool for early detection of PrCa.
- Due to its low accuracy, the PSA test leads to a number of biopsies that harbor indolent cancers.
- Diagnosis of indolent and insignificant cancers leads to overdiagnosis and possible overtreatment.
- Expressed prostatic fluid in urine following attentive DRE and prostate massage is enriched with prostate-specific biomarkers including PCA3, TMPRSS-ERG, HOXC6, DLX1, TDRD1, AMACR, PSMA, and Exosomal cargo.
- Some of these biomarkers have been validated and developed into commercially available PrCa tests.
- Emerging PrCa biomarkers include miRNAs such as miR-141 and miR-375.
- Commercially available PrCa proximal fluid biomarker tests include Progensa® (targets PCA3 transcripts), SelectMDx (targets HOXC6 and DLX1 transcripts), and ExoDx (targets exosomal PCA3, SPDEF, and ERG transcripts).

References

1. Thompson IM, Klein EA, Lippman SM, et al. Prevention of prostate cancer with finasteride: US/European perspective. Eur Urol. 2003;44:650–5.
2. Goessl C, Krause H, Muller M, et al. Fluorescent methylation-specific polymerase chain reaction for DNA-based detection of prostate cancer in bodily fluids. Cancer Res. 2000;60:5941–5.
3. Goessl C, Muller M, Heicappell R, et al. DNA-based detection of prostate cancer in urine after prostatic massage. Urology. 2001;58:335–8.
4. Goessl C, Muller M, Heicappell R, et al. DNA-based detection of prostate cancer in blood, urine, and ejaculates. Ann N Y Acad Sci. 2001;945:51–8.
5. Cairns P, Esteller M, Herman JG, et al. Molecular detection of prostate cancer in urine by GSTP1 hypermethylation. Clin Cancer Res. 2001;7:2727–30.
6. Woodson K, O'Reilly KJ, Hanson JC, et al. The usefulness of the detection of GSTP1 methylation in urine as a biomarker in the diagnosis of prostate cancer. J Urol. 2008;179:508–11; discussion 511-502
7. Wu T, Giovannucci E, Welge J, et al. Measurement of GSTP1 promoter methylation in body fluids may complement PSA screening: a meta-analysis. Br J Cancer. 2011;105:65–73.
8. Ge YZ, Xu LW, Jia RP, et al. The association between RASSF1A promoter methylation and prostate cancer: evidence from 19 published studies. Tumour Biol. 2014;35:3881–90.
9. Tomlins SA, Rhodes DR, Perner S, et al. Recurrent fusion of TMPRSS2 and ETS transcription factor genes in prostate cancer. Science. 2005;310:644–8.
10. Laxman B, Tomlins SA, Mehra R, et al. Noninvasive detection of TMPRSS2:ERG fusion transcripts in the urine of men with prostate cancer. Neoplasia. 2006;8:885–8.
11. Garcia-Perdomo HA, Chaves MJ, Osorio JC, Sanchez A. Association between TMPRSS2:ERG fusion gene and the prostate cancer: systematic review and meta-analysis. Cent Eur J Urol. 2018;71:410–9.
12. Hagglof C, Hammarsten P, Stromvall K, et al. TMPRSS2-ERG expression predicts prostate cancer survival and associates with stromal biomarkers. PLoS One. 2014;9:e86824.
13. Wei JT, Feng Z, Partin AW, et al. Can urinary PCA3 supplement PSA in the early detection of prostate cancer? J Clin Oncol. 2014;32:4066–72.
14. Cornu JN, Cancel-Tassin G, Egrot C, et al. Urine TMPRSS2:ERG fusion transcript integrated with PCA3 score, genotyping, and biological features are correlated to the results of prostatic biopsies in men at risk of prostate cancer. Prostate. 2013;73:242–9.
15. Leyten GH, Hessels D, Jannink SA, et al. Prospective multicentre evaluation of PCA3 and TMPRSS2-ERG gene fusions as diagnostic and prognostic urinary biomarkers for prostate cancer. Eur Urol. 2014;65:534–42.
16. O'Malley PG, Nguyen DP, Al Hussein Al Awamlh B, et al. Racial variation in the utility of urinary biomarkers PCA3 and T2ERG in a large multicenter study. J Urol. 2017;198:42–9.
17. Zhu Y, Ren S, Jing T, et al. Clinical utility of a novel urine-based gene fusion TTTY15-USP9Y in predicting prostate biopsy outcome. Urol Oncol. 2015;33(384):e389–20.
18. Leyten GH, Hessels D, Smit FP, et al. Identification of a candidate gene panel for the early diagnosis of prostate cancer. Clin Cancer Res. 2015;21:3061–70.
19. Hamid AR, Hoogland AM, Smit F, et al. The role of HOXC6 in prostate cancer development. Prostate. 2015;75:1868–76.
20. Bussemakers MJ, van Bokhoven A, Verhaegh GW, et al. DD3: a new prostate-specific gene, highly overexpressed in prostate cancer. Cancer Res. 1999;59:5975–9.
21. Hansen J, Auprich M, Ahyai SA, et al. Initial prostate biopsy: development and internal validation of a biopsy-specific nomogram based on the prostate cancer antigen 3 assay. Eur Urol. 2013;63:201–9.
22. Greene DJ, Elshafei A, Nyame YA, et al. External validation of a PCA-3-based nomogram for predicting prostate cancer and high-grade cancer on initial prostate biopsy. Prostate. 2016;76:1019–23.

23. Aubin SM, Reid J, Sarno MJ, et al. PCA3 molecular urine test for predicting repeat prostate biopsy outcome in populations at risk: validation in the placebo arm of the dutasteride REDUCE trial. J Urol. 2010;184:1947–52.
24. Jiang Z, Zhao Y, Tian Y. Comparison of diagnostic efficacy by two urine PCA3 scores in prostate cancer patients undergoing repeat biopsies: a meta-analysis. Minerva Urol Nefrol. 2018; https://doi.org/10.23736/S0393-2249.18.03093-X.
25. Luo Y, Gou X, Huang P, Mou C. Prostate cancer antigen 3 test for prostate biopsy decision: a systematic review and meta analysis. Chin Med J. 2014;127:1768–74.
26. Cui Y, Cao W, Li Q, et al. Evaluation of prostate cancer antigen 3 for detecting prostate cancer: a systematic review and meta-analysis. Sci Rep. 2016;6:25776.
27. Xue WJ, Ying XL, Jiang JH, Xu YH. Prostate cancer antigen 3 as a biomarker in the urine for prostate cancer diagnosis: a meta-analysis. J Cancer Res Ther. 2014;10(Suppl):C218–21.
28. Ruiz-Aragon J, Marquez-Pelaez S. Assessment of the PCA3 test for prostate cancer diagnosis: a systematic review and meta-analysis. Actas Urol Esp. 2010;34:346–55.
29. Prensner JR, Iyer MK, Sahu A, et al. The long noncoding RNA SChLAP1 promotes aggressive prostate cancer and antagonizes the SWI/SNF complex. Nat Genet. 2013;45:1392–8.
30. Mehra R, Udager AM, Ahearn TU, et al. Overexpression of the long non-coding RNA SChLAP1 independently predicts lethal prostate cancer. Eur Urol. 2016;70:549–52.
31. Prensner JR, Zhao S, Erho N, et al. RNA biomarkers associated with metastatic progression in prostate cancer: a multi-institutional high-throughput analysis of SChLAP1. Lancet Oncol. 2014;15:1469–80.
32. Koppers-Lalic D, Hackenberg M, de Menezes R, et al. Noninvasive prostate cancer detection by measuring miRNA variants (isomiRs) in urine extracellular vesicles. Oncotarget. 2016;7:22566–78.
33. Stuopelyte K, Daniunaite K, Bakavicius A, et al. The utility of urine-circulating miRNAs for detection of prostate cancer. Br J Cancer. 2016;115:707–15.
34. Osisami M, Keller ET. SPDEF: a molecular switch for E-cadherin expression that promotes prostate cancer metastasis. Asian J Androl. 2013;15:584–5.
35. McKiernan J, Donovan MJ, O'Neill V, et al. A novel urine exosome gene expression assay to predict high-grade prostate cancer at initial biopsy. JAMA Oncol. 2016;2:882–9.
36. Chan DW, Hui WW, Wang JJ, et al. DLX1 acts as a crucial target of FOXM1 to promote ovarian cancer aggressiveness by enhancing TGF-beta/SMAD4 signaling. Oncogene. 2017;36:1404–16.
37. Van Neste L, Hendriks RJ, Dijkstra S, et al. Detection of high-grade prostate cancer using a urinary molecular biomarker-based risk score. Eur Urol. 2016;70:740–8.
38. Tomlins SA, Day JR, Lonigro RJ, et al. Urine TMPRSS2:ERG plus PCA3 for individualized prostate cancer risk assessment. Eur Urol. 2016;70:45–53.

Chapter 10
Ovarian Cancer Biomarkers in Proximal Fluids

10.1 Introduction

Globally, 295,414 women were estimated to be diagnosed with OvCa (OvCa) in 2018, while in the same year, as many as 184,799 women died from the disease. This mortality rate is on the rise, because the 2012 (140,000) and 2018 (184,000) estimates are up from 113,000 in 1990. OvCa is the most lethal gynecological cancer and, globally, is the eighth cause of cancer-related deaths in women. In 2018, the US estimated cases were 22,240 with 14,070 deaths. There are geographic variations in the incidence rates, with rates being higher in the more developed than the less developed parts of the world. For example, the rate of 11.7/100,000 women in the UK contrasts sharply with that of 4.1/100,000 for other parts of the world.

The 5-year survival rate for women diagnosed with OvCa has increased over the past decades due to improved gynecologic surgical techniques, coupled with combination therapies, but not due to early detection. While established that early detection of organ-confined tumor (stage I) has the best prognosis, OvCa is rarely detected early. Indeed, only about 15% are localized cancers, with the vast majority presenting with some regional spread (about 18%) or worse still distant metastasis (about 60%). The survival rate can be as high as 92% for organ-confined early-stage disease. This survival rate drops significantly to under 30%, when cancers spread to the peritoneum or distant organs. The need for early detection biomarkers is thus obvious. Because there are no recommended screening procedures, coupled with the need for early and appropriate treatment, the "risk malignancy index" (RMI) was established in 1990. This risk index includes ultrasound detection of pelvic masses, elevated serum CA125, and menopausal status. While RMI has a good sensitivity (71–88%) and a high specificity (74–97%), only women considered to be of above-average risk receive such periodic screening, leaving many, especially premenopausal women without any screening, though OvCa occurs in about 30% of this population. Indeed, while commonly diagnosed in women above age 55 years, the incidence rises from about age 35 to 39 years.

G. D. Dakubo, *Cancer Biomarkers in Body Fluids*,
https://doi.org/10.1007/978-3-030-24725-6_10

CA125 is the most commonly used noninvasive screening biomarker for OvCa. Overall, CA125 is elevated in about 80% of women with OvCa. This rate is about 60% in stage I and up to 90% in advanced-stage III/IV diseases. Thus, its use in early detection has shortcomings. However, because it has established utility in monitoring chemotherapy response, the US FDA has approved this biomarker for such intended use. However, the CA125 assay has limitations. Endometriosis, menstruation, and benign uterine lesions in premenopausal women can elevate circulating levels of CA125. There is still therefore a need for better noninvasive biomarkers with increased accuracy and companion diagnostic ability for OvCa.

Ovarian ascites represent the OvCa microenvironment. Indeed there is evidence on the potential use of ovarian ascites and its biomarkers as a representation of the tumor microenvironment in order to augment early detection as well as therapeutic efforts in OvCa.

10.2 The Peritoneal Cavity

Gross anatomically, the peritoneum is a serous membrane that covers the abdominal and pelvic cavities, as well as the intra-abdominal organs. It is composed of two layers: an outer parietal layer that lines the walls of the abdominal and pelvic cavities and an inner visceral layer that wraps around visceral organs such as the stomach, liver, and intestines. The space between the two layers is the peritoneal cavity, which usually contains about 50 ml of serous fluid that facilitates easy sliding of the two layers. In addition to providing support for the many abdominal organs, the peritoneum also brings in blood vessels, lymphatics, and nerves needed to maintain the physiologic functions of the organs.

At the fine anatomic level, the peritoneal membrane is made of five layers; the capillary endothelial cells with their sub-glycocalyx, endothelial basement membrane, the interstitial space, the sub-mesothelial basement membrane, and mesothelial cells. The function of this structure serves to prevent macromolecular exit from the capillaries into the interstitium. First, the endothelium of continuous capillaries does not allow macromolecular passage. Second, anionic charges of the endothelial cells and sub-glycocalyx as well as basement membrane proteoglycans prevent macromolecules such as albumin from exiting the vasculature. In malignant ascites, this physiologic function that allows only about 50 ml of serous fluid in the peritoneal cavity is disrupted leading to excess accumulation of ascitic fluid in the peritoneal space. This imbalance in fluid dynamics is due to peritoneal invasion by OvCa cells, increased net filtration, and/or impaired fluid clearance.

10.3 Formation of Malignant Ovarian Ascites

At least three factors contribute to formation of malignant ovarian ascites: peritoneal invasion by cancer cells, increased blood vessel permeability, and impaired lymphatic clearance.

OvCa cells have an innate propensity for transcoelomic invasion. Following ovulation, with oocyte release and injury to epithelium of the ovary, the epithelial cells undergo epithelial-to-mesenchymal transition (EMT) to facilitate repair of the surface epithelium. Thus, epithelial OvCa (EOC) cells have an innate program to undergo EMT, engendering in them the increased proliferation and motility to invade surrounding structures. OvCa cells express β integrins, CA125, and CD44 that enable their adhesion to hyaluronan and mesothelin on mesothelial cells. This process enhances OvCa cell proliferation and invasion of mesothelium that is associated with transcoelomic metastasis and formation of malignant ascites.

Several factors contribute to increased fluid exudation into the peritoneal cavity during formation of ovarian malignant ascites. VEGF production, which increases in EOC, is associated with formation of malignant ascites and poor prognosis. VEGF, which accumulates at much higher levels in ascites from EOC, causes increased vascular permeability with formation of ascites. Consistent with this, inhibition of VEGF functions suppresses the formation and accumulation of ascitic fluids in mouse models of intraperitoneal OvCa [1, 2]. The elevated VEGF production in EOC ascites is due to multiple factors including the actions of lysophosphatidic acid (LPA), TNF, endothelin 1, EGF, PDGF, MMPs, cyclooxygenase 1, IL-1β, insulin-like growth factor 1 (IGF1), and hypoxia. For example, in othotopic human OvCa models, blockage of TNF-β inhibited VEGF expression, which reduced production of malignant ascites [3]. Moreover, LPA levels in ascites and serum are much high in women with OvCa. LPA is an active phospholipid produced extracellularly by the actions of phosphodiesterase autotaxin (ATX). LPA signals via G-protein-dependent receptors leading to diverse cellular activities including transcriptional activation of VEGF, IL-6, IL-8, and urokinase plasminogen activator (uPA). The next effect is increased endothelial permeability. VEGF downregulates tight junction protein, claudin 5, in peritoneal endothelium and also mediates tyrosine phosphorylation of cadherin-catenin complexes resulting in decreased junctional strength associated with increased permeability. In addition to their role in cancer cell invasion, MMPs (especially MMP9) induce the release of VEGF that mediates formation of ascites. Other factors that may contribute to formation of ascites in EOC include CXCL4 that is elevated in ascitic fluid due to OvCa. Of interest, CXCL4, CXCL6, CXCL8, CXCL14, and CCL13 were upregulated in peritoneal specimens from OvCa patients compared to patients with benign ovarian conditions, despite the absence of cancer cells in the peritoneum [4].

The increased capillary permeability leads to macromolecular escape into malignant ascitic fluid, which increases the colloid osmotic pressure to draw more fluid from the microcirculation. Malignant spread, from any source, to the abdominal cavity causes an increase in the cross-sectional area of microvessels lining the peritoneal cavity, which translates into increased surface area for fluid filtration.

In addition to fluid exudate into the peritoneal cavity, there is reduced fluid clearance during formation of malignant ascites. The rich lymphatics of the peritoneal membrane drain residual fluid, proteins, and other macromolecules back into the blood circulation. The subdiaphragmatic and omental peritoneal membranes are particularly rich in lymphatic vessels, and their obstruction is implicated in the formation of malignant ascites. A number of experimental evidences have been provided to support this conclusion. In mouse models of malignant ascites, there was a failure of lymphatic clearance of intraperitoneally injected Indian ink. In another mouse model of malignant ascites from ovarian tumor, intraperitoneal injection of radioactive erythrocytes could not be detected in the blood stream within 5 h. Furthermore, clearance of radioactive albumin was impaired after intraperitoneal injection [5]. On the contrary, ascites could form in the absence of peritoneal lymphatic obstruction by tumor cells [6]. Thus, increased peritoneal membrane permeability, actions of cytokines, and chemokines in the OvCa microenvironment appear to play a major role in the formation of malignant ascites.

10.3.1 Composition of Malignant Ovarian Ascites

The malignant ovarian ascitic fluid represents the OvCa microenvironment. Consistent with cancer cell microenvironmental composition, malignant ovarian ascites is made up of cellular and acellular elements including extracellular vesicles.

10.3.1.1 Cellular Composition

In addition to cancer cells, malignant ascites is rich in immune cells, as well as cancer-associated fibroblasts (CAFs), endothelial cells, human peritoneal mesothelial cells, adipocytes, bone marrow-derived cells, and adipose tissue-derived stromal cells. All these cells are reactive cells in ascites that subserve either pro-tumoral or antitumoral functions.

OvCa cells in ascites occur as single adherent cells and as aggregates of nonadherent cells called spheroids. Subsets of these metastatic cells in ascites are important to disease recurrence. Spheroids also contribute to chemoresistance due to inefficient drug delivery to inner cells. Due to the fact that OvCa cells in ascites might have undergone EMT, two types of adherent cells have been isolated in ovarian malignant ascites: those with features of mesenchymal and epithelial morphologies [7]. Both cell types express cancer stem cell markers including $CD24^{low}$, $CD44^{high}$, and AC133, as well as TGFβ, EGFR, BMP2, BMP4, and integrin $\alpha_2\beta_1$. Wintzell et al. characterized the phenotypes of these cells [8]. They uncovered high levels of tumor-initiating cells in ovarian malignant ascitic fluid that expressed $Nanog^{high}$ and $EpCAM^{high}$, which could either exist as monolayer single cell suspension (epithelial phenotype) or adherent spheres (mesenchymal phenotype). The single cell suspension of OvCa ascitic fluid cells was more tumorigenic and expressed CD44, Oct4A, and CAF markers including α-SMA. The less tumorigenic sphere-forming cells expressed high levels of E-cadherin and no to little vimentin, integrin β3, or Oct4A. However, Latifi et al. found that ascitic fluids from women with chemoresistant OvCa contained predominantly nonadhesive cell population that expressed E-cadherin, STAT3, and Oct4A. The few adherent cells expressed CD44, MMP9, and Oct4 [9]. These findings demonstrate the level of heterogeneity of cancer cells in ascites. Characterization of these cells in every patient could help inform treatment options, in the age of personalized medicine.

Malignant ascites is rich in lymphocytes and other cells that secrete cytokines and chemokines into the fluid. The concentration of cytokines including IL-1β, IL-6, IL-8, and IL-10 are in the order of 2–3 logs greater than serum levels [10]. There may be selective release of IL-6 into ascites secondary to OvCa because ascites from this tumor harbors higher levels of this cytokine than ascites from primary tumors [11]. IL-6 enhances tumor growth, invasion, angiogenesis, and chemoresistance. Thus, elevated IL-6 and IL-10 levels in ascites are correlated with shorter PFS, poor initial response to chemotherapy, poor OS, and drug resistance.

CAFs secrete factors that act in both autocrine and paracrine fashions in ascitic fluid to drive OvCa cell growth, proliferation, migration, and chemoresistance. Human peritoneal mesothelial cells secrete similar tumor-promoting factors including lysophosphatidic acid, VEGFs, and dipeptidyl peptidase IV that also promote tumor cell growth, adhesion, migration, invasion, and chemoresistance.

10.3.1.2 Acellular Composition

The acellular components in ascites are extracellular vesicles, proteins, metabolites, and nucleic acids. Consistent with other body fluids, ascites contain extracellular vesicles (e.g., exosomes) used for intercellular communication. OvCa exosomes in ascites harbor miRNAs (miR-141 and miR-200c family) [12] as well as MUC1, CD24, and CA125.

The inflammatory process in ascitic fluid is associated with different cytokine profiles. An immunosuppressive ascitic fluid is indicated by the significantly elevated levels of IL-6, IL-8, IL-10, IL-15, as well as MIP-1β, IP-10, VEGF, and MCP-1, in association with significantly decreased levels of IL-2, IL-5, IL-7, RANTES, and PDGFR-BB.

The proteome of ascites has been characterized [13, 14]. Of the >2000 proteins in ascites, the levels of proteins involved in RNA splicing were ≤ sevenfold in fluids from women with EOC compared to cirrhotic ascites [13]. Also significantly elevated in ascites from women with EOC compared to those with benign ovarian tumors are pyruvate kinase isoenzymes M1/M2, mesothelin, and GAPDH.

The ascitic fluid metabolome has also been fairly well characterized [13, 15]. Shender et al. found significantly decreased levels of glucose, fructose, glycolate, and furanose, in association with elevated levels of cholesterol, glycerol-3-phosphate, ceramide, and monoacylglycerol in ascites from women with OvCa [13]. Of interest, this study found LPA, ceramide, and derivatives of fatty acids only in malignant ascites. In another study that compared ovarian malignant to cirrhotic ascites, differential levels of glucose, glucose-3-phosphate, fatty acids, cholesterol, ceramide, and glycerol-3-phosphate were revealed. The most elevated and reduced were glucose-1-phosphate and 2-hydroxyisovalerate, respectively [15]. These metabolite findings suggest active amino acid catabolism as well as increased glucose utilization in ascitic fluid.

10.4 Signaling in Malignant Ovarian Ascites

Signaling pathways activated in OvCa ascitic fluid include the PI3K, NF-κB, and STAT3-JAK2 pathways. Activation of the PI3K pathway through activating PTEN mutations and/or amplification of PIK3CA and AKT occurs in >70% of OvCa [16]. AKT-mediated BMP signaling is involved in adhesion and dispersion of OvCa spheroids [17]. Importantly, AKT as well as ERK1 or ERK2-ELK1 signaling provides survival signals to OvCa cells by conferring in them resistance to TRAIL-induced apoptosis [18–20]. Also commonly dysregulated in >50% of OvCa is the NF-κB pathway. EGFR activation induces NF-κB signaling to establish pro-inflammatory state in ascites through upregulation of several genes including IL-6 and IL-8 [21]. Consistent with its pro-tumorigenic activity, inhibition of NF-κB signaling in mice resulted in significant reduction in IL-8 and VEGF levels that were associated with reduced formation of malignant ascites and prolonged survival [22]. Moreover, stimulation of IL-6 receptor of OvCa cells activated STAT3-JAK2 signaling to mediate angiogenesis and cancer cell survival [23, 24].

10.5 Ovarian Cancer Biomarkers in Proximal Fluids

10.5.1 Ovarian Cancer miRNA Biomarkers in Proximal Fluid

Large-scale profiling (754 human miRNAs) of ascitic fluid from women with high-grade serous OvCa enabled identification of 153 miRNAs with significant differential levels [12]. Seven miRNAs (miR-200a, miR-200b, miR-200c, miR-141, miR-429, miR-1290, miR-30a-5P) were further validated in samples from women with serous endometrioid and mucinous subtypes of OvCa. As a diagnostic, the AUROCC was 1.00 for the panel of miR-200a, miR-200c, miR-141, miR-429, and miR-1290 and 0.996 and 0.885 for only mR-200b and miR-30a-5p, respectively. Preliminary survival analysis implicated elevated ascitic fluid miR-200b with poor OS (HR = 4.04). Comparison of ascites from women with high-grade serous OvCa to those with benign cysts and endometriomas uncovered differential levels of miR-23b, miR-29a, miR-30d, miR-205, miR-720, and let-7b between the two groups [25].

10.5.2 Ovarian Cancer Protein Biomarkers in Proximal Fluid

In a pilot peptidomic study to identify low molecular weight molecules as OvCa biomarkers in ascites, ultrafiltration was used to remove high molecular weight proteins before further analysis [26]. Orbitrap MS analysis identified 2000 unique peptides from 259 proteins including vitronectin, transketolase, and haptoglobin, of which 777 peptides were cataloged. Ascitic profiling uncovered 4388 nonredundant peptides associated with OvCa [27]. Significant differential levels (>twofold change) of 104 peptides (52 decreased and 52 increased) were found between OvCa patients and women with benign gynecological conditions. Another proteomic profile uncovered 2096 and 1855 proteins in OvCa and cirrhotic ascites, respectively, of which 424 were specific to malignant ascites [13]. The major difference between the two fluids was in spliceosomal proteins in malignant ascites. In addition, splicing RNAs in protein complexes were exclusively observed in malignant ascites.

Glycoproteomic analysis of ascites identified 579 glycosylation sites in 333 proteins [28]. Thirteen were exclusive to OvCa, while another eight were shared with OvCa cell line supernatant. Separate glycomic, proteomic, and glycopeptide analysis uncovered OvCa biomarkers in ascites [29]. N-glycan analysis revealed large, highly fucosylated and sialylated complexes, as well as hybrid glycans in malignant ascites. More abundant in OvCa ascites were the following: haptoglobin, fibronectin, lumican, fibulin, hemopexin, ceruloplasmin, α-1-antitrypsin, and α-1-antichymotrypsin. Glycopeptide analysis also identified N- and O-glycans (some of which were unusual) in clusterin, hemopexin, and fibulin. Another N-glycome profiling using MALDI-TOF MS of ascites from women with primary serous EOC uncovered increased antennarity, branching, sialylation, and LewisX motives compared to serum from healthy controls [30]. The degree of sialylation correlated with the volume of ascites. Features of inflammation were revealed in ascites and sera from EOC women compared to serum samples from healthy controls.

Prognostic biomarkers identified in ascitic fluid include VEGF, IFNγ, TNFα, sEpCAM, and the volume of ascitic fluid. VEGF-C levels in serum and ascites are much higher in women with OvCa than those with benign gynecological conditions [31]. The elevated levels in both fluids significantly correlated with FIGO stage, tumor grade, lymph node metastasis, and OS. Multivariate analysis uncovered elevated serum and ascites VEGF-C levels to be an independent predictor of shorter OS. Quantitative measurement of malignant ascitic fluid VEGF revealed levels to be as high as 676 ± 303.86 pg/ml compared to 218.37 ± 98.15 pg/ml in benign ascites [32]. Of interest, levels of ascitic fluid VEGF were much higher in OvCa patients than patients with other cancers. High ascitic fluid VEGF was an independent prognostic factor of OS in multivariate Cox regression analysis. Cytokine profiling of ascites has identified IFNγ, TNFα, and IL-6 as potential prognostic biomarkers of OvCa. High levels of IFNγ were significantly associated with advanced stage disease, high tumor histologic grade, and suboptimal surgical resection. In multivariate analysis, a tenfold increase in ascites IFNγ was associated with shorter disease-free survival (DFS, HR = 2.74) and OS (HR = 1.72) [33]. High levels of TNFα and IL-6 in ascites have been associated with poor DFS in women with advanced EOC [34]. Soluble EpCAM in malignant ascites may be predictive of treatment with anti-EpCAM antibody, catumaxomab. Additionally, ascites sEpCAM was significantly associated with OS, especially in OvCa patients [35]. Profiling of tumor-associated macrophages (TAM) in ascites has identified subgroups of OvCa women with different outcomes based on gene expression [36]. Markers of unfavorable outcomes included high levels of CD163, PCOLCE2, IL-6, and IL-10 that are associated with anti-inflammatory, enhanced extracellular matrix (ECM) organization, OvCa aggressiveness, and immunosuppressive states, respectively. Genes linked to immune defense mechanisms and interferon signaling characterized patients with favorable outcomes. In this cohort of women, the suppressive effects of OvCa ascites on IL-12β expression and IL-12 secretion that are important in cytotoxicity were abrogated by IFNγ administration.

Ascites volume is a prognostic factor in women with OvCa [37]. It has been demonstrated that each liter of ascites was associated with shorter PFS (HR = 1.12) and OS (HR = 1.12). Ascites volume > 2000 ml was significantly associated with PFS and OS. Acellular ascites contain factors responsible for disease progression because intraperitoneal injection of cell-free ascites could accelerate OvCa progression in mice. Of relevance to disease progression, proteomic profiling of ascites uncovered six α-1-isoform and one α-2 isoform of haptoglobin to be associated with OvCa [38]. Increased levels of fucosylated haptoglobin isoforms correlated with advanced-stage OvCa. Immunohistochemical analysis further confirmed the levels of fucosylated haptoglobin with OvCa progression. Another proteomic profiling of ascites identified differential levels of ceruloplasmin in fluids from women with chemoresistant and chemosensitive OvCa [39]. The elevated levels of ascites ceruloplasmin could be a predictive biomarker of chemoresistance in women with serous EOC.

10.5.3 Ovarian Cancer Extracellular Vesicle Biomarkers in Proximal Fluid

Levels of extracellular vesicles (EVs) are much higher in ascites from women with low/high-grade serous OvCa (>1010 particles/ml) than control peritoneal fluid from women with benign cysts or endometriomas [25]. EV transcripts of CA11, MEDAG, LAMA4, SPINT2, and NANOG were differential between cases and controls. SPINT2 and NANOG mRNAs were 100-fold elevated, while CA11 was 0.5-fold decreased in conditioned media of cancer cells compared to immortalized ovarian surface and fallopian tube epithelial cells. Exosomes derived from malignant ovarian ascites promote tumor progression in vivo. Moreover, exosomes have direct and indirect effects on the immune ascites microenvironment, because B and NK cells could interact with them [40, 41].

10.6 Therapeutic Biomarkers of Malignant Ascites

Ascites is managed non-pharmacologically (such as paracentesis and catheter drainage to temporarily relieve symptoms) or with pharmacologic agents including immunotherapy. Biomarkers in ovarian ascites have been explored as targets for treating malignant ascites. These targets include immune cells (B and T lymphocytes, NK cells, TAMs, Tregs, and MDSCs), CAFs, angiogenesis (mainly targeting VEGF), and expressed molecules that enable adhesion of OvCa cells to the mesothelium. Multiple therapeutic strategies have been developed and tested for prevention of OvCa dissemination to the peritoneal cavity and subsequent formation of secondary tumors.

10.6.1 VEGF and Angiogenesis as Ovarian Cancer Ascites Therapeutic Target

Tumor and stromal cells secrete proangiogenic factors that are involved not only in promoting tumor progression but also in the formation of ascites. Ascites angiogenic factors include VEGF, PDGF, angiopoietin (NG), IL-6, and IL-8. However, the most extensively studied in OvCa ascites is VEGF. Because VEGF-A has been proven to be associated with increased microvascular density and BRCA-mutated OvCa [42], therapeutic targeting of this molecule to improve survival of OvCa patients has been explored in clinical trials.

The secreted glycoprotein, VEGF-A, belongs to a family of growth factors including VEGF-B, VEGF-C, VEGF-D, VEGF-E, and placental growth factor (PLGF) involved in angiogenesis. The interaction of VEGF with its tyrosine kinase receptors, VEGFR1 (Flt-1) and VEGFR2 (KDR/Flk-1), causes receptor dimerization and cellular activation that results in endothelial cell proliferation, differentiation, migration, and survival [43, 44]. Therapies targeting this pathway have been focused on ligand or receptor inhibition. The human monoclonal anti-VEGF antibody, bevacizumab (Avastin, Roche), which inactivates VEGF, has been shown to be successful as a single agent or in combination with other agents in the treatment of women with high-grade serous OvCa. It is a US FDA-approved agent for treating initial or recurrent disease [45, 46]. Multiple clinical trials including ICON7, GOG218, AURELIA, OCEANS, and GOG213 phase III trials have been conducted to test the efficacy of Avastin in women with OvCa.

In the initial GOG trial (protocol GOG170D) of bevacizumab on patients with recurrent or platinum-resistant OvCa, objective clinical response was achieved in 21%, while PFS for at least 6 months was achieved in 40.3% of patients. Of relevance, median PFS and OS were 4.7 and 17 months, respectively [47]. The ICON7 phase III trial included bevacizumab in combination with platinum and paclitaxel in women with metastatic epithelial OvCa following cytoreductive surgery. At 42 months follow-up, PFS was 24.1 months in the treatment arm compared to 22.4 months for those on only chemotherapy ($P = 0.04$). This modest survival benefit of the combination therapy was more pronounced in women at high risk for disease progression [48]. The GOG218 trial considered patients on chemotherapy alone vs. chemotherapy and bevacizumab initiation vs. chemotherapy and bevacizumab throughout treatment in patients newly diagnosed with stage III and IV OvCa following cytoreduction surgery. Again while marginal, bevacizumab plus chemotherapy followed by maintenance bevacizumab therapy improved PFS compared to patients on only platinum and paclitaxel chemotherapy [49]. In the AURELIA randomized phase III trial, bevacizumab in combination with chemotherapy was assessed in women with recurrent platinum-resistant OvCa. Once more, there was a marginal improvement with median PFS extended by 3.3 months (3.4 to 6.7 months) and OS from 13.3 to 16.6 months for patients on bevacizumab plus chemotherapy [50]. Similarly, the median PFS improved from 8.4 to 12.4 months in women on bevacizumab plus chemotherapy in the OCEANS phase III trial, while the median OS was 37.3 vs. 42.2 months in favor of women on bevacizumab plus chemotherapy in the GOG213 trial [51]. These modest outcomes led to the approval of this targeted therapy of the ovarian malignant microenvironment to improve disease outcome.

Other agents such as decoy receptors and tyrosine kinase inhibitors used to block angiogenesis have shown promise. Aflibercept, a recombinant fusion protein that targets the extracellular domains of VEGFR1 and VEGFR2, has demonstrated potential for treating malignant ascites. Aflibercept is a decoy receptor that blocks VEGF signaling by targeting VEGF-A, VEGF-B, and PLGFs 1 and 2. Following successful demonstration that aflibercept could decrease ascites formation and reduce peritoneal spread in OvCa xenograft models, a phase II clinical trial on women with advanced platinum-resistant OvCa with ascites that required ≥3 paracentesis per month was conducted [52]. The patients were given 4 mg/kg IV aflibercept biweekly, and the primary endpoint was repeat paracentesis response rate (RPRR). A minimum of twofold increase in time to repeat paracentesis compared to baseline interval was considered a response. Of the 16 women enrolled in this phase II study, 10 (62.5%) achieved a response. The median time to repeat paracentesis (76.0 days) was 4.5 times longer than baseline interval of 16.8 days [53, 54].

Tyrosine kinase receptor inhibitors, cediranib, nintedanib, and pazopanib, have demonstrated potential as anti-angiogenic therapeutic agents of OvCa. Cediranib (AZD2171, AstraZeneca) blocks VEGFR1–3, c-kit, and PDGFRα and PDGFRβ. A phase II clinical trial recruited 46 women with gynecological malignancies and who had received less than two lines of platinum-based chemotherapy. While none achieved complete response (CR) in this cohort, partial response (PR) and stable disease (SD) were observed in 17% and 13%, respectively [55]. Another phase II study of cediranib involved 74 women with recurrent or persistent OvCa who had received one round of platinum-based chemotherapy. Data analysis dichotomized the patients into platinum-sensitive (PLS) and platinum-resistant (PLR) groups. The primary endpoint to examine the efficacy of single-agent cediranib was objective response rate at 16 weeks of treatment. Among the PLS group, 26% achieved PR and 51% had SD. While there were no partial responders in the PLR group, 66% had SD. Both PFS and OS were better in the PLS than PLR group, being 7.2 vs. 3.7 months and 27.7 vs. 11.9 months, respectively [56]. Pazopanib (GW786034) inhibits similar targets as cediranib. Pazopanib in conjunction with paclitaxel appear to offer some survival benefits in women with refractory or platinum-resistant OvCa. In a phase II trial (MITO-11), both PFS and OS improved in patients on paclitaxel plus pazopanib compared to paclitaxel monotherapy, being 6.3 vs. 3.5 months and 18.7 vs. 14.8 months, respectively [57]. Nintedanib also inhibits VEGFR1–3 and PDGFRα and PDGFRβ, in addition to FGFR1–3. In a randomized trial of nintedanib as a maintenance therapy following chemotherapy, a promising survival benefit was uncovered at 36 weeks, with PFS being 5.0% for placebo and 16.3% for the targeted group. However, a follow-up phase III trial (AGO-OVAR12) failed to reveal significant benefit for this therapy. Median PFS was 16.6 vs. 17.2 months for placebo and cases, respectively. However, nintedanib may improve PFS in women with non-high-risk OvCa [58].

10.6.2 Cancer-Associated Fibroblasts as Ovarian Cancer Ascites Therapeutic Target

CAFs in the tumor microenvironment (TME) drive tumorigenesis through multiple interacting networks with several cell types. While most CAFs differentiate from fibroblasts, other cell types including endothelial cells, pericytes, epithelial cells, adipocytes, and bone marrow-derived mesenchymal cells can transdifferentiate into CAFs. The macromolecules involved in intercellular communications to increase CAFs in ovarian ascites include VEGF, βFGF, TGFβ, PDGF-BB, MMPs, ROS, miRNAs, extracellular vesicles, and fibroblast activation protein (FAP). All these molecules are potential therapeutic targets of CAF molecules that could be explored. Due to the involvement of tyrosine kinase receptor ligands such as VEGF, PDGF, and FGF in CAF signaling in the ovarian microenvironment, efforts have been made to treat patients with pathway inhibitors. While outcomes are still awaited, concrete evidence has been provided to support a role for imatinib, a PDGFR inhibitor, in suppressing OvCa cell growth, which is likely through its anti-angiogenic effects. Dasatinib, and anti-PDGFR TKI, is a US FDA-approved agent for targeting CAF. This agent might be relevant for targeting CAFs in malignant ovarian ascites. Another anti-PDGFR, sorafenib, together with imatinib appears to have clinical activity in women with recurrent platinum-resistant OvCa.

Fibroblasts secrete TGFβ into ascites that promote tumorigenesis. It has therefore been a target for development of several agents that show promise in preclinical studies. For example, the TGFβ inhibitor, A-83-01, could improve survival of mouse models of peritoneal metastasis. Another TGFβ agent, LY2109761, could possibly synergize with cisplatin to inhibit growth of cisplatin-resistant OvCa xenografts. Additionally, galunisertib, an inhibitor of TGFβ receptor I, could counter tumor growth in various PDX tumors. These molecules await clinical translational studies.

CAFs also secrete FAB that drive cancer cell proliferation, invasive propensity, immunosuppression, and associated poor prognosis. Cancer cell death was enhanced in mouse models with targeted deletion of FAB-expressing CAFs. This effect possibly relies on effects of TNFα and IFNγ in cancer cell cytotoxicity via CD8+ lymphocytes [59]. In support of this mechanism, vaccines targeting FAB-expressing CAFs significantly suppressed tumor growth through CD8+ and CD4+ cell responses [60, 61]. While studies showed that the enzymatic activity of FAB promoted tumor cell proliferation, inhibition of FAB activity with small molecules failed in clinical trials [62].

10.6.3 Ovarian Cancer Cell Adhesion to Mesothelium as Therapeutic Target

Adherence of OvCa spheroids to the mesothelium is a prerequisite to formation of secondary deposits and disease relapse. This process involves downregulation of E-cadherin and upregulated expression of a number of molecules including α5 and α1 integrins, CD44, fibronectin, and tissue transglutaminase (TG2). The adhesion of OvCa cell to FN matrix of mesothelial cell requires TG2-mediated induction of α5β1 integrin complex formation and recruitment of talin to stabilize the adhesion [63]. Additionally, TG2 helps tether FN to β1 integrin. This interaction also activates RhoA and suppression of Src-p190RhoGAP signaling. All these molecular interactions are therefore therapeutic targets for preventing secondary tumor formation in ovarian ascites. Consistent with this macromolecular interaction in ascites, TG2 knockdown in the TG2-β1-FN complex blocked peritoneal spread of OvCa, and the mechanism was dependent on β1 integrin-mediated cell adhesion and downstream signaling [64, 65]. Expectedly, targeting integrins, FN, and TG2-FN complex has been a focus of therapeutic developments.

Moreover, both OvCa and neovascular endothelial cells express α5β1 integrins in ovarian ascites. Thus, this complex has also been targeted therapeutically. Several anti-integrin molecules, including inotuzumab and cilengitide (target αvβ3 and αvβ5), etaracizumab (targets αvβ3), and volociximab (targets α5β1), have been developed. Unfortunately, these molecules are yet to produce convincing clinical evidence of efficacy. For example, inotuzumab demonstrated antitumor and anti-angiogenic activity in breast cancer xenografts, but in a phase I trial, only one OvCa patient demonstrated stable disease for 6 months [66]. Similarly, cilengitide failed to improve OS of glioblastoma patients in a phase II trial, and etaracizumab showed little benefit [67]. Volociximab could block growth and dissemination of OvCa in xenograft models but failed to benefit patients with recurrent platinum-resistant OvCa in phase II trials [68].

FN also plays an important role in attachment of spheroids to mesothelial cells and thus is an attractive therapeutic target. As a proof of principle, an antibody that disrupts β1 integrin-TG2-FN complex by targeting FN-binding domain on TG2 could block OvCa spheroid proliferation and ability to form tumors [69]. Current efforts are ongoing to discover and develop small molecules that disrupt the FN-TG2 complex to prevent OvCa spheroid adhesion to the mesothelium [70].

10.6.4 Immune Targeting in Ovarian Cancer Ascites

The immune microenvironment is proven to be critical to survival of women with OvCa. Multiple studies support the association of antitumor immunoreactive cells such as effector CD8+, CD4+, and CD3+ tumor-infiltrating lymphocytes (TILs) with improved patient survival. TILs from ascites secrete antitumor factors such as

TNFα and GM-CSF. T-cell-rich tumors express high levels of IFNγ, IL-2, and factors such as CCL21, CCL22, and CXCL9 that attract more lymphocytes. On the contrary, decreased survival is correlated with tumors that possess immunosuppressive cells such as MDSCs, M2 subtype of TAMs, Th2 subtype of CD4+ cells, and Tregs. Several immunotherapy strategies have thus been successfully tested in women with OvCa [71]. Targeting the immune system in OvCa microenvironment has focused on cellular components such as TAMs and MDSCs, as well as other factors such as PD1/PD-L1 signaling, and tumor neoantigen load.

TAMs have been well characterized in OvCa microenvironment. In OvCa, these are predominantly M2 subtype that promotes tumorigenesis via secretion of cytokines such as IL-6 and IL-8. They have also been located in the centers of spheroids where they stimulate OvCa cell proliferation, migration, and invasiveness via NF-κB, JNK, and EGF signaling pathways [72–74]. A number of agents targeting TAMs have been developed and tested in preclinical models. These include monoclonal antibodies such as catumaxomab and alemtuzumab and epigenetic modulators including bromodomain inhibitor, JQ1, and folate receptor 2. The humanized antibody, catumaxomab, targets EpCAM on tumor cells, CD3 on T cells, and Fcγ receptors (I, IIa and III) on macrophages, dendritic cells, and NK cells. This multitargeting generates multiple effects in the tumor microenvironment. The efficacy of catumaxomab on malignant ascites led to its approval in Europe for treating EpCAM+ malignant ascites. It is delivered intraperitoneally [75]. Alemtuzumab is another monoclonal that targets CD52+ leukocytes and Tie2+ monocytes to reduce tumor growth. It also demonstrates anti-angiogenic and anti-myeloid activities in mouse models of OvCa [76].

The epigenome of TAMs, myeloid cells, and other immune cells have been targeted in the OvCa microenvironment [77, 78]. In preclinical models, the combination of inhibitors of DNA methyltransferase and HDAC could delay tumor progression by decreasing the numbers of TAMs while activating immune cells (T and NK cells). An ongoing clinical trial examines a combination therapy of these two inhibitors together with inhibitor of PD1 in women with recurrent OvCa. Another epigenetic modulator, the bromodomain inhibitor, JQ1, could suppress OvCa growth by significantly reducing PD-L1 on TAMs and dendritic cells, as well as increasing T-cell cytotoxicity.

TAMs in the tumor microenvironment express high levels of folate receptor 2, which makes it an attractive therapeutic target. Thus, methotrexate-loaded G5-dendrimer nanoparticles targeting folate receptor 2 on TAMs could reverse anti-VEGF-A therapy-resistance in preclinical OvCa models [79].

MDSCs are potent inhibitors of T-cell functions in stroma of various tumors. These are bone marrow-derived cells of the myeloid lineage that include immature macrophages, dendritic cells, and granulocytes, as well as other myeloid precursors. Lin^-/CD45+/CD33+ MDSCs comprised 37% of stromal cells in OvCa microenvironment and were demonstrated to impair T-cell proliferation and effector functions [80]. Thus, increased MDSCs are associated with decreased CD8+ TILs and poor outcomes in women with advanced OvCa. Multiple strategies have been developed to therapeutically target MDSCs. These include use of inhibitors of immune suppression such as COX2 inhibitors, triterpenoids, sildenafil, and inducible NO; agents that promote MDSC apoptosis; agents that block immature myeloid cell differentiation such as vitamin D3, HDACi, and retinoic acid; agents targeting chemokines or their receptors to block MDSC recruitment or proliferation; and antibodies that induce MDSC depletion in the TME.

Other soluble and cell surface receptors targeted in OvCa microenvironment for immunotherapy of OvCa are PD1 and PD-L1. In normal immune regulatory functions, PD1 signaling plays an immunosuppressive role by preventing naïve T-cell activation. The role of this pathway in OvCa, however, appears complex. The ligands of PD1, PD-L1 and PD-L2, are upregulated in tumor and immune cells. PD-L1 expression in OvCa microenvironment is associated with increased presence of TILs and better survival [81, 82]. Previous studies provide contradictory results. Increased PD-L1 expression in OvCa was associated with decreased intratumoral CD8+ T cells and poor survival [83]. Additionally, PD1+ dendritic cells in OvCa microenvironment were associated with decreased TILs and suppressed T-cell functions. However, blockage of PD1 signaling could restore antitumor immune response in xenograft models of OvCa [84], and in clinical trials, PD1 inhibitory antibody, pembrolizumab, achieved response and stable disease in 11% and 23%, respectively, in women with recurrent OvCa. Similarly, the anti-PD-L1 monoclonal, avelumab, achieved a response in 10% and stable disease in 40% of recurrent OvCa women. The complex role of PD1/PD-L signaling in OvCa microenvironment needs further clarification to inform efficient therapeutic targeting.

Immunotherapy of the OvCa microenvironment has also relied on tumor neoantigen load. Blockage of immune checkpoint factors including PD1, PD-L, and CTLA-4 have been effective immunotherapy targets associated with neoantigen burden. However, OvCa cells harbor intermediate neoantigen load. Thus, only a small percentage of patients harbor 20 or more mutations per Mb genome, which is significant enough for favorable response to immunotherapy [85]. Clinical trials with nivolumab and pembrolizumab that target PD1, ipilimumab that targets CTLA-4, and avelumab and MS936559 that target PD-L1 have achieved response rate in just 5–20% of patients [86, 87].

The numerous biomarkers in OvCa ascites being targeted offer promise in patient management. However, there is the need to uncover optimal targets that improve patient survival and quality of life.

10.7 Summary

- OvCa is a common gynecological malignancy that is age-associated.
- Diagnosis of OvCa is often late, making it the leading cause of gynecological cancer-related deaths.
- Various modalities aimed at early detection, including serum CA125 measurement and the "risk malignancy index," are available.

- While sensitive at detection of advanced-stage disease, CA125 has shortcomings in early OvCa detection.
- The ovary has no proximal fluid amenable to noninvasive sampling.
- OvCa biomarkers are, however, abundant in malignant ovarian ascites, which is considered OvCa microenvironment or interstitial fluid.
- Biomarkers discovered in OvCa peritoneal fluid could be leveraged in blood for screening and disease management.
- The reactive malignant ovarian ascites is rich in inflammatory and other immune mediators, as well as numerous signaling molecules that promote OvCa growth and progression.
- Thus, in addition to early detection biomarkers, the malignant ovarian ascites also contains therapeutic biomarkers such as VEGF, CAFs, TAM, and MDSCs.

References

1. Mesiano S, Ferrara N, Jaffe RB. Role of vascular endothelial growth factor in ovarian cancer: inhibition of ascites formation by immunoneutralization. Am J Pathol. 1998;153:1249–56.
2. Yukita A, Asano M, Okamoto T, et al. Suppression of ascites formation and re-accumulation associated with human ovarian cancer by an anti-VPF monoclonal antibody in vivo. Anticancer Res. 2000;20:155–60.
3. Liao S, Liu J, Lin P, et al. TGF-beta blockade controls ascites by preventing abnormalization of lymphatic vessels in orthotopic human ovarian carcinoma models. Clin Cancer Res. 2011;17:1415–24.
4. Wang E, Ngalame Y, Panelli MC, et al. Peritoneal and subperitoneal stroma may facilitate regional spread of ovarian cancer. Clin Cancer Res. 2005;11:113–22.
5. Nagy JA, Herzberg KT, Dvorak JM, Dvorak HF. Pathogenesis of malignant ascites formation: initiating events that lead to fluid accumulation. Cancer Res. 1993;53:2631–43.
6. Garrison RN, Kaelin LD, Galloway RH, Heuser LS. Malignant ascites. Clinical and experimental observations. Ann Surg. 1986;203:644–51.
7. Ho CM, Chang SF, Hsiao CC, et al. Isolation and characterization of stromal progenitor cells from ascites of patients with epithelial ovarian adenocarcinoma. J Biomed Sci. 2012;19:23.
8. Wintzell M, Hjerpe E, Avall Lundqvist E, Shoshan M. Protein markers of cancer-associated fibroblasts and tumor-initiating cells reveal subpopulations in freshly isolated ovarian cancer ascites. BMC Cancer. 2012;12:359.
9. Latifi A, Luwor RB, Bilandzic M, et al. Isolation and characterization of tumor cells from the ascites of ovarian cancer patients: molecular phenotype of chemoresistant ovarian tumors. PLoS One. 2012;7:e46858.
10. Penson RT, Kronish K, Duan Z, et al. Cytokines IL-1beta, IL-2, IL-6, IL-8, MCP-1, GM-CSF and TNFalpha in patients with epithelial ovarian cancer and their relationship to treatment with paclitaxel. Int J Gynecol Cancer. 2000;10:33–41.
11. Kryczek I, Grybos M, Karabon L, et al. IL-6 production in ovarian carcinoma is associated with histiotype and biological characteristics of the tumour and influences local immunity. Br J Cancer. 2000;82:621–8.
12. Zavesky L, Jandakova E, Weinberger V, et al. Ascites-derived extracellular microRNAs as potential biomarkers for ovarian Cancer. Reprod Sci. 2019;26:510–22.
13. Shender VO, Pavlyukov MS, Ziganshin RH, et al. Proteome-metabolome profiling of ovarian cancer ascites reveals novel components involved in intercellular communication. Mol Cell Proteomics. 2014;13:3558–71.

14. Gortzak-Uzan L, Ignatchenko A, Evangelou AI, et al. A proteome resource of ovarian cancer ascites: integrated proteomic and bioinformatic analyses to identify putative biomarkers. J Proteome Res. 2008;7:339–51.
15. McMillan A, Rulisa S, Sumarah M, et al. A multi-platform metabolomics approach identifies highly specific biomarkers of bacterial diversity in the vagina of pregnant and non-pregnant women. Sci Rep. 2015;5:14174.
16. Bast RC Jr, Hennessy B, Mills GB. The biology of ovarian cancer: new opportunities for translation. Nat Rev Cancer. 2009;9:415–28.
17. Peart TM, Correa RJ, Valdes YR, et al. BMP signalling controls the malignant potential of ascites-derived human epithelial ovarian cancer spheroids via AKT kinase activation. Clin Exp Metastasis. 2012;29:293–313.
18. Lane D, Robert V, Grondin R, et al. Malignant ascites protect against TRAIL-induced apoptosis by activating the PI3K/Akt pathway in human ovarian carcinoma cells. Int J Cancer. 2007;121:1227–37.
19. Lane D, Matte I, Rancourt C, Piche A. The prosurvival activity of ascites against TRAIL is associated with a shorter disease-free interval in patients with ovarian cancer. J Ovarian Res. 2010;3(1):1.
20. Goncharenko-Khaider N, Matte I, Lane D, et al. Ovarian cancer ascites increase Mcl-1 expression in tumor cells through ERK1/2-Elk-1 signaling to attenuate TRAIL-induced apoptosis. Mol Cancer. 2012;11:84.
21. Alberti C, Pinciroli P, Valeri B, et al. Ligand-dependent EGFR activation induces the co-expression of IL-6 and PAI-1 via the NFkB pathway in advanced-stage epithelial ovarian cancer. Oncogene. 2012;31:4139–49.
22. Huang S, Robinson JB, Deguzman A, et al. Blockade of nuclear factor-kappaB signaling inhibits angiogenesis and tumorigenicity of human ovarian cancer cells by suppressing expression of vascular endothelial growth factor and interleukin 8. Cancer Res. 2000;60:5334–9.
23. Niu G, Wright KL, Huang M, et al. Constitutive Stat3 activity up-regulates VEGF expression and tumor angiogenesis. Oncogene. 2002;21:2000–8.
24. Rosen DG, Mercado-Uribe I, Yang G, et al. The role of constitutively active signal transducer and activator of transcription 3 in ovarian tumorigenesis and prognosis. Cancer. 2006;107:2730–40.
25. Yamamoto CM, Oakes ML, Murakami T, et al. Comparison of benign peritoneal fluid- and ovarian cancer ascites-derived extracellular vesicle RNA biomarkers. J Ovarian Res. 2018;11:20.
26. Bery A, Leung F, Smith CR, et al. Deciphering the ovarian cancer ascites fluid peptidome. Clin Proteomics. 2014;11:13.
27. Huang X, Zhou J, Tang R, et al. Potential significance of Peptidome in human ovarian Cancer for patients with ascites. Int J Gynecol Cancer. 2018;28:355–62.
28. Kuzmanov U, Musrap N, Kosanam H, et al. Glycoproteomic identification of potential glycoprotein biomarkers in ovarian cancer proximal fluids. Clin Chem Lab Med. 2013;51:1467–76.
29. Miyamoto S, Ruhaak LR, Stroble C, et al. Glycoproteomic analysis of malignant ovarian Cancer ascites fluid identifies unusual Glycopeptides. J Proteome Res. 2016;15:3358–76.
30. Biskup K, Braicu EI, Sehouli J, et al. The ascites N-glycome of epithelial ovarian cancer patients. J Proteome. 2017;157:33–9.
31. Liang B, Guo Z, Li Y, Liu C. Elevated VEGF concentrations in ascites and serum predict adverse prognosis in ovarian cancer. Scand J Clin Lab Invest. 2013;73:309–14.
32. Zhan N, Dong WG, Wang J. The clinical significance of vascular endothelial growth factor in malignant ascites. Tumour Biol. 2016;37:3719–25.
33. Chen YL, Cheng WF, Chang MC, et al. Interferon-gamma in ascites could be a predictive biomarker of outcome in ovarian carcinoma. Gynecol Oncol. 2013;131:63–8.
34. Kolomeyevskaya N, Eng KH, Khan AN, et al. Cytokine profiling of ascites at primary surgery identifies an interaction of tumor necrosis factor-alpha and interleukin-6 in predicting reduced progression-free survival in epithelial ovarian cancer. Gynecol Oncol. 2015;138:352–7.

35. Seeber A, Braicu I, Untergasser G, et al. Detection of soluble EpCAM (sEpCAM) in malignant ascites predicts poor overall survival in patients treated with catumaxomab. Oncotarget. 2015;6:25017–23.
36. Adhikary T, Wortmann A, Finkernagel F, et al. Interferon signaling in ascites-associated macrophages is linked to a favorable clinical outcome in a subgroup of ovarian carcinoma patients. BMC Genomics. 2017;18:243.
37. Szender JB, Emmons T, Belliotti S, et al. Impact of ascites volume on clinical outcomes in ovarian cancer: a cohort study. Gynecol Oncol. 2017;146:491–7.
38. Garibay-Cerdenares OL, Hernandez-Ramirez VI, Osorio-Trujillo JC, et al. Proteomic identification of fucosylated haptoglobin alpha isoforms in ascitic fluids and its localization in ovarian carcinoma tissues from Mexican patients. J Ovarian Res. 2014;7:27.
39. Huang H, Li Y, Liu J, et al. Screening and identification of biomarkers in ascites related to intrinsic chemoresistance of serous epithelial ovarian cancers. PLoS One. 2012;7:e51256.
40. Keller S, Konig AK, Marme F, et al. Systemic presence and tumor-growth promoting effect of ovarian carcinoma released exosomes. Cancer Lett. 2009;278:73–81.
41. Peng P, Yan Y, Keng S. Exosomes in the ascites of ovarian cancer patients: origin and effects on anti-tumor immunity. Oncol Rep. 2011;25:749–62.
42. Ruscito I, Cacsire Castillo-Tong D, Vergote I, et al. Characterisation of tumour microvessel density during progression of high-grade serous ovarian cancer: clinico-pathological impact (an OCTIPS consortium study). Br J Cancer. 2018;119:330–8.
43. Neufeld G, Cohen T, Gengrinovitch S, Poltorak Z. Vascular endothelial growth factor (VEGF) and its receptors. FASEB J. 1999;13:9–22.
44. Gupta K, Kshirsagar S, Li W, et al. VEGF prevents apoptosis of human microvascular endothelial cells via opposing effects on MAPK/ERK and SAPK/JNK signaling. Exp Cell Res. 1999;247:495–504.
45. Burger RA, Brady MF, Bookman MA, et al. Risk factors for GI adverse events in a phase III randomized trial of bevacizumab in first-line therapy of advanced ovarian cancer: a gynecologic oncology group study. J Clin Oncol. 2014;32:1210–7.
46. Coleman RL, Brady MF, Herzog TJ, et al. Bevacizumab and paclitaxel-carboplatin chemotherapy and secondary cytoreduction in recurrent, platinum-sensitive ovarian cancer (NRG oncology/gynecologic oncology group study GOG-0213): a multicentre, open-label, randomised, phase 3 trial. Lancet Oncol. 2017;18:779–91.
47. Burger RA, Sill MW, Monk BJ, et al. Phase II trial of bevacizumab in persistent or recurrent epithelial ovarian cancer or primary peritoneal cancer: a gynecologic oncology group study. J Clin Oncol. 2007;25:5165–71.
48. Perren TJ, Swart AM, Pfisterer J, et al. A phase 3 trial of bevacizumab in ovarian cancer. N Engl J Med. 2011;365:2484–96.
49. Burger RA, Brady MF, Bookman MA, et al. Incorporation of bevacizumab in the primary treatment of ovarian cancer. N Engl J Med. 2011;365:2473–83.
50. Pujade-Lauraine E, Hilpert F, Weber B, et al. Bevacizumab combined with chemotherapy for platinum-resistant recurrent ovarian cancer: the AURELIA open-label randomized phase III trial. J Clin Oncol. 2014;32:1302–8.
51. Aghajanian C, Blank SV, Goff BA, et al. OCEANS: a randomized, double-blind, placebo-controlled phase III trial of chemotherapy with or without bevacizumab in patients with platinum-sensitive recurrent epithelial ovarian, primary peritoneal, or fallopian tube cancer. J Clin Oncol. 2012;30:2039–45.
52. Moroney JW, Sood AK, Coleman RL. Aflibercept in epithelial ovarian carcinoma. Future Oncol. 2009;5:591–600.
53. Colombo N, Mangili G, Mammoliti S, et al. A phase II study of aflibercept in patients with advanced epithelial ovarian cancer and symptomatic malignant ascites. Gynecol Oncol. 2012;125:42–7.
54. Byrne AT, Ross L, Holash J, et al. Vascular endothelial growth factor-trap decreases tumor burden, inhibits ascites, and causes dramatic vascular remodeling in an ovarian cancer model. Clin Cancer Res. 2003;9:5721–8.

55. Matulonis UA, Berlin S, Ivy P, et al. Cediranib, an oral inhibitor of vascular endothelial growth factor receptor kinases, is an active drug in recurrent epithelial ovarian, fallopian tube, and peritoneal cancer. J Clin Oncol. 2009;27:5601–6.
56. Hirte H, Lheureux S, Fleming GF, et al. A phase 2 study of cediranib in recurrent or persistent ovarian, peritoneal or fallopian tube cancer: a trial of the Princess Margaret, Chicago and California phase II consortia. Gynecol Oncol. 2015;138:55–61.
57. Pignata S, Scambia G, Katsaros D, et al. Carboplatin plus paclitaxel once a week versus every 3 weeks in patients with advanced ovarian cancer (MITO-7): a randomised, multicentre, open-label, phase 3 trial. Lancet Oncol. 2014;15:396–405.
58. du Bois A, Kristensen G, Ray-Coquard I, et al. Standard first-line chemotherapy with or without nintedanib for advanced ovarian cancer (AGO-OVAR 12): a randomised, double-blind, placebo-controlled phase 3 trial. Lancet Oncol. 2016;17:78–89.
59. Kraman M, Bambrough PJ, Arnold JN, et al. Suppression of antitumor immunity by stromal cells expressing fibroblast activation protein-alpha. Science. 2010;330:827–30.
60. Zhang Y, Ertl HC. Starved and asphyxiated: how can CD8(+) T cells within a tumor microenvironment prevent tumor progression. Front Immunol. 2016;7:32.
61. Wen Y, Wang CT, Ma TT, et al. Immunotherapy targeting fibroblast activation protein inhibits tumor growth and increases survival in a murine colon cancer model. Cancer Sci. 2010;101:2325–32.
62. Cheng JD, Valianou M, Canutescu AA, et al. Abrogation of fibroblast activation protein enzymatic activity attenuates tumor growth. Mol Cancer Ther. 2005;4:351–60.
63. Iwanicki MP, Davidowitz RA, Ng MR, et al. Ovarian cancer spheroids use myosin-generated force to clear the mesothelium. Cancer Discov. 2011;1:144–57.
64. Satpathy M, Cao L, Pincheira R, et al. Enhanced peritoneal ovarian tumor dissemination by tissue transglutaminase. Cancer Res. 2007;67:7194–202.
65. Shao M, Cao L, Shen C, et al. Epithelial-to-mesenchymal transition and ovarian tumor progression induced by tissue transglutaminase. Cancer Res. 2009;69:9192–201.
66. Mullamitha SA, Ton NC, Parker GJ, et al. Phase I evaluation of a fully human anti-alphav integrin monoclonal antibody (CNTO 95) in patients with advanced solid tumors. Clin Cancer Res. 2007;13:2128–35.
67. Hersey P, Sosman J, O'Day S, et al. A randomized phase 2 study of etaracizumab, a monoclonal antibody against integrin alpha(v)beta(3), + or - dacarbazine in patients with stage IV metastatic melanoma. Cancer. 2010;116:1526–34.
68. Bell-McGuinn KM, Matthews CM, Ho SN, et al. A phase II, single-arm study of the anti-alpha5beta1 integrin antibody volociximab as monotherapy in patients with platinum-resistant advanced epithelial ovarian or primary peritoneal cancer. Gynecol Oncol. 2011;121:273–9.
69. Condello S, Sima L, Ivan C, et al. Tissue Transglutaminase regulates interactions between ovarian Cancer stem cells and the tumor niche. Cancer Res. 2018;78:2990–3001.
70. Yakubov B, Chen L, Belkin AM, et al. Small molecule inhibitors target the tissue transglutaminase and fibronectin interaction. PLoS One. 2014;9:e89285.
71. Kandalaft LE, Powell DJ Jr, Chiang CL, et al. Autologous lysate-pulsed dendritic cell vaccination followed by adoptive transfer of vaccine-primed ex vivo co-stimulated T cells in recurrent ovarian cancer. Oncoimmunology. 2013;2:e22664.
72. Wang X, Deavers M, Patenia R, et al. Monocyte/macrophage and T-cell infiltrates in peritoneum of patients with ovarian cancer or benign pelvic disease. J Transl Med. 2006;4:30.
73. Yin M, Li X, Tan S, et al. Tumor-associated macrophages drive spheroid formation during early transcoelomic metastasis of ovarian cancer. J Clin Invest. 2016;126:4157–73.
74. Hagemann T, Wilson J, Kulbe H, et al. Macrophages induce invasiveness of epithelial cancer cells via NF-kappa B and JNK. J Immunol. 2005;175:1197–205.
75. Burges A, Wimberger P, Kumper C, et al. Effective relief of malignant ascites in patients with advanced ovarian cancer by a trifunctional anti-EpCAM x anti-CD3 antibody: a phase I/II study. Clin Cancer Res. 2007;13:3899–905.
76. Pulaski HL, Spahlinger G, Silva IA, et al. Identifying alemtuzumab as an anti-myeloid cell antiangiogenic therapy for the treatment of ovarian cancer. J Transl Med. 2009;7:49.

77. Zhu H, Bengsch F, Svoronos N, et al. BET Bromodomain inhibition promotes anti-tumor immunity by suppressing PD-L1 expression. Cell Rep. 2016;16:2829–37.
78. Stone ML, Chiappinelli KB, Li H, et al. Epigenetic therapy activates type I interferon signaling in murine ovarian cancer to reduce immunosuppression and tumor burden. Proc Natl Acad Sci U S A. 2017;114:E10981–90.
79. Penn CA, Yang K, Zong H, et al. Therapeutic impact of nanoparticle therapy targeting tumor-associated macrophages. Mol Cancer Ther. 2018;17:96–106.
80. Horikawa N, Abiko K, Matsumura N, et al. Expression of vascular endothelial growth factor in ovarian Cancer inhibits tumor immunity through the accumulation of myeloid-derived suppressor cells. Clin Cancer Res. 2017;23:587–99.
81. Darb-Esfahani S, Kunze CA, Kulbe H, et al. Prognostic impact of programmed cell death-1 (PD-1) and PD-ligand 1 (PD-L1) expression in cancer cells and tumor-infiltrating lymphocytes in ovarian high grade serous carcinoma. Oncotarget. 2016;7:1486–99.
82. Webb JR, Milne K, Kroeger DR, Nelson BH. PD-L1 expression is associated with tumor-infiltrating T cells and favorable prognosis in high-grade serous ovarian cancer. Gynecol Oncol. 2016;141:293–302.
83. Hamanishi J, Mandai M, Iwasaki M, et al. Programmed cell death 1 ligand 1 and tumor-infiltrating CD8+ T lymphocytes are prognostic factors of human ovarian cancer. Proc Natl Acad Sci U S A. 2007;104:3360–5.
84. Duraiswamy J, Freeman GJ, Coukos G. Therapeutic PD-1 pathway blockade augments with other modalities of immunotherapy T-cell function to prevent immune decline in ovarian cancer. Cancer Res. 2013;73:6900–12.
85. Chalmers ZR, Connelly CF, Fabrizio D, et al. Analysis of 100,000 human cancer genomes reveals the landscape of tumor mutational burden. Genome Med. 2017;9:34.
86. Hamanishi J, Mandai M, Ikeda T, et al. Safety and antitumor activity of anti-PD-1 antibody, Nivolumab, in patients with platinum-resistant ovarian Cancer. J Clin Oncol. 2015;33:4015–22.
87. Hodi FS, Butler M, Oble DA, et al. Immunologic and clinical effects of antibody blockade of cytotoxic T lymphocyte-associated antigen 4 in previously vaccinated cancer patients. Proc Natl Acad Sci U S A. 2008;105:3005–10.

Chapter 11
Brain Cancer Biomarkers in Proximal Fluids

11.1 Introduction

Nervous system (NS) tumors are a conglomerate of neoplastic transformation of cells that constitute the nervous system. While there are numerous types, gliomas are the commonest NS tumors. Gliomas constitute a group of central NS (CNS) tumors further subdivided based on putative cell of origin into astrocytomas, oligodendrogliomas, and oligoastrocytomas. The 2018 estimated global incidence, mortality, and 5-year prevalence of brain and nervous system tumors were 296,851, 241,037, and 771,110, respectively. While not as common as other solid tumors such as colon cancer, the prognosis of glioma is very dismal. The recurrence rate is high, with usually emergence of high-grade tumors. The median survival is 12–18 months for WHO grade IV glioblastoma (GBM). Even supposedly early-stage grade II patients have just 5–10 years, while grade III oligodendroglioma and astrocytoma patients survive for 3–10 years and 2 years, respectively. The need for early detection and importantly predictive biomarkers for this tumor is thus urgently needed.

For personalized medicine, accurate classification of CNS tumors is needed. Thus, biomarkers that inform tumor behavior or biology ushers in this paradigm shift in management of BrTms. As is established, co-deletion of chromosomes 1p and 19q in grade III anaplastic oligodendrogliomas has a better prognosis than other glioma subtypes. Similarly, isocitrate dehydrogenase 1 (NADP+) *IDH1* mutations in grade III glioblastoma are associated with better prognosis than patients with *IDH1* wild-type tumors. There are currently emerging biomarkers such as noncoding RNAs, proteomics, and metabolomics that should enhance our knowledge and management of gliomas. Being able to assay these biomarkers noninvasively and longitudinally will definitely improve glioma early detection and optimal patient care.

G. D. Dakubo, *Cancer Biomarkers in Body Fluids*,
https://doi.org/10.1007/978-3-030-24725-6_11

11.2 Cerebrospinal Fluid

Normal CSF is a clear and colorless fluid that percolates the brain and spinal cord and is continuously produced by specialized ependymal cells of the choroid plexus in the lateral, third, and fourth ventricles. This body fluid circulates in the ventricles, cisterns, the subarachnoid space, and over the brain cortices before being absorbed in the arachnoid granulations. It nourishes the brain and spinal cord and removes waste products from these tissues. Because of this circulatory path, CSF is in contact with the entire CNS and hence serves as a minimally invasive sample for diagnosis and management of CNS pathologies including neurological disorders, infections, and cancer. CSF is produced at a rate of 0.3–0.4 ml min^{-1}, and the total volume is 65–150 ml in children and 90–150 ml in adults. The normal CSF contains 0–5 mononuclear cells/ml, 50–80 mg/dl glucose, and 15–45 mg/dl proteins. These parameters change in various CNS pathologies including cancer.

Brain cancer biomarkers reach the CSF by direct release or shedding of cancer cells from tumors that are in contact with the fluid and also via the blood-brain barrier from brain metastasis. CSF is acquired for diagnosis and management of brain diseases including cancer. It is usually obtained via a lumbar puncture, whereby a needle is inserted in between the third and fourth lumbar vertebrae to obtain about 20 ml of fluid for analysis. Various techniques and technologies are employed for biomarker analysis of CSF. Cytology (the gold standard), flow cytometry, and various molecular techniques enable detection of cancer signatures in CSF.

11.2.1 Cytoanalysis of Cerebrospinal Fluid for Brain Cancer Cells

CSF cytology and flow cytometry augment each other in detecting cancer cells. Cytology is clinically the gold standard for diagnosing leptomeningeal spread of primary brain cancer as well as cancer metastasis to the brain. CSF cytology involves acquisition of CSF, primarily via lumbar puncture, followed by immediate centrifugation to avoid cell lysis with prolonged storage, slide preparation, staining, and examination for neoplastic cells. Another procedure is thin layer preparation (ThinPrep), which is being advocated because it improves malignant cell detection by preserving cell morphology. Despite being highly specific and the gold standard, CSF cytology suffers from a number of limitations. It is a qualitative analysis of CSF by pathologists, and therefore inter-observer variability is unavoidable. Moreover, because cancer cells are shed intermittently, multiple sampling will be required to increase sensitivity. Thus, depending on the number of sampling, sensitivity could be as low as 45% and false-negative rates as high as 10–20% [1]. In a review of diagnosis of CNS lymphoma between 1966 and 2011, sensitivity of cytology was 2–32%, which was augmented by incorporating flow cytometry [2]. But performance of cytology increased to a sensitivity of 58–85% at a specificity of 85%

when combined with analysis of proteins such as β2-microglobulin, immunoglobulin heavy chain rearrangement, and LDH isoenzyme 5. Moreover, this analysis observed the superiority of miRNA that had a specificity of 95% in diagnosis of CNS lymphoma.

11.3 Brain Cancer Biomarkers in Proximal Fluid

11.3.1 Brain Cancer miRNA Biomarkers in Proximal Fluid

The stability of miRNA in body fluids has made them targets of exploration in CSF as brain cancer biomarkers. Several CSF miRNAs including miR-10b, miR-15b, miR-21, miR-92a, miR-125b, miR-200 family, miR-223, miR-451, miR-711, and miR-935 have been associated with different CNS tumors. For example, miR-15b and miR-21 are glioma (GBM) biomarkers, while miR-19, miR-21, and miR-92a are diagnostic biomarkers of primary central nervous system lymphoma (PCNSL).

In 2012, Baraniskin et al. examined the role of miRNAs in CSF from brain cancer patients [3]. Of six miRNAs of interest, miR-15b and miR-21 were associated with glioma because they could distinguish glioma patients from even patients with other BrTms including PCNSL and BrTms from metastasis at a sensitivity of 90% and perfect specificity. miRNA analysis of CSF from patients with GBM, metastatic brain cancer, and non-cancer controls enabled discriminatory miRNAs between the two brain cancers to be uncovered [4]. A panel of seven miRNAs achieved 90% accuracy in this regard. Of interest, both GBM and metastatic brain cancer patients' CSF harbored elevated miR-10b and miR-21, while miR-200 was elevated in CSF from patients with only brain metastasis. Apart from the diagnostic potential, the three miRNAs could be useful in monitoring disease burden and treatment response. In patients with recurrent glioma, CSF miR-21 was demonstrated to have diagnostic and prognostic utility. Elevated levels were associated with poor prognosis and disease recurrence [5].

Baraniskin et al. uncovered significantly increased levels of miR-19, miR-21, and miR-92a in CSF from patients with primary central nervous system lymphoma (PCNSL) compared to control patients with other neurological disorders [6]. This miRNA panel achieved a sensitivity and specificity of 96.7% and 96.7%, respectively, in diagnosis of PCNSL. CSF samples from neoplastic (PCNSL, GBM, MB, brain metastasis) and nonneoplastic (benign and normal) patients were subjected to miRNA profiling [7]. Significant differential levels of miR-125b, miR-223, miR-451, miR-711, and miR-935 were uncovered that could stratify some tumors. Following RT-PCR and in situ hybridization validation, a diagnostic chart was constructed for CNS malignancies based on CSF miRNAs. A meta-analysis of 23 studies (13 glioma and 10 PCNSL studies) involving 299 cases and 418 controls considered the diagnostic accuracy of circulating miRNAs (CSF and blood) for these tumors. CSF miRNAs, especially for PCNSL, achieved higher sensitivity than blood [8].

Medulloblastoma cell lines released miRNAs into culture medium that could discriminate between the cell lines. The tested MB cell lines were D341 (metastatic-related group 3 MB subtype), D283 (metastasis-related group 4 MB subtype), and DAOY (Sonic Hedgehog-related subtype). Each cell line released >1000 miRNAs into the medium, of which a panel was specific to the metastatic-related group 3 and 4 subtypes. Sixty miRNAs of the panel were increased, while 52 were decreased compared to DAOY miRNAs. miR-125a, miR-125b, and miR-1290 that were elevated in culture medium of the metastasis-related cell lines were significantly enriched in CSF from a MB patient [9].

11.3.2 Brain Cancer Protein Biomarkers in Proximal Fluid

Numerous proteins have been identified in CSF from brain cancer patients. While some are used in clinical practice, the vast majority remains to be validated.

Several studies have examined for differential protein levels in CSF from glioma patients. A study measured VEGF levels in CSF from 27 patients with high-grade astrocytoma, 39 with non-astrocytoma CNS neoplasia, and 14 normal controls [10]. The findings suggest VEGF as a biomarker for high-grade astrocytoma because levels were significantly elevated in 89% of CSF from malignant astrocytoma than those with non-astrocytic tumors. Another protein significantly altered in CSF from GBM compared to astrocytoma (grade II) patients is gelsolin [11]. In a pilot study (n = 2 each of cases and controls), decreased gelsolin levels were associated with histologic grades. To investigate the possible prognostic value of gelsolin, 41 formalin-fixed and paraffin-embedded (FFPE) astrocytoma tissues of different grades were examined for gelsolin expression. Consistent with their discovery phase data, levels of gelsolin were significantly lower in high- than low-grade astrocytomas, and this was significantly associated with OS, which was poorer in patients with low-expressing gelsolin in their tumors.

Distinction between primary brain tumors and metastasis from elsewhere is important in disease management. CEA levels in CSF could be used to differentiate between the two [12, 13], and this augmented diagnosis of meningeal carcinomatosis [14], e.g., from the lung [15].

Proteomic analysis of CSF has also enabled discovery of brain tumor biomarkers. CSF proteomic signature could differentiate malignant patients from nonmalignant controls, and this analysis uncovered carbonic anhydrase as a potential brain tumor prognostic biomarker [16]. 2-DGE and cleavable isotope-coded affinity tag (ICAT) was used to uncover brain tumor-associated proteins in CSF. The samples included WHO grade II, III, and IV astrocytomas, metastatic brain tumors, schwannomas, inflammatory disease conditions, and normal controls. Analysis of 60 samples enabled identification of 103 potential brain tumor biomarkers. Twenty of these including CEGFB, FGF14, β2M, and SPARCL1 were specific to high-grade astrocytoma [17]. MS-based proteomic analysis of CSF from GBM patients and controls detected 2000 peptides of which 4 could significantly differentiate patients from controls. The four peptides, osteopontin, transthyretin, N-terminal residue of albumin, and C-terminal fragment of a-1-antichymotrypsin, are constituents of normal CSF but are elevated in CSF from GBM patients [18]. In a review by Shen et al., 19 proteins with differentially altered levels in CSF from glioma patients were reported [19]. The majority including CA2, CA12, CALD1, MYCN, SERPINA3, SPARCL1, DDAH1, PPIA, VEGFB, SP1, MAPT, and ALB were elevated, while GSN was lower in glioma patients.

Both targeted protein measurement and proteomic approaches have been used to uncover medulloblastoma (MB) biomarkers in CSF. Treatment monitoring and recurrence detection may be possible by determining the levels of polysialic acid-neural cell adhesion molecule (PSA-NCAM), because levels were significantly higher in CSF from MB patients refractory to treatment and relapsed patients than those in remission [20]. Rajagopal et al. used 2-DGE to analyze proteins in CSF from 33 MB patients and 25 age-matched controls [21]. This enabled the identification of prostaglandin D2 synthase, which was significantly decreased (sixfold) in CSF from patients compared to controls. Another proteomic analysis of CSF from 14 pediatric patients with posterior fossa tumors, including 5 MBs, 6 pilocytic astrocytomas, and 3 ependymomas, in comparison to 5 non-tumoral controls uncovered hemoglobin subunit fragments (VV- and LVV-hemorphin-7 peptides) as potential biomarkers. While both peptides were present in control CSF samples, they were undetectable in CSF from cases [22]. As a potential biomarker for postsurgical monitoring, relapsed patients had been undetectable of the peptides in CSF collected 6 days after surgery.

Biomarkers in CSF play important roles in the clinical management of intracranial malignant germ cell tumors (IMGCTs). Germ cell tumors comprise of gonadal and extragonadal tumors that are derived from primordial germ cells during embryonic development. The pineal gland and suprasellar region are common intracranial sites of extragonadal GCTs, which comprise about 3% of all childhood brain tumors. Consistent with their origin, IMGCTs express embryonic markers such as βHCG and β-FP (AFP), and therefore their levels are markedly elevated in CSF of patients [23, 24]. These biomarkers are thus clinically employed for diagnosis and treatment response monitoring of IMGCTs. Serum and CSF measurements of AFP and total βHCG are used to distinguish between non-germinoma and germinoma GCTs. Prognostic wise, age (< 6 years) and CSF AFP levels >1000 ng/ml at diagnosis are considered high-risk for disease and require more aggressive treatment. Additionally, following surgical resection, IMGCT patients with increasing CSF βHCG and/or AFP are deemed to have relapsed. Other CSF protein biomarkers for management of IMGCTs are LDH isoenzymes, PLAP, and soluble c-kit receptor (s-kit). Although less specific than AFP and βHCG, PLAP and isozymes of LDH in CSF are also used for diagnosis and management of IGCTs. Patients with IGCTs have elevated CSF levels of s-kit, and this has been demonstrated to be a reliable biomarker for disease diagnosis, as well as detection of recurrence and dissemination into the subarachnoid space [25].

CSF from patients with PCNSL harbors differential levels of some proteins. Many investigators suggest that elevated levels of antithrombin III in CSF form

PCNSL patients have clinical utility. In a prospective validation study, CSF levels of antithrombin III > 1.2 g/ml enabled disease diagnosis at a sensitivity and specificity of >70% and 99%, respectively [26]. Moreover, the elevated CSF levels of antithrombin III have been associated with decreased response to chemotherapy and shorter patient survival. However, Kuusisto et al. suggest the elevated antithrombin III levels in CSF are due to compromised blood-brain barrier, and hence may not be a suitable biomarker for PCNSL [27].

Because of its irresectability, and hence paucity of tissue samples for study, CSF has been an attractive sample for analysis of diffuse intrinsic pontine glioma (DIPG) biomarkers. To this end, MS proteomics was used to interrogate CSF from DIPG patients and controls. This approach led to the identification of cyclophilin A (CypA) and N(G), N(G)-dimethylarginine dimethylaminohydrolase 1 (DDAH1) as being elevated in CSF from patients [28]. Immunohistochemistry and Western blot analysis were used to validate these biomarkers in CSF, brain tissue, and serum samples. By immunohistochemistry, it was uncovered that the elevated DDAH1 and CypA levels were due to secreted and not cytosolic levels. Measurement of serum and/or CSF levels of these biomarkers may be clinically useful in treatment response and recurrence monitoring.

While rare, atypical teratoid/rhabdoid tumor (AT/RT) is a highly aggressive pediatric tumor commonly diagnosed in children <5 years of age. Osteopontin (OPN) is a biomarker of AT/RT because levels are significantly elevated in these tumors. Kao et al. used ELISA and immunohistochemistry to analyze OPN levels in CSF from 39 patients with AT/RT (8), MB (16), hydrocephalus (9), and epilepsy (6) [29]. CSF and plasma levels of OPN were much higher in AT/RT patients than patients with the other pathologies. The elevated levels significantly correlated with disease relapse, while treatment was associated with decreased CSF levels.

11.3.3 Brain Cancer Metabolomics Biomarkers in Proximal Fluid

Analysis of meningioma, neuroblastoma, and glioblastoma cell lines yielded metabolic profiles that differentiated histologic subtypes of cancers. The metabolites were alanine, glutamine, creatine, phosphorylcholine, and threonine.

11.4 Summary

- While not among the top 10 cancers diagnosed globally, the prognosis of WHO grade IV glioblastoma is dismal with median survival of 12–18 months.
- The gold standard for diagnosing leptomeningeal spread of primary and metastatic brain cancer is cytologic analysis of CSF.
- CSF cytology, while highly specific, suffers from sensitivity, which is as low as 45% depending on a number of samples and false-negative rates of 10–20%.

- Flow cytometry enhances CSF cytoanalysis in BrTm detection.
- A role for molecular analysis of CSF is the enhanced sensitivity and specificity achieved by incorporating proteins.
- Commonly investigating CSF of BrTm patients are miRNAs and proteins.

References

1. Ahluwalia MS, Wallace PK, Peereboom DM. Flow cytometry as a diagnostic tool in lymphomatous or leukemic meningitis: ready for prime time? Cancer. 2012;118:1747–53.
2. Scott BJ, Douglas VC, Tihan T, et al. A systematic approach to the diagnosis of suspected central nervous system lymphoma. JAMA Neurol. 2013;70:311–9.
3. Baraniskin A, Kuhnhenn J, Schlegel U, et al. Identification of microRNAs in the cerebrospinal fluid as biomarker for the diagnosis of glioma. Neuro-Oncology. 2012;14:29–33.
4. Teplyuk NM, Mollenhauer B, Gabriely G, et al. MicroRNAs in cerebrospinal fluid identify glioblastoma and metastatic brain cancers and reflect disease activity. Neuro-Oncology. 2012;14:689–700.
5. Shi R, Wang PY, Li XY, et al. Exosomal levels of miRNA-21 from cerebrospinal fluids associated with poor prognosis and tumor recurrence of glioma patients. Oncotarget. 2015;6:26971–81.
6. Baraniskin A, Kuhnhenn J, Schlegel U, et al. Identification of microRNAs in the cerebrospinal fluid as marker for primary diffuse large B-cell lymphoma of the central nervous system. Blood. 2011;117:3140–6.
7. Drusco A, Bottoni A, Lagana A, et al. A differentially expressed set of microRNAs in cerebrospinal fluid (CSF) can diagnose CNS malignancies. Oncotarget. 2015;6:20829–39.
8. Wei D, Wan Q, Li L, et al. MicroRNAs as potential biomarkers for diagnosing cancers of central nervous system: a meta-analysis. Mol Neurobiol. 2015;51:1452–61.
9. Shalaby T, Grotzer MA. Tumor-associated CSF MicroRNAs for the prediction and evaluation of CNS malignancies. Int J Mol Sci. 2015;16:29103–19.
10. Sampath P, Weaver CE, Sungarian A, et al. Cerebrospinal fluid (vascular endothelial growth factor) and serologic (recoverin) tumor markers for malignant glioma. Cancer Control. 2004;11:174–80.
11. Ohnishi M, Matsumoto T, Nagashio R, et al. Proteomics of tumor-specific proteins in cerebrospinal fluid of patients with astrocytoma: usefulness of gelsolin protein. Pathol Int. 2009;59:797–803.
12. Batabyal SK, Ghosh B, Sengupta S, et al. Cerebrospinal fluid and serum carcinoembryonic antigen in brain tumors. Neoplasma. 2003;50:377–9.
13. Moldrich G, Lange P, Strik H. Carcinoembryonic antigen in the CSF of cancer patients--the value of intrathecal synthesis and correlation with IgA-diffusion dynamics. Acta Neurol Belg. 2010;110:314–20.
14. Nakagawa H, Kubo S, Murasawa A, et al. Measurements of CSF biochemical tumor markers in patients with meningeal carcinomatosis. No Shinkei Geka. 1991;19:1135–41.
15. Wang P, Piao Y, Zhang X, et al. The concentration of CYFRA 21-1, NSE and CEA in cerebrospinal fluid can be useful indicators for diagnosis of meningeal carcinomatosis of lung cancer. Cancer Biomark. 2013;13:123–30.
16. Khwaja FW, Nolen JD, Mendrinos SE, et al. Proteomic analysis of cerebrospinal fluid discriminates malignant and nonmalignant disease of the central nervous system and identifies specific protein markers. Proteomics. 2006;6:6277–87.
17. Khwaja FW, Reed MS, Olson JJ, et al. Proteomic identification of biomarkers in the cerebrospinal fluid (CSF) of astrocytoma patients. J Proteome Res. 2007;6:559–70.

18. Schuhmann MU, Zucht HD, Nassimi R, et al. Peptide screening of cerebrospinal fluid in patients with glioblastoma multiforme. Eur J Surg Oncol. 2010;36:201–7.
19. Shen F, Zhang Y, Yao Y, et al. Proteomic analysis of cerebrospinal fluid: toward the identification of biomarkers for gliomas. Neurosurg Rev. 2014;37:367–80. discussion 380
20. Figarella-Branger D, Dubois C, Chauvin P, et al. Correlation between polysialic-neural cell adhesion molecule levels in CSF and medulloblastoma outcomes. J Clin Oncol. 1996;14:2066–72.
21. Rajagopal MU, Hathout Y, MacDonald TJ, et al. Proteomic profiling of cerebrospinal fluid identifies prostaglandin D2 synthase as a putative biomarker for pediatric medulloblastoma: a pediatric brain tumor consortium study. Proteomics. 2011;11:935–43.
22. Desiderio C, D'Angelo L, Rossetti DV, et al. Cerebrospinal fluid top-down proteomics evidenced the potential biomarker role of LVV- and VV-hemorphin-7 in posterior cranial fossa pediatric brain tumors. Proteomics. 2012;12:2158–66.
23. Nishizaki T, Kajiwara K, Adachi N, et al. Detection of craniospinal dissemination of intracranial germ cell tumours based on serum and cerebrospinal fluid levels of tumour markers. J Clin Neurosci. 2001;8:27–30.
24. Qaddoumi I, Sane M, Li S, et al. Diagnostic utility and correlation of tumor markers in the serum and cerebrospinal fluid of children with intracranial germ cell tumors. Childs Nerv Syst. 2012;28:1017–24.
25. Miyanohara O, Takeshima H, Kaji M, et al. Diagnostic significance of soluble c-kit in the cerebrospinal fluid of patients with germ cell tumors. J Neurosurg. 2002;97:177–83.
26. Gomes HR. Cerebrospinal fluid approach on neuro-oncology. Arq Neuropsiquiatr. 2013;71:677–80.
27. Kuusisto ME, Haapasaari KM, Remes AM, et al. Antithrombin III is probably not a suitable biomarker for diagnosis of primary central nervous system lymphoma. Ann Hematol. 2015;94:1167–74.
28. Saratsis AM, Yadavilli S, Magge S, et al. Insights into pediatric diffuse intrinsic pontine glioma through proteomic analysis of cerebrospinal fluid. Neuro-Oncology. 2012;14:547–60.
29. Kao CL, Chiou SH, Ho DM, et al. Elevation of plasma and cerebrospinal fluid osteopontin levels in patients with atypical teratoid/rhabdoid tumor. Am J Clin Pathol. 2005;123:297–304.

Chapter 12
Hematologic Malignancy Biomarkers in Proximal Fluids

12.1 Introduction

Collectively, the global incidence, mortality and 5-year prevalence for hematologic malignancies in 2018 were 1,186,598, 690,002, and 3,179,658, respectively (GLOBOCAN 2018). The majority in terms of these statistics was non-Hodgkin lymphoma and leukemia, but the mortality appears disproportionately high among cases of multiple myeloma. Abnormal proliferation and unwary expansion of hematopoietic lineage cells give rise to hematologic malignancies. Thus, these cancers most commonly occur in hematopoietic tissues such as the bone marrow or tissues of the immune system such as the lymph nodes. Normal hematopoiesis involves stem cell proliferation and dichotomized differentiation into the myeloid or lymphoid lineage. Myeloid stem cells give rise to granulocytes, monocytes, basophils, mast cells, eosinophil's, erythrocytes, platelets, and monocytoid dendritic cells, while T and B lymphocytes, natural killer (NK) cells, and plasmacytoid dendritic cells originate from the lymphoid lineage. Therefore hematologic malignancies can be viewed as diseases from the myeloid or lymphoid lineages. Because of the numerous lineage relationships of these cells during hematopoiesis, there can be considerable overlap in hematopoietic diseases (e.g., myelodysplastic/myeloproliferative overlap syndromes, chronic lymphocytic leukemia/small lymphocytic lymphoma overlap). Moreover, these overlaps and molecular phenotypes can lead to more complex classification of hematologic malignancies that are beyond this text.

Signs and symptoms of hematologic cancer can be obtained from patients, or suspicion can be made based on routine peripheral blood examination (e.g., low cell counts) or for myeloma, abnormally high immunoglobulin (Ig) protein levels. Definite diagnosis of hematologic malignancy, however, requires bone marrow aspiration and tumor or bone marrow biopsy. With lymphomas however, core needle biopsy is reserved for inaccessible nodes, while preference is given to excisional biopsy. Samples obtained are subjected to a number of diagnostic procedures

G. D. Dakubo, *Cancer Biomarkers in Body Fluids*,
https://doi.org/10.1007/978-3-030-24725-6_12

including morphologic examination, flow cytometry, histochemistry, cytogenetics, and targeting specific gene mutations. Because all these procedures are invasive and can be costly, and yet biopsy tends to sample only tumor tissue at specific anatomical site, it is unable to be representative of all clones of any particular tumor. Body fluid biopsy offers such advantage and hence is preferred for holistic disease profiling. Because hematologic malignancy is largely a genetic disease, there are numerous biomarkers amenable to body fluid biopsy applications, and these have been extensively explored.

12.2 Classification of Hematologic Malignancies

Neoplastic proliferation of white blood cells in the bone marrow, immune system, or other tissues such as the brain falls under three distinct categories: (i) lymphoid neoplasm, (ii) myeloid neoplasm, and, rarely, (iii) histiocytic neoplasm. Tumors from hematopoietic progenitor cells that expand uncontrollably to replace normal repertoire of bone marrow cells (myeloid neoplasms) fall under three main categories, namely, (i) acute myeloid leukemia (AML) whereby neoplastic cells are arrested at early stages of myeloid cell development and hence blast cells replace the normal marrow cells; (ii) myeloproliferative disorders (MPD) whereby neoplastic cells have increased growth and proliferation, but proceed to differentiate as red blood cells (RBCs), granulocytes, and/or platelets in circulation; and (iii) myelodysplastic syndromes (MDS) whereby neoplastic cells undergo abnormal differentiation to generate increased dysplastic precursor cells in the bone marrow, hence leading to cytopenias. Note there are considerable overlaps between MPD and MDS, and both could proceed to AML. The other major category of hematologic malignancy is lymphoid neoplasm. This large category includes (i) acute lymphocytic/lymphoblastic leukemia (ALL), which includes precursor B- and T-cell lymphoblastic leukemia/lymphoma; (ii) chronic lymphocytic leukemia (CLL), which includes chronic lymphocytic leukemia/small lymphocytic lymphoma; (iii) follicular lymphoma; (iv) diffuse large B-cell lymphoma; (v) mantle cell lymphoma; (vi) Burkitt lymphoma; (vii) Hodgkin (HL) and non-Hodgkin lymphoma (NHL); and (viii) multiple myeloma. Langerhans cell histiocytosis constitutes histiocytic neoplasm.

12.3 Biology of Noncoding RNAs in Hematologic Malignancies

Noncoding transcripts appear to have a profound role in normal hematopoiesis and hematologic malignancy. The authentic characterization of these functions should usher in a new understanding of how hematopoietic cells diversify and how dysregulation of these molecules cause blood cancers.

12.3.1 Role of Long Noncoding RNA in Hematopoiesis

A role for long noncoding RNA (lncRNA) in normal hematopoiesis and hematologic malignancy has been demonstrated in a number of studies. In general, it appears their role do not necessarily overlap, such that the lncRNA regulating hematopoiesis are not necessarily the same dysregulated in hematologic neoplasm.

Erythroid lineage cell diversification is partly controlled by lncRNA. Developmentally, erythroid prosurvival intergenic lncRNA, lincRNA-EPS, regulate erythroid differentiation. This lncRNA is highly expressed in erythroid precursors, and its knockdown inhibited erythroid precursor differentiation in association with apoptosis, which could be rescued by ectopic expression [1]. A number of lncRNAs targeted by GATA1, TAL1, and KLF1 (erythroid transcription factors) were uncovered by RNA-sequencing [2]. Silencing of these RNAs impaired erythroid maturation with reduced cell sizes. One of these lncRNA, EC7, activates expression of a neighboring gene, BAND3.

Some lncRNAs also modulate myeloid lineage cell development. Highly expressed in the bone marrow and matured eosinophil is lncRNA eosinophil granule ontogeny (EGO). Identified in eosinophil differentiation of CD34+ progenitor cells, EGO regulates major basic protein (MBP) and eosinophil-derived neurotoxin (EDN) expression [3]. An essential regulator of hematopoiesis, which when dysregulated leads to leukemia and lymphoma development (PU.1), is negatively regulated by lncRNA PU.1-AS [4]. Another lncRNA expressed in myeloid lineage cells, especially at the terminal stages of granulocyte differentiation, HOX antisense intergenic RNA myeloid 1 (HOTAIRM1), attenuates expression of HOXA1 and HOXA4 and selectively impairs expression of CD11b, CD18, and CD11c, which are myeloid differentiation markers.

Similarly, some lymphoid functions are regulated by lncRNAs. LncRNAs NRON, Thy-ncR1, linc-MAF-4, and TMEVPG1 are involved in T-cell development. Lymphocyte functions may be controlled by noncoding RNA repressor of NFAT (lincRNA NRON), because its knockdown caused NFAT1 dephosphorylation and nuclear translocation with induced expression of NFAT-dependent genes [5]. Highly expressed in the thymus and possibly involved in T-cell differentiation is Thy-ncR1. This lncRNA might regulate T-cell selection and maturation by directly targeting MFAP4 [6]. Located adjacent to IFNγ gene is lincRNA TMEVPG1 that drives Th1 differentiation and IFNγ expression [7]. Linc-MAF-4 targets the Th2-associated transcription factor, MAF, to promote Th1 CD4+ T-cell differentiation. Thus, knockdown of lincRNA-MAF4 was associated with Th2 transcription profile [8].

12.3.2 Role of Long Noncoding RNA in Myeloid Neoplasm

A number of lncRNAs have been linked to the initiation and progression of myeloproliferative diseases. The lncRNA, X-inactive specific transcript (XIST), involved in X-chromosome inactivation might control MPDs. Deletion of XIST after

X-chromosome inactivation in vivo caused development of highly aggressive and lethal myeloproliferative neoplasm (MPN) and MPS [9]. Putatively, loss of XIST resulting in X-reactivation caused dysregulation of oncogenes and tumor suppressor genes involved in myeloproliferative disorders. H19 is a maternally expressed imprinted gene transcribed from the H19/IGF2 cluster. This gene appears to have diverse and complex roles in hematologic malignancy, because it is downregulated in AML, CML, polycythemia vera, essential thrombocythemia, primary myelofibrosis, and chronic myelomonocytic leukemia [10, 11]. On the contrary, loss of imprinting and elevated expression is demonstrated in T-cell leukemia/lymphoma cell line [12]. The upregulation in CML and Bcr-Abl-positive K562 cell line was dependent on Bcr-Abl kinase activity, suggesting H19 and Bcr-Abl might cooperate in development of chronic myeloproliferative diseases. The lncRNA, β-globin locus 3 (BGL3), might function as a tumor suppressor during Bcr-Abl-mediated transformation. Loss of Bcr-Abl expression or kinase activity in K562 cell line and primary CML samples caused upregulation of BGL3, and its ectopic expression inhibited Bcr-Abl-mediated tumor formation in xenograft mouse model, as well as sensitization of K562 leukemic cells to imatinib-induced apoptosis. BGL3 might be a target of a set of miRNAs known to repress PTEN [13]. IRAIN is a maternally expressed imprinted lncRNA within the IGF1R locus. IRAIN promotes cell growth dependent on PI3K/Akt signaling. A role for IRAIN in AML is its demonstrated downregulation in leukemic cell lines and individuals at high risk for developing AML [14]. This downregulation might contribute to activation of oncogenic IGF1R, because of its involvement in the transcriptional control of IGF1R. Another lncRNA, maternally expressed gene 3 (MEG3), is a tumor suppressor under epigenetic control. MEG3 is downregulated in several neoplasms including AML, MDS, and myeloid leukemia, and promoter methylation is associated with poor patient survival [15–18]. BEG3 might contribute to hematologic malignancy through control of *RB* and *CDKN2A/INK4A*. A set of lncRNAs has been associated with common recurrent mutations involving FLT3-ITD, NPM1, CEBP, IDH2, and RUNX1 in AML. Strongest expression of some of these lncRNAs that are antisense to HOX genes such as MEIS1-AS and HOXB-AS3 was particularly associated with NPM1 mutations. Of interest, HOTAIRM1 involved in myeloid lineage differentiation was upregulated in a large series of AML patients [19, 20]. The biomarker potential of these lncRNAs in myeloid disorders requires further elucidation.

12.3.3 Role of Long Noncoding RNA in Lymphoid Neoplasm

In hematologic malignancy, the biology of lncRNA has been most extensively studied in multiple myeloma. Single-gene targets and global gene-profiling studies have both been applied with preliminary interesting results.

In regard to single-gene studies, the roles of MALAT1, MEG3, CRNDE, UCA1, and OIP5-AS1 have specifically been addressed. MALAT1 functions as an oncogenic lncRNA as it is overexpressed in many solid tumors as well. In hematologic malignancy, Cho et al. first examined the expression of MALAT1 in bone marrow mononuclear cells from multiple myeloma patients [21]. Compared to normal control samples, MALAT1 was significantly overexpressed in samples from multiple myeloma patients with different disease statuses. In a large cohort study of patients with different plasma cell dyscrasias, microarray expression analysis further confirmed the elevated expression of MALAT1 in plasma cell tumors. Of interest, the overexpression of MALAT1 was associated with molecular pathways involved in p53-mediated DNA damage response, mRNA maturation, and cell cycle control [22]. The increased levels of MALAT1 in multiple myeloma are from different sources because elevated levels were found in both bone marrow mononuclear cells from untreated patients with different disease statuses and multiple myeloma cell lines [23, 24]. Interestingly, patients in complete remission demonstrated significant reduction of its expression. MALAT1 may promote multiple myeloma development and progression via downstream effectors such as high-mobility group box 1 (HMGB1). Thus, the expression of MALAT1 showed a strict correlation with HMGB1 that mediates autophagy [25]. Not only is it overexpressed, but HMGB1 also sustains the growth, survival, and proliferation of myeloma cells [26]. Reduced levels of HMGB1 were associated with decreased levels of autophagy molecules (Beclin 1 and LC3B) in MALAT1 knockdown multiple myeloma cell lines and animal models [25]. In another experiment, MALAT1 knockdown led to significant reduction in viable multiple myeloma cells in association with increased apoptosis, which could be rescued with concomitant MALAT1 knockdown and HMGB1 overexpression. In addition to HMGB1, MALAT1 appears to modulate molecules involved in cell cycle and apoptosis. Experimental findings suggest that the induction of apoptosis in multiple myeloma cells with MALAT1 knockdown might involve coordinated downregulation of cyclins D1 and E, activation of proapoptotic caspases 3 and 9, and increased levels of BAX, in concert with reduced levels of anti-apoptotic BCL2 [23]. Extramedullary spread of multiple myeloma cells often develops following several cycles of chemotherapy and is a worse prognostic factor. It has been demonstrated that substantially high levels of MALAT1 was present in extramedullary multiple myeloma cells. Additionally, MALAT1 levels were higher in extramedullary compared to matched intramedullary plasma cells from the same patients [24]. This finding validates a previous study, thus supporting a role for MALAT1 in promoting extramedullary spread of multiple myeloma cells. A prognostic role of MALAT1 has also been suggested by the correlation of higher levels with worse OS and PFS. In particular, it was an independent predictor of PFS and possibly mediates drug resistance. The elevated MALAT1 expression in multiple myeloma cells might be associated with chemotherapeutic stress, because a positive correlation between the expression of MALAT1 and HSP90 (a stress induced protein) was demonstrated, and also in vitro experiments indicate upregulation of MALAT1 following treatment with proteasome inhibitors and doxorubicin [24]. Another plausible role for MALAT1 is in blockage of terminal differentiation of osteoblasts as occurs in multiple myeloma patients. Overexpression of MALAT1 in mesenchymal stromal cells caused transcriptional activation of nearby antisense protein-coding gene, latent TGFβ-binding protein 3 (LTBP3). LTBP3 regulates

TGFβ, which in turn might inhibit osteoblastogenesis in multiple myeloma [27]. In support of this role, MALAT1 could recruit the transcription factor SP1 to LTBP3 promoter and thus increase its expression. Expectedly, knockdown of MALAT1 caused significant reduction in LTBP3 transcription.

Another putative oncogenic lncRNA of interest in multiple myeloma is colorectal neoplasia differentially expressed (CRNDE), located at 16q12.2. It was initially demonstrated to be upregulated in colorectal cancer, but later shown to equally be elevated in several solid tumors, hematologic malignancies, and early stage of human development. Meng et al. found a link between CRNDE, miR-451, and multiple myeloma [28]. Increased expression of CRNDE was demonstrated in multiple myeloma cell lines and patient samples, and the elevated levels were associated with poor OS. To uncover the mechanism of this finding, CRNDE was knocked down in U266 and RPMI-8226 cell lines, and the effects were inhibition of colony formation and cellular proliferation in association with increased apoptosis and G0/G1 cell arrest. An additional finding in the CRNDE knockdown cells was increased expression of miR-451 that is normally downregulated in multiple myeloma patients. Meng et al. were able to determine a binding site for miR-451 on the 3'-UTR of CRNDE using bioinformatic analysis and dual luciferase assay. This negative correlation between CRNDE and miR-451 suggests the upregulation of CRNDE in multiple myeloma might regulate multiple myeloma pathogenesis via miR-451.

Maternally expressed gene 3 (MEG3), located at 14q32.2, acts as a tumor-suppressive lncRNA through p53-dependent and p53-independent mechanisms, and its expression is epigenetically controlled [15, 29]. Benetatos et al. studied the effects of MEG3 in multiple myeloma. Hypermethylation of the "differentially methylated region" (DMR) of MEG3 promoter was demonstrated in 60% of their patients, and this correlated with both disease stage and subtype [17]. The epigenetic regulation was dependent on Ig subtype multiple myeloma, because 66% of IgG and all IgM multiple myeloma patients demonstrated hypermethylation of the DMR, while no IgA multiple myeloma patient had hypermethylation. Because gene promoter methylation is associated with gene silencing, the investigators reasoned reduced expression of MEG3 in multiple myeloma. Expression analysis of MEG3 in MSCs from normal donors (ND-MSCs) and multiple myeloma patients (multiple myeloma-MSCs) revealed reduced expression throughout osteogenic differentiation in multiple myeloma-MSCs compared to ND-MSCs [30]. Overexpression of MEG3 in multiple myeloma-MSCs caused osteogenic differentiation. Further exploration uncovered bone morphogenetic protein 4 (member of the TGF family) as a target of MEG3. Mechanistically, MEG3 binds and removes SOX2 from bone morphogenetic protein 4 promoter enabling its transcriptional activation.

At 19p13.12 is located an lncRNA referred to as urothelial cancer-associated 1 (UCA1) that was initially shown to be highly expressed in transitional cell carcinoma of the bladder. Further studies linked UCA1 to CAMP response element-binding protein (CREB) and cell cycle control via PI3K-AKT pathway. UCA1 might have a prognostic role in multiple myeloma. In a comparison of bone marrow plasma cells from newly diagnosed multiple myeloma patients and healthy controls, 27 out of 83 candidate lncRNAs were differentially expressed between the two groups. UCA1 was significantly downregulated in multiple myeloma compared to healthy control samples. Moreover, the levels of UCA1 in multiple myeloma samples showed a positive correlation with serum levels of monoclonal Ig, but negative with albumin. Higher levels of UCA1 were associated with poor OS of multiple myeloma patients and also correlated with known poor multiple myeloma prognostic karyotype, t(4;14) [31].

In newly diagnosed multiple myeloma patients, the levels of another lncRNA OIP5 antisense RNA 1 (OIP5-AS1) at 15q15.1 were found to negatively correlate with miR-410 expression [32]. Overexpression in NCI-H929 and RPMI-8226 cell lines suggested OIP5-AS1 could modulate miR-410 expression to orchestrate its oncogenic effects including cell proliferation, cell cycle progression, and inhibition of apoptosis. Kruppel-like factor 10 (KLF10), a member of the PTEN-AKT signaling pathway, is a direct downstream target of miR-410 in multiple myeloma. Thus, further experimental evidence indicated OIP5-AS1 could negatively regulate miR-410 to activate the KLF10-PTEN-AKT signaling axis in multiple myeloma cells. Thus, the oncogenic effects of miR-410 in multiple myeloma cells due to OIP5-AS1 are through KLF10-PTEN-AKT signaling.

Global lncRNA expression analysis in multiple myeloma has also been conducted using publicly available microarray data on 559 multiple myeloma patients and next-generation RNA-sequencing. Two studies examined the same microarray datasets (GSE24080) and were able to identify lncRNAs with prognostic relevance. One study re-annotated the dataset and interrogated 2330 lncRNAs, which enabled identification of 4 lncRNAs with prognostic utility in predicting multiple myeloma patient survival. Functional analysis indicated these four lncRNAs might be involved in known genetic and epigenetic events in multiple myeloma. Of interest, two of these RNAs, RP1-43E13.2 and RP4-803I11.2, that are frequently altered in multiple myeloma were associated with poor prognosis [33]. Increased expressions were associated with high-risk group of patients, who also demonstrated downregulation of lncRNAs, RP11-533-L6.5 and ZFY-AS1. The other study focused on custom lncRNA-oriented annotation files of the same microarray dataset. This study identified 176 lncRNAs that could cluster patients into two groups with significant differences in OS [34]. They could also predict patient prognosis independent of serum LDH, albumin, and β2-microglobulin levels.

Ronchetti et al. performed a number of studies on global expression of lncRNA in multiple myeloma patients [22]. In one study, samples from 269 patients that presented with the major progressive forms of plasma cell dyscrasias including monoclonal gammopathy of undetermined significance (MGUS), asymptomatic smoldering multiple myeloma (SMM), symptomatic multiple myeloma, extramedullary multiple myeloma or plasma cell leukemia, and normal plasma cells were studied using whole transcript arrays containing 1852 lncRNA unique probes. This approach enabled identification of 230 lncRNAs that differentiated normal from pathological samples, as well as the different types of plasma cell dyscrasias. A specific set of 31 lncRNAs including MALAT1 were dysregulated in pathological samples compared to normal bone marrow plasma cells. Another set of 21 lncRNAs demonstrated progressive dysregulation consistent with disease progression from normal plasma cells to plasma cell leukemia. In 19 multiple myelomas, 3 lncRNAs, lnc-LRRC47.1, lnc-CPSF2.2, and lnc-SENP5-4, showed significant differential expression with disease relapse (plasma cell leukemia patients). Other interesting findings from this study included identification of growth arrest-specific 5 (GAS5) to be among the 21 deregulated RNAs. GAS5 is involved in cell cycle arrest and apoptosis and was significantly upregulated in multiple myeloma with 1q gains. Deleted in lymphocytic leukemia 2 (DLEU2) was significantly downregulated in patients with del13, a chromosomal locus (13q14.3) that also contains cell cycle inhibitory miR-15a and miR-16-1, and there was significant correlation between expression of DLEU2 and these miRNAs. In an attempt to study the pathophysiology of lncRNA dysregulation in plasma cell dyscrasias, Ronchetti et al. examined the associations between lncRNAs and miRNAs in multiple myeloma, plasma cell leukemia, and normal plasma cells [35]. This analysis led to the identification of the following lncRNA/miRNA pairs, lnc-DLEU2/miR-3175, LINC00173/miR-221, lnc-MCL1-2/miR-17 gene family, and lnc-AGBL1-4/miR-185-5 that have important functions in the pathogenesis of multiple myeloma.

In another study by Ronchetti et al., lncRNAs were investigated in 30 multiple myeloma patients using RNA-sequencing based on the 9540 lncRNAs (among the 14,202 in GENCODE encyclopedia) that were detectable upon removal of those unexpressed across the whole dataset [36]. Among the highly expressed with read counts of >500 were NFAT1, MALAT1, MIAT, and TUG1, which are frequently dysregulated in malignant B-cell neoplasms. Using unsupervised learning method, cluster of global lncRNAs could identify major multiple myeloma subgroups with prognostic associations including t(11;19), t(4;14), MAF gene translocation, or hyperdiploidy status. Overall, 391 unique lncRNAs were differentially expressed among the 4 multiple myeloma subgroups; 150, 118, 96, and 42 dysregulated lncRNAs characterized hyperdiploidy status, t(11;14), t(4;14), and MAF gene translocation, respectively. Further analysis associated some dysregulated lncRNAs with genetic alterations in multiple myeloma patients. Twelve lncRNAs were significantly modulated in multiple myeloma patients with 1q gains, 2 of which are located on chromosome 1q; 109 lncRNAs characterized del (13)-positive multiple myeloma patients, of which 7 downregulated lncRNAs are located on chromosome 13; 2 lncRNAs were downregulated in del (17) patients; and 97 upregulated lncRNAs were associated with DIS3 mutated samples.

12.3.4 miRNAs in B-Cell Lymphoma

A number of miRNAs, including miR-155, miR-17-92 cluster, miR-34a, miR-125b, and miR-21, have been implicated in pathogenesis of B-cell lymphomas.

miR-155 regulates normal lymphocyte functions; however, dysregulation of this miRNA is associated with hematologic pathologies. To study the role of miR-155 in germinal center B-cell responses, Thai et al. analyzed miRNA-deficient and knock-in mice [37]. The deficient mice demonstrated reduced total number of germinal center B cells, and the converse was true for the knock-in mice. These observations could partly be accounted for by direct targeting of SPI1 transcription factor [38]. Activation of wild-type B cells in vitro caused strong upregulation of miR-155 expression and activation of CD4+ T lymphocytes, while only a third of the normal levels of TNF and lymphotoxin, as well as Th2 CD4+ T-cell differentiation, were observed with activation of B cells deficient in miR-155. Additionally, miR-155 deficiency resulted in immunodeficiency as B cells produced significantly low levels of Igs and T cells also produced low levels of IFNγ and IL-2 in response to antigen challenge. Dagan et al. demonstrated that miR-155 increased germinal center lymphocytes and motility of germinal center-derived lymphomas by directly targeting and suppressing the expression of germinal center-specific GCSAM (HGAL) and Rhotekin-2 [39].

Kluiver et al. first demonstrated a role for miR-155 in pathogenesis of lymphomas, when they observed its downregulation in Burkitt lymphoma [40]. Implicated in this pathology is a critical regulator of somatic hypermutation in germinal center, the activation-induced cytidine deaminase (AICDA) gene. Thus, Dorsett et al. observed that mice with mutations in the 3′-UTR of miR-155, in the AICDA gene, had increased levels of AICDA, which could increase translocation of MYC-IGH, a genetic feature of Burkitt lymphoma [41]. However, it had been demonstrated that mice overexpressing AICDA failed to develop overt Burkitt lymphoma [42], which might be due to compensation from miR-181 that also targets AICDA [43]. Of interest, miR-181 is an independent prognostic biomarker of survival in DLBCL patients on rituximab, cyclophosphamide, doxorubicin, vincristine, and prednisone (R-CHOP) therapy.

While the mechanism in Burkitt lymphoma was decreased expression of miR-155 in concert with increased AICDA expression, in several other lymphomas, miR-155 is overexpressed. This is an example of the dualistic roles of some miRNAs that can function as oncogenes and tumor suppressors under different circumstances. Downstream of miR-155 are key signaling mediators of malignancy including PI3K-AKT, SMAD5, bone morphogenetic proteins 2/bone morphogenetic protein 4, TGFβ1, TNFα, SPI1, and SHIP1. It is at least established that in the development of DLBCLs, miR-155 targets Src homology 2 domain-containing inositol-5-phosphatase-1 (INPP5D or SHIP1) [44–46]. Thus, in in vitro and in vivo xenotransplant models, miR-155 promoted TNFα-dependent growth of DLBCL cells by direct modulation of INPP5D levels [44]. The levels of INPP5D were also different between activated B-cell-like (ABC-like) and germinal center B-cell-like (GCB-like) subtypes of DLBCLs, which supports earlier findings of differential levels of miR-155 expression between the two DLBCL subtypes [47, 48]. Putatively, the molecular mechanism may be related to SPI1 and the molecular markers of the two subtypes, CD10 for GCB-like and NF-κB for ABC-like. Thompson et al. had linked these markers: miR-155/CD10/SPI1 pathway for GCB-like and miR-155/NF-κB/SPI1 for ABC-like subtypes [49]. In addition, miR-155 targets SMAD5, and therefore the ectopic expression suppressed the in vitro growth inhibitory effects of TGFβ1 and bone morphogenetic proteins 2/bone morphogenetic protein 4 in DLBCL cells [50].

It has also been demonstrated that miR-155 could target PIK3R1 to activate the PI3K-AKT pathway in DLBCLs.

The contribution of miR-155 dysregulation during B-cell development and lymphoma pathogenesis has been explored. Expression of miR-155 at the stage of hematopoietic stem cell (HSC) development resulted in myeloproliferative type disease without overt B-cell lymphomas [51]. However, mice overexpressing miR-155 at the late pro-B-cell stage progressed to proliferative pre-B cells followed by the development of B-cell malignancy identical to high-grade lymphoma after 6 months [52]. This finding was mechanistically probably due to dysregulated IL-6 signaling from direct targeting of INPP5D and CEBPB, with subsequent increases in the number of large pre-B cells and acute lymphoblastic leukemia/high-grade lymphoma [53]. With miR-155 at its highest level, INPP5D and CEBPB proteins were much reduced at the pre-B-cell stage where further development was arrested.

Dysregulated miR-155 is also associated with lymphomas caused by some viruses. These include EBV, Kaposi's sarcoma-associated herpes virus (KSHV), and Marek disease virus (MDV). Though the entire mechanism by which these viruses activate miR-155 expression is unclear, persistent lymphocyte infection might explain the eventual dysregulation of miR-155. For instance, KSHV and MDV generate miR-155 orthologues, while EBV transactivate LMP1 in infected lymphocytes [54–56].

It appears continuous miR-155 overexpression is needed for sustained growth of lymphoma. To address this requirement, Babar et al. generated inducible miR-155 knock-in model that enabled induction of its expression in lymphoid tissues [57]. Induction caused disseminated lymphomas in the mice that were quickly reduced in sizes following withdrawal of miR-155 induction, and the mice were tumor free after a week of being deprived of miR-155 overexpression. Supporting evidence was provided by treating explant tumors with miR-155 antagomir nanoparticles, which resulted in significant reductions in tumor growth.

Other miRNAs with roles in pathogenesis DLBCL and possible other lymphomas/leukemias are miR-17-92 cluster (miR-17HG), miR-34a, miR-125, and miR-21. Located at 13q31-q32 that is frequently amplified in lymphomas, especially GCB-like DLBCL, is miR-17HG [58, 59]. miR-17HG is similar to miR-155 in controlling lymphocyte biology and pathology. Targeted deletion of this miRNA cluster caused increased B-cell expression of proapoptotic BCL2L11 (BIM), as well as blockage of transition from pro- to pre-B-cell development [60]. Its oncogenic features were demonstrated by overexpression in lymphocytes, which caused increased proliferation, decreased apoptosis, and development of lymphoproliferative and autoimmune diseases [61]. The mechanism involves a number of downstream mediators including downregulation of PTEN tumor suppressor with activation of oncogenic PI3K-AKT pathway. miR-17HG synergizes with MYC in lymphoid malignancy because co-overexpression (Eu-Myc mice) caused an increase in the rate of lymphoid malignancy development and aggressiveness [58, 62]. This effect is suggested to be via a MYC/miR-17HG/E2F axis [63]. Mechanistically, MYC upregulates miR-17HG, which then targets destruction of proapoptotic E2F1. Additionally, E2F3, a pro-proliferation factor, regulates miR-17HG expression [64]. A component of miR-17-92 cluster is miR-19a that was demonstrated in the Eu-Myc mice to activate AKT1-mTOR signaling by antagonizing PTEN [65]. Another target of miR-17HG is protein phosphatase PHLPP2, which is an important regulator of the PI3K-AKT1 pathway. In mantle cell lymphoma xenotransplant model, inhibition of miR-17HG suppressed PIK3CA-AKT1 signaling associated with reduced tumor growth [66].

miR-34a is a tumor-suppressive miRNA connected with the *TP53* signaling network. As a tumor suppressor, the locus of miR-34a, 1p36, is reportedly frequently lost in a number of solid tumors [67] and is epigenetically silenced in many hematologic malignancies [68, 69]. P53 induces miR-34a expression, which in turn activates p53 by inhibiting SIRT1 [70]. On the contrary, MYC downregulates miR-34 expression [71]. Craig et al. studied the in vivo effects of miR-34a in lymphoma biology using NOD/SCID/IL2RG−/− mice [72]. Tumors were generated in these mice by inoculation with an ABC-like cell line (U2932) that has minimal endogenous levels of miR-34a. Tumor-bearing mice received intratumoral or intravenous miR-34a, which caused significant decreases in apoptotic-mediated tumor growth. In vitro, siRNA targeting of FOXP1, a component of MYC-mediated miR-34a repression in transformation of high-grade lymphomas, produced similar results to miR-34a injection [73].

miR-125b has been implicated in both lymphoid and myeloid malignancies because of its association with chromosomal abnormalities in these tumors [74, 75]. Evidence has been provided through ectopic expression of miR-125b in hematopoietic stem cells that led to the development of hematologic malignancies [76, 77]. Identified miR-125b downregulated downstream targets include PRDM1 and IRF4 [78]. Transgenic mice that constitutively expressed miR-125b under the Eu promoter developed IgM+ or IgM- lethal B-cell malignancies [79]. The NF-κB pathway was implicated in the development of DLBCL caused by miR-125b because a negative pathway regulator, TNFATIP3, is a direct target of miR-125a/b. Thus, a strong correlation has been observed between the expression of miR-125a/b and NF-κB activity in primary DLBCL cases. Moreover, overexpression of either of these miRNAs increased the aggressiveness of DLBCL cell lines [80].

miR-21 is an oncomir that is overexpressed in several solid tumors as well as hematologic malignancies. It is overexpressed in HL and NHL [48, 81]. miR-21 has numerous targets that may differ with the type of cancer. In regard to hematologic malignancies, it targets TPM1, PDCD4, SERPINB5, PTEN, ANP32A, and SMARCA4 in lymphomas. In multiple myeloma, STAT3 activated miR-21 expression in IL-6-dependent fashion. Also, miR-21 mediates bortezomib resistance in multiple myeloma cells [82]. Various molecules involved in hematopoietic lineage differentiation such as AP-1, ETS1/SPI1, and CEBPA have binding sites in miR-21 promoter, suggestive of regulatory roles on miR-21 by these transcription factors. Medina et al. demonstrated the in vivo role of miR-21 in hematologic malignancy by developing and analyzing inducible transgenic knock-in mouse model of miR-21 [83]. Mice with induction of miR-21 spontaneously developed lymphomas that resembled precursor B-cell lymphoblastic leukemia. In mice with significant tumor load, doxycycline-induced removal of miR-21-inducible stimulus caused complete tumor disappearance via apoptosis within a week.

Also implicated in B-cell transformation is miR-217 [84]. miR-217 is specifically upregulated in germinal center B cells and is a positive modulator of the germinal center response that increases the generation of class-switched antibodies as well as the frequency of somatic hypermutation. miR-217 downregulates expression of DNA damage response and repair gene network and stabilizes Bcl6 expression in germinal center B cells. miR-217 overexpression promotes mature B-cell lymphomagenesis and is overexpressed in aggressive human B-cell lymphomas.

12.3.5 Hodgkin Lymphoma

Some miRNAs are implicated in the pathogenesis of Hodgkin lymphoma. Hodgkin lymphoma cell profiling studies identified miR-9 and Let-7a to be most abundantly expressed [85]. These miRNAs directly target and downregulate PRDM1 (BLIMP1), which is an important regulator of B-cell differentiation. Expectedly, inhibition of these miRNAs in HL cell lines caused decreased levels of PRDM1, which was suggested to contribute to the development of HL via blockage of GC B-cell differentiation into plasma cells. Of note, miR-30 that inhibits a GC marker, BCL6, also targets PRDMI in DLBCL [86]. Other targets of miR-9 in HL are ELAVL1 (HuR) and DICER1, the levels of which are increased in association with decreased cytokine production and inflammation by inhibition of this miRNA in HL cell lines [87]. Supporting evidence was provided by observed decreased tumor growth from ectopic delivery of miR-9 antagomirs to xenotransplants.

JAK/STAT signaling is altered in myeloid neoplasm due to frequent JAK2 mutations. On the contrary, despite constitutive activation of STAT3 in lymphoid malignancies, such mutations have not been uncovered [88]. It was subsequently observed that the altered JAK/STAT signaling in lymphomas was due to direct targeting and downregulation of JAK2 by miR-135a [89]. Thus, there were increased apoptotic cell death and decreased cell growth mediated by BCL2L1 when miR-135a was overexpressed in HL cell lines, and low level of this miRNA is a poor prognostic predictor for HL patients.

miRNAs also regulate some NHL. miR-150 targets MYB to regulate B-cell development and NK cell functions [90]. Moreover, it targets NOTCH3 to regulate other T-cell subsets [91]. Thus, downregulation of miR-150 might be involved in pathogenesis of NK/T-cell lymphoma [92]. Transduction and increased expression of miR-150 in NK/T-cell lymphoma cells caused increased apoptosis, decreased proliferation, but rather decreased telomerase activity. These antitumoral effects were mediated by direct targeting of DKC1 and AKT2 in concert with decreased anti-apoptotic BCL2L11.

12.3.6 Chronic Lymphocytic Leukemia

miR-15a and miR-16-1 are frequently dysregulated in CLL. Calin et al. initially provided this evidence in 2002, by observing the association of a frequently deleted locus (13q14) in CLL with downregulation of miR-15a/16-1 cluster encoded within this locus [93]. Identified downstream targets of these miRNAs include *BCL2*, *CDK6*, *MCL1*, and *TP53* [94, 95]. The regulation of *TP53* exists as a positive feedback loop whereby p53 also regulates these miRNAs via direct interaction.

Functional studies have attempted to unravel the relationships between del 13q14 and miR-15a/16-1 cluster in CLL. The first study was analysis of the nongenetically engineered New Zealand Black (NZB) mouse strain that has an elevated risk of developing a human CLL-like disease. A genome-wide linkage study identified a locus on chromosome 14 linked to lymphoproliferative disease in mice, and this locus was syntenic with human chromosome 13q14 locus. Corroborative evidence for the involvement of this locus with miR-15a/16-1 cluster was decreased level of miR-16 in lymphoid tissues from these mice. Moreover, in vitro treatment of NZB-derived CLL cell line with exogenous miR-16 caused increased apoptosis with decreased G1-S phase transition [96]. A recurrent point mutation was later identified in a flanking region of miR-15a/16-1 cluster precursor miRNA in the NZB strain that was absent in closely related strains. This mutation was also similar to a mutation found in two CLL patients with family histories of CLL and breast cancer [97]. To more closely study the contribution of miR-15a/16-1 cluster to the development of CLL, transgenic mouse models carrying various conditional alleles of this locus were generated and analyzed [98]. Two models were initially developed with conditional alleles that targeted deletion of (i) the minimal deleted region (MDR) of 13q14 locus inclusive of miR-15a/16-1 cluster and DLEU2 and (ii) only miR-15a/16-1 cluster. Homozygous mice from both deletions developed human CLL-like diseases, but the disease was more aggressive in mice with deleted MDR. These findings suggest the presence of other factors in the MDR that contribute to miR-15a/16-1-mediated CLL severity. The third mouse strain they developed offered corroborative evidence for the presence of additional disease loci in this region. This third strain extended the MDR to include deletion of DLEU7 and RNASEH2B, which is the commonly deleted region in CLL [99]. Phenotypically, these mice developed more aggressive tumors than the previous two strains, and there were more CLL than lymphomas. Thus, the role of miR-15a/16-1 cluster in CLL pathogenesis requires further clarification. Indeed, a number of 13q14 deletion CLL cases have no involvement of this cluster, and studies have found no significant correlation between 13q14 deletion status of CLL patients and miR-15a/16-1 expression [100–102]. In anaplastic lymphoma kinase (ALK)-positive anaplastic large cell lymphomas, the mechanism appears to be downregulation of HIF1α by ALK [103]. However, several other lymphomas including mantle cell lymphomas are linked to miR-15a/16-1 cluster [104, 105].

12.4 Hematologic Malignancy Biomarkers in Proximal Fluids

12.4.1 Cell-Free DNA Biomarkers in Hematologic Malignancy

Cell-free DNA (cfDNA) is a noninvasive sample suitable for the diagnosis and monitoring of disease progression and relapse or presence of minimally residual disease in hematologic malignancy patients.

12.4.1.1 Myelodysplastic Syndrome

The levels of cfDNA are much higher in patients with MDS and correlate with disease status, LDH levels, and number of blast cells in peripheral blood (PB). Reports of the feasibility of detecting MDS genetic alterations in cfDNA date back to 1994 when *NRAS* point mutation detectable in bone marrow samples was equally detectable in PB cfDNA from patients with MDS and AML [106]. More recent studies are attempting to determine the possible clinical relevance of these genetic alterations in patient management. One study focused on detecting both mutations and CpG island methylation in LINE1 promoter in cfDNA from MDS patients [107]. Mutations in TET2 uncovered in bone marrow blast cells from MDS patients could be detected in cfDNA. Of clinical interest were the better sensitivity of detecting LINE1 methylation in serially collected cfDNA samples than bone marrow cells and the decrease in levels of methylation following treatment. Before allogeneic transplantation, mutations in NRAS, *IDH2*, *SETBP1*, *U2AF1*, and *SRSF2* were detectable in PB cfDNA from MDS patients [108]. However, after transplantation, these mutations were undetectable, which could possibly be used as a measure of the effectiveness of the treatment. Confirmatory detection of molecular alterations in cfDNA from MDS patients was uncovered using NGS [109]. This approach that could identify one or more MDS mutations in cfDNA enabled diagnosis of all MDS patients. Indeed, in five samples, NGS could detect some mutations in cfDNA that were undetectable by conventional Sanger sequencing of cellular DNA. It appears cfDNA could serve as accurate substitute sample for molecular analysis when biopsy cannot be performed. A panel of 55 genes recurrently mutated in MDS was subjected to analysis in serially collected samples [110]. In follow-up, there was a significant correlation between mutations detected in bone marrow and cfDNA samples.

12.4.1.2 Myeloid Leukemia

Specific gene mutations and cytogenetic abnormalities have been examined in cfDNA from AML and MDS patients [111]. In 45 patients with confirmed cytogenetic abnormalities at 5q-, 7q-, +8, 17p-, and 20q-, LOH was equally confirmed in

100% of cfDNA samples. Detection of MSA in cfDNA was more sensitive than in bone marrow samples where the rates of detection were 70% in AML and 89% in MDS patients. Quantification of copies of the most commonly mutated gene (nucleophosmin – NPM) in AML was performed using cfDNA [112]. NPM1 mutations were detectable at comparable frequencies in cfDNA and DNA from peripheral blood cells (37% vs. 35%). Copies of mutant NPM1 were significantly associated with high WBC and platelet counts and percentage of blast cells in the bone marrow.

12.4.1.3 Lymphoid Leukemia

Many more studies have been performed on cfDNA in lymphoid than myeloid malignancies. Schwarz et al. explored the rational to possibly use measurements of cfDNA in monitoring minimal residual disease (MRD) in pediatric ALL cases [113]. In a study of ALL patients compared to controls comprised of patients with other malignancies and healthy individuals, cfDNA was significantly higher in ALL patients (277 ng/ml) than control malignant group (76 ng/ml) and healthy controls (57 ng/ml). Of clinical relevance, the levels of cfDNA dropped to within normal range of 62 ng/ml on the fourth day after treatment, and this drop correlated with decreased numbers of circulating leukocytes. Serial sampling of cfDNA and leukocytes showed concordance of 86.7% in MRD detection. Another study also indicated treatment monitoring by assessing tumor-specific mutations in cfDNA [114]. Mutations in CRDIII of IgH were detectable in 54% of cfDNA samples from ALL and NHL patients, and these levels were altered by therapy. Mutational evaluation due to acquired resistance to treatment with BTK inhibitors could be sensitively detected using plasma cfDNA [115]. While undetectable in untreated patients, mutations were uncovered in 11 plasma cfDNA (7 BTK and 4 PLCγ2), in 9 cellular DNA (7 BTK and 2 PLCγ2), and in only 2 serum cfDNA (1 each of BTK and PLCγ2). Because some mutations detected in plasma were undetectable in cellular gDNA, it was concluded that plasma cfDNA was more reliable for mutation detection.

12.4.1.4 Lymphoma

CfDNA levels are significantly elevated in patients compared to healthy controls. In DLBCL, HL, and NHL patients, the elevated levels (targeting β-globin gene) correlated with advanced-stage disease, poor prognosis, and other clinical parameters including fever, night sweats, weight loss, elevated LDH levels, and age above 60 years [116]. Another study determined levels of cfDNA in pediatric HL cases by targeting POLR2 and demonstrated levels of 122 ng/ml in patients compared to 5.5 ng/ml in controls [117]. Upon follow-up after first-round chemotherapy, many demonstrated reduced cfDNA levels; however, in a subset of patients, the levels rather increased, and this was associated with disease relapse or progression. Targeting POLR2 in pediatric lymphoma and NPM-ALK fusion in ALCL patients demonstrated elevated cfDNA levels in patients (median 46 ng/ml) compared to controls (median 1.6 ng/ml) [118]. Poor prognostic correlation was also uncovered for pediatric HL patients. However, in ALCL patients, the large tumor size appeared to have induced cfDNA release from surrounding normal cells, such that about 80% of cfDNA was not of tumor origin and hence had no association with clinical parameters.

Detection of mutations associated with aggressive NHL using plasma cfDNA was comparable and possibly more sensitive than using biopsy samples. Thus, IgH and TCRγ rearrangements were detected in 81% of plasma cfDNA vs. 77% of biopsy sample for IgH and 44% plasma cfDNA vs. 39% biopsy samples for TCRγ [119]. Because circulating tumor cells (CTCs) are rare in DLBCL patients, cytogenetic monitoring for MRD is only possible in just a few patients. Thus, other means and biomarkers have been explored for this utility. In a cohort of newly diagnosed DLBCL patients, IgH rearrangements were detectable in plasma cfDNA of 69% of patients compared to 50% using gDNA from CTCs [120]. Following successful therapy, only one of the 16 patients demonstrated this mutation in cfDNA, suggesting this sample is more accurate at disease monitoring than other methods, albeit this is a pilot study.

TP53 exons 5–9 mutations (Arg-176, phe-238, Ser-249, Lys-249, and Phe-250) were uncovered in 30% of NHL patients, and these were associated with resistance to treatment and poor prognosis [121]. Single nucleotide variants in *MYD88*, *CD79A/B*, or *CARD11* were detected in cfDNA from a vast majority of DLBCL patients (11/12), and these variants were similar to those detected in DNA from matched tumor cells [122].

Rare mutations in *XPO1, EZH2,* and *MYD88* that are useful biomarkers for patient selection for targeted therapy could be detected by digital PCR (dPCR) in cfDNA at an analytical sensitivity of 0.05% mutant concentration [123]. Of interest, there was 100% concordance between mutations detected by dPCR and NGS methods, which suggests dPCR suffices accurate mutation detection in cfDNA for such clinical utility. Another evidence for use of cfDNA mutational analysis for disease detection and monitoring for relapse was demonstrated in HL patients [124]. A recurrent hotspot mutation in *XPO1* (E571K) was detectable in both cfDNA and gDNA from tissue biopsy. Of note, 29% of *XPO1* mutations in cfDNA were not demonstrable in biopsy specimens. Of the patients who relapsed, 54% harbored these mutations detectable in cfDNA after cessation of therapy.

In conclusion, cfDNA levels are much higher in lymphoma patients than controls, and the levels may have prognostic value. Moreover, cfDNA appear to be a suitable noninvasive surrogate sample for mutational analysis, especially in patients whereby biopsy is not possible.

12.4.1.5 Multiple Myeloma

CfDNA analysis seems to have complementary role in the management of multiple myeloma patients, given the genetic heterogeneity, multifocality, and multiclonality of this disease. In a pilot study, allele-specific oligonucleotide (ASO)-PCR was used to characterize VDJ of IgH sequence variations specific for each patient in peripheral blood mononuclear cells (PBMNCs), bone marrow MNCs (BMMNCs), and CD20+ CD38- B cells [125]. Circulating cfDNA samples were also interrogated for these rearrangements. As evidence of circulating clonogenic plasma cells, the results of PBMNCs and BMMNCs were correlated. The levels of mutant clones decreased in PBMNCs after treatment. Identical bone marrow sequence variations were found in cfDNA at diagnosis and follow-up. A similar study characterized bone marrow plasma cell clonotypic VDJ rearrangements and used it to evaluate their presence in cfDNA [126]. PB samples for analysis were obtained before and after treatment with a variety of drugs including bortezomib, panobinostat, and lenalidomide, as well as allogeneic transplantation. The detection rate of VDJ variants was 71% and 100% in PB and cfDNA, respectively, at baseline. On follow-up, however, the detection rates were 40% for PB and 34% for cfDNA samples. Detection of the rearrangement in PB or cfDNA was 91% of non-responders and 41% of responders. While VDJ sequence variation was significantly concordant between the two sample sets, discordance was present in 30% of cases, which suggests the complementary utility of both samples to more completely capture these sequence variations in patients. While further evidence is required to ascertain the clinical utility, these findings suggest the potential of genetic analysis of VDJ of IgH variants in cfDNA for patient management.

Another study revealed the complex evolution of mutations detectable in cfDNA with multiple myeloma progression [127]. cfDNA analysis supports the anatomic site heterogeneity of multiple myeloma growth. This study targeted activating mutations in *KRAS*, *NRAS*, *BRAF*, and *TP53* in paired DNA samples from CD138+ bone marrow plasma cells and cfDNA in circulation of newly diagnosed multiple myeloma patients in comparison with the healthy controls. The elevated cfDNA levels in patients correlated only with disease stage. The most common genetic alteration was in *KRAS*. While in total 53.9% of mutations were detected in cfDNA, 24.2% were detected only in cfDNA. Mutation frequency was higher in relapsed than newly diagnosed patients. Also high frequency of mutations was found in only cfDNA from relapsed compared to newly diagnosed patients (27.2% vs. 6.6%). In newly diagnosed patients, *NRAS* and *KRAS* mutations were common, but in relapsed patients, *KRAS* mutations (56) were more common than *NRAS* (27 mutations). *TP53* mutations were exclusive to relapsed patients. Attesting to cost-effective disease management, digital droplet PCR (ddPCR) was used for disease monitoring, which was evidenced by clonal changes indicative of disease progression.

12.4.2 Extracellular Vesicles as Biomarkers in Hematologic Malignancy

Extracellular vesicles (EVs), including exosomes and their cargo, in particular miRNAs have been extensively investigated in hematologic malignancy in regard to their functional biology, as well as biomarker and therapeutic potential. The increased levels of serum EV counts in patients with CLL, NHL, HL, Waldenstrom's macroglobulinemia, multiple myeloma, AML, MPN, and MDS compared to healthy controls suggest a general biomarker of hematologic malignancy. This feature should also increase the sensitivity of sampling for these EVs in body fluids of patients. These particles and molecules are implicated in cancer microenvironmental reprogramming, angiogenesis, drug resistance, and immunosuppression (immunomodulation) and can be therapeutic targets or vehicles for drug delivery. In order to bring focus to the clinical relevance, this section addresses the roles of these molecules in reference to the major types of hematologic malignancies.

12.4.2.1 Acute Myeloid Leukemia

The bone marrow could provide a permissive microenvironment for leukemogenesis and disease progression. Exosomes released from AML cells could alter proliferative and migratory abilities of stromal and hematopoietic progenitor cells in co-culture. Thus, the microenvironment could be reprogrammed to favor invasion of the bone marrow by AML cells. AML exosomes transferred mRNA of human *CXCR4* and *IGF-IR* to murine bone marrow stromal cells. The exosomal transfer of IGF-IR could modulate the proliferation of neighboring cells as well as promote the expression of VEGF by these cells [128].

Increased angiogenesis is a feature of hematologic malignancies including AML. The release of EVs from AML cells has been demonstrated in vitro and in sera from patients. In co-culture experiments of stromal and hematopoietic progenitor cells, AML exosome trafficking could alter the angiogenic responses to augment bone marrow invasion.

Hong et al. demonstrated that in AML patients, exosomal protein levels might reflect the extent of disease and also correlate with relapse after therapy [129]. Because the authors observed large differences in exosomal protein levels in patients with AML at diagnosis, they hypothesized that this could be a prognostic biomarker, whereby patients with low protein levels should have prolonged survival. Also suggested was that changes in exosomal protein levels may predict response to chemotherapy and presence of residual disease in patients in complete remission. In this study, the authors focused on biologically active TGFβ1 levels in exosomes from AML patients undergoing treatment. TGFβ1 levels were higher in AML-derived exosomes than normal control exosomes, and upon treatment, levels significantly decreased. For patients in long-term complete remission, the levels were even much lower. Thus, changes in exosomal TGFβ1 levels may reflect response of AML patients to chemotherapy. Hong et al. also observed that AML patients at diagnosis had elevated plasma levels of blast-derived CD34+, CD117+, and CD33+ exosomes [129]. Indeed, AML-derived exosomes protect AML blast and ensure their survival [130].

While cancer-derived exosomes could stimulate the immune system, many exosomes derived from hematologic malignancy microenvironment are immunosuppressive to favor cancer cell survival. Tumor-derived exosomes use diverse mechanisms including inhibition of effector immune cell differentiation, antileukemic functions, induction of CD8+ T-cell apoptosis, delivery of tolerogenic signals, and enhanced Treg and MDSC production to achieve immunosuppression. Thus, cancer-derived exosomal interactions with T/B cells, NK cells, monocytes, or granulocytes result in immune-inhibition and therefore escape of leukemic cells from immune destruction. In AML patients, NK cell frequency is low in addition to significantly depressed NK cell activity in the peripheral circulation. Moreover, the few NK cells present have decreased expression of activating NK cell cytotoxic receptors including NKp30, NKp44, NKp46, as well as C-type lectin receptors such as NKG2D and NKG2C [131]. AML patients have increased Tregs that mediate immune suppression. Indeed, exosomes isolated at time of AML diagnosis carry activated TGFβ1, which, upon co-culture with normal human NK cells, were able to reduce NKG2D expression and cytotoxicity. These activities of AML-derived exosomes were confirmed by antibody neutralization of TGFβ1, which interrupted their immunosuppressive activities. In a similar experiment, co-culture of plasma exosomes from AML patients in complete remission with normal NK cells could downregulate NKG2D expression and NK cell cytotoxicity. Thus, elevated levels of biologically active exosomes in AML patients contribute to disease relapse [129]. Additionally, AML-derived exosomes are enriched in immunosuppressive molecules including TGFβ1, Fas/FasL/PD-1/PD-L1, CD39/CD73, and MICA/MICB that could signal to NK cells to reduce their functions [131, 132]. Adoptively transferred activated NK cells and engineered CAR T cells or vaccine-induced CD8+ T cells may encounter tumor exosomes carrying immunoinhibitory cargo. Such effector cells may become functionally ineffective or undergo apoptosis. Thus, in an experimental model, adoptive transfer of NK-92 cells to relapsed AML patients failed to provide significant benefit, presumably because they encountered preexisting AML-derived exosomes with immunosuppressive cargo [133].

EVs from leukemic stem cells could promote the proliferation and migration of AML cells [134]. AML-derived exosomes suppressed residual hematopoietic stem and progenitor cell functions by decreasing clonogenicity and also by reprogramming the stroma [135, 136]. Bone marrow AML-EVs could promote the survival of healthy hematopoietic stem cells (HPCs), with no effect on colony formation or phenotypic changes in the maturity, but these appear to induce leukemic-like features on the HSCs by overexpression of miR-21 and miR-29 [137]. A role for vacuolar protein sorting 33b (VPS33b) in HSC exosome functions and initiation of leukemia has been demonstrated [138]. VPS33b deletion in an in vivo AML model caused impairment of exosomal maturation and secretion, as well as delay in the onset of AML.

It has been demonstrated that leukemic cell-derived EVs were efficiently transferred into MSCs [139]. EV miR-7977 from AML/MDS CD4+ cells were transferred into bone marrow MSCs resulting in their reduced ability to support the CD4+ cells. Muntion et al. (118) also demonstrated that MSC-derived EVs from MDS patients strongly modified CD4+ cell properties by promoting their viability and clonogenic potential and altered expression profiles of miRNA and mRNA [140].

Stromal exosome trafficking could be a mechanism for extrinsic drug resistance in AML patients by increasing TKI resistance [141]. When an AML cell line carrying FLT3 internal tandem duplication mutation was exposed to exosomes derived from normal or AML-BMSC, both types of exosomes protected AML cells against cytarabine treatment; however, only AML-BMSC-derived exosomes protected AML cells from FLT3 inhibitor treatment [142]. Apoptosis resistance is transferable via exosomes. Thus, apoptosis-resistant AML cells could use EVs to modulate the expression profiles of apoptosis-related proteins in blast cells that were sensitive to chemotherapy [143]. Additionally, a multiresistant AML cell line could transfer its chemoresistance via EVs to chemosensitive promyelocytic leukemia cells.

The demonstrated changes and unique markers of AML-EVs could have biomarker potential for patient management. As potential diagnostic biomarkers, AML-EVs are enriched with CD13, CD34, and CD117, and plasma exosomes from AML patients harbor greater levels of proteins than controls [141]. Analysis of these proteins uncovered TGFβ1 that could serve as a biomarker of response to therapy, as well as inform the presence or not of residual disease after treatment [144]. Huan et al. uncovered AML-EV mRNAs of potential utility in patient management [128]. Transcripts of *FLT3-ITD* and *NPM1* could be of prognostic relevance, and *FLT-ITD*, *IGF-IR*, and *CXCR4* could be used for treatment selection and monitoring, while leukemia microenvironmental reprograming biomarkers included MMP4, CXCR4, and IGF-IR. In addition, serum EV miR-155 levels were much higher in AML patients than controls, and the elevated levels correlated with WBC counts, complex karyotypes [145], and could also serve as a biomarker of residual disease. Circulating EVs were much higher in MDS patients than controls, and in high-risk patients, the levels were comparable to those of AML patients.

12.4.2.2 Chronic Myeloid Leukemia

CML-derived exosomes could stimulate bone marrow stromal cells to release IL-8, which provided prosurvival signals in vitro and in vivo to CML cells. The blockage of IL-8 receptor with SB225002 prevented the IL-8-mediated CML cell survival in vitro and in vivo growth of CML xenograft. These and other findings uncovered key roles for CXCL18/CXCR1-2 signaling in CML cell growth [146]. Leukemic cells and normal neutrophils could communicate to enhance tumor development. The Bcr/Abl fusion gene in CML could be transferred through K562-derived EVs to neutrophils. Incubation of these neutrophils with K562-EVs for 24 h resulted in expression of the hybrid gene in 20% of neutrophils [147]. These K562-EVs could induce formation of CML, because injections via tail veins into Sprague-Dawley rats or NOD/SCID mice caused several CML-like symptoms such as loss of weight, weakness, splenomegaly, and neutrophilia with reduced phagocytic abilities. These rats and mice expressed the Bcr/Abl gene with disease development. These findings suggest that transfer of Bcr/Abl gene from CML-derived EVs to neutrophils might induce in vivo transformation of normal cells [148].

Angiogenesis is an important factor in tumor microenvironment that promotes tumor growth and metastasis. EVs play a central role in promoting the development of tumor angiogenesis depending on their origin and cargo. EVs can deliver angiogenic factors such as proteins, mRNA, or miRNAs and can also induce changes in target cells to modulate endothelial cell (EC) environment. Several hematologic malignancies including AML, CML, ALL, multiple myeloma, and lymphomas are associated with increased angiogenesis [149]. Indeed, bone marrow microvessel density is greater in patients with advanced MDS than normal individuals, suggestive of the importance of angiogenesis in hematologic malignancies. Exosomes derived from CML cells promote angiogenesis by directly influencing ECs. They modulate the neovascularization process by inducing ECs to release proangiogenic factors such as IL-8 [150]. This same group also demonstrated that imatinib-resistant CML cells release exosomes with proangiogenic abilities [151]. Exosomes released by K562 CML cells could be internalized by ECs during the process of tubular differentiation on Matrigel. Moreover, these exosomes could be transferred to nearby cells through formation of nanotubular structures that connect the cells. These exosomes stimulate tube formation in ECs partly through Src activation [152]. Moreover, several angiogenic miRNAs (miR-92a, miR-126, miR-135b, and miR-210) have been identified that are delivered to tumor microenvironment via EVs. One of these angiogenic miRNAs, miR-126, was expressed sixfold more in LAMA84 exosomes compared to parental cells. The transfer of miR-126 via exosomes to ECs led to direct targeting of the 3′-UTR of CXCL12 and VCAM1 mRNA, which could modulate adhesion and migration of CML cells [153]. Umezu et al. demonstrated that K562-derived miR-92 could be transferred to ECs via exosomes to mediate endothelial cell migration and tube formation [154]. These studies are quite confirmatory as other groups have shown similar effects of K562-derived exosomal miRNAs in promoting EC migration and tube formation [155]. Another feature of tumor growth is increasing hypoxia in the tumor microenvironment, which promotes angiogenesis. Hypoxia promotes EV release, and both microarray and proteomic studies have shown that these hypoxic EVs are loaded with proangiogenic factors [155, 156]. Thus, the hypoxic human leukemic cell line, K562, secretes exosomes containing miRNAs. These miRNAs, specifically miR-210, enhanced tube formation in human umbilical vein ECs by inhibiting receptor tyrosine kinase ligand EPHRIN-A3.

EVs from CML cells interact with stromal cells to influence malignant behavior. EVs from CML cells contained cancer cell transcripts that were transferred to healthy MSCs to increase their proliferation [157]. CML EVs containing Bcr/Abl fusion genes could induce malignant transformation of normal mononuclear cells through induction of genome instability, associated with DNA strand breaks and recombination [158]. Telomerase (hTERT) mRNA could be transferred via exosomes from CML and T-cell leukemic cells to hTERT-negative fibroblasts. The hTERT transcripts were translated into active forms that transformed the cells into telomerase-positive cells [159]. MSC-derived EVs from patients with myeloproliferative neoplasms were enriched with miR-155 that could induce increased granulocyte colony-forming units from CD4+ neoplastic cells.

A differential miRNA signature between K562 cell exosomes and K562 cells has been uncovered [160], and preliminary analysis suggests miR-215 may be a biomarker for determining CML patients who can discontinue imatinib therapy [161]. Circulating CD13+ MVs are higher in CML and primary myelofibrosis patients than healthy controls [162].

12.4.2.3 Acute Lymphocytic/Lymphoblastic Leukemia

Exosomes from pre-B acute lymphoblastic leukemia cell line grown at high density could induce proliferation and survival of neighboring low-density cells. Similarly, exosomes from ALL cells promoted proliferation of both leukemic and non-leukemic B-cell lines in autocrine and paracrine fashions (74).

EVs are involved in stromal cell communication in ALL. B-cell precursor ALL-derived EVs containing galectin-3 (GAL-3) could protect stromal cells [163]. GAC-3 internalized by ALL cells stimulated transcription of endogenous GAL-3, which provided protection against treatment of ALL. Stromal cell exosomes captured by ALL cells could induce metabolic switch from oxidative phosphorylation to aerobic glycolysis [144]. Adult T-cell leukemia/lymphoma (ATL) cell-derived exosomes transferred miR-21 and miR-155 to promote proliferation and morphological changes in human MSCs, which enabled the creation of conducive microenvironment for the cancer cells [164].

12.4.2.4 Chronic Lymphocytic Leukemia

EVs are involved in modulating CLL microenvironment, drug resistance, and immune evasion and also serve as biomarkers. EVs isolated from plasma of patients with B-cell CLL could interact with BMSCs to modulate their functions in preparing a conducive microenvironment for the B-CLL cells. These functions of CLL-derived exosomes partly depend on the AKT/mTOR/p7056K/HIF1α signaling axis, as they could maintain the activation of this pathway in a sustained state. Another potential pathway used by these exosomes is AKT/GSK3β/β-catenin signaling. Activation of the AKT signaling axis induced the production of VEGF, which is a survival signal for CLL cells. CLL exosomes also induced a transition of ECs and MSCs toward cancer-associated fibroblast phenotype and also promoted cell migration and angiogenesis in vitro and in vivo. Moreover, CLL exosomes were enriched with miR-202-3p [165, 166]. miR-155 that has functional roles in the development of lymphomas is also a potential biomarker for patients with monoclonal B-cell lymphocytosis as well as those with B-cell lymphocytic leukemia. Moreover, high levels of miR-155 were associated with patients who failed to respond to chemotherapy compared to those who achieved complete response. miR-155 was associated with EVs in circulation of these patients [167].

NK cell dysfunction is a feature of CLL. Reiners et al. demonstrated that plasma-soluble ligand, BAG6, inactivated NK cell function by binding to their NKp30 receptors [168]. However, BAG6-positive exosomes activated NK cells that could kill tumor cells. These findings have two implications: (i) in the natural state, it appears immunosuppression, or immunostimulation is determined by the balance between the levels of soluble BAG6 and BAG6 exosomes, and (ii) BAG6 exosomes could be engineered and used as immunotherapeutic agents for CLL patients.

Patients with hematologic malignancies have high levels of circulating EVs, which serve as biomarkers. In a study whereby the size, number, and phenotypic profiles of EVs from sera of patients with CLL, as well as HL, NHL, Waldenstrom's macroglobulinemia, multiple myeloma, AML, MPN, and MDS, and normal controls, levels of EVs were significantly higher in patients than controls. Phenotypically, the cancer cells expressed tumor-associated antigens (TAAs) including CD33, in myeloid tumors, CD30 in HL, CD19 in B-cell neoplasm, and CD38 in multiple myeloma. Of interest, the number of circulating EVs correlated with clinical features of the patients [162]. In addition to the increased levels of CLL-EVs in patients, the total number of EVs positively correlated with advanced clinical stages and OS. The levels also correlated with time to treatment in patients presenting with early-stage disease. These serum CLL-EVs were CD19 and CD37 positive [169]. A DotScan antibody microarray analysis uncovered a number of markers in plasma CLL-EVs to include moderate to high levels of CD5, CD19, CD31, CD44, CD55, CD62L, CD82, HLA-A, HLA-B, HLA-C, and HLA-DR, with low levels of CD21, CD49c, and CD63. Preferential release of CD52-positive EVs from CLL cells was uncovered to be potential predictive biomarker of disease progression [170]. miR-155 is a potential prognostic biomarker of CLL patients independent of clinical stage [145, 171].

12.4.2.5 Multiple Myeloma

Multiple myeloma-bone marrow mesenchymal stromal cell (MM-BMSC)-derived exosomes could transfer miR-15a into multiple myeloma cells to induce their proliferation and survival. However, normal bone marrow MSC exosomes inhibited growth of multiple myeloma cells [172]. Bone marrow angiogenesis also favors multiple myeloma growth and progression. Multiple myeloma RPMI-8226 cells could secrete MVs containing oncogenic and angiogenic regulator, CD138. EC uptake of these EVs reprogrammed them to promote their proliferation, invasion, and secretion of proangiogenic VEGF and IL-6 [173]. An in vitro system of hypoxic-resistant multiple myeloma (HR-MM) cell line was established as a model of therapy-resistant multiple myeloma cells for study. It was demonstrated that HR-MM cells released more exosomes than parental cells, and these exosomes contained specific miRNAs. Oncogenic miR-135b, secreted by HR-MM cells, facilitated hypoxia-driven tube formation. The mechanism for this is the direct targeting of an asparaginyl hydroxylase enzyme, FIH-1, that binds to HIF1α to inhibit its transactivation. Thus, miR-135b promoted HIF1α transactivation by inhibiting FIH-1.

Murine model and human multiple myeloma cells treated with bone marrow MSC exosomes were resistant to bortezomib therapy. In these cells, activation of several pathways involved in drug resistance and multiple myeloma cell survival was uncovered. These include NOTCH1, STAT3, NF-κB, AKT, JNK, p38, and p53 pathways [174]. Multiple myeloma cells play a role in promoting plasma cell proliferation. Exosomes from multiple myeloma cells overexpressing CD147, an extracellular matrix metalloproteinase inducer, enhanced neoplastic proliferation more than EVs from cells with downregulated CD147 [175]. Multiple myeloma EVs carrying angiogenic proteins enhanced angiogenesis by modulating STAT3 pathway.

ECs stimulated with these multiple myeloma-MVs secreted IL-6 and VEGF [173]. Exosomes from multiple myeloma cells and multiple myeloma patient sera interacted with osteoclasts to support their growth, migration, and differentiation into multinucleated osteoclasts, which eroded dentine cells [176]. Bcl-xL was present in bone marrow-derived fibroblast exosomes, and cleavage of BcL-xL (clBcl-xL) exposed on the surface was required for EV uptake by both multiple myeloma and aggressive lymphoma cells [177].

A mechanism for exosome-mediated cross talk by multiple myeloma cells with the ECM has been demonstrated. Surface heparan sulfate (sHS)-positive exosomes could bind to fibronectin to act as ligands for sHS-positive target cells. Thus, the interaction between fibronectin-sHS-positive exosomes and multiple myeloma cells induced activation of p38 and pERK, and the production of DKK1 and multiple myelomaP9 required for multiple myeloma cell invasion [178].

Multiple myeloma exosomes could modulate tumor immune microenvironment by reducing cytotoxicity of NK cells against multiple myeloma cells (95). Both multiple myeloma cells and BMSC exosomes promoted growth and enhanced MDSC immunosuppressive functions in vitro and in multiple myeloma xenografts [179]. Ectoenzyme, CD38, on multiple myeloma EVs could mediate anergic immune environment by converting nucleotides to immunosuppressive adenosine. CD8-positive multiple myeloma EVs could bind to mAb (daratumumab) and be internalized by FcR-positive immune cells such as monocytes, NK cells, and MDSCs [180]. The effects of EV uptake by immune cells remain to be clarified.

Markers of multiple myeloma EVs with clinical relevance include CD38, CD44, CD138, CD147, and superficial HSP70. The number of serum CD38-positve EVs correlated with clinical international staging system, and plasma CD138-positive EVs were associated with disease phase and treatment response. Moreover, increased levels of plasma CD147-positive EVs were detected at disease progression. Multiple myeloma EV cargo may also serve as biomarkers. Uncovered in circulating multiple myeloma EVs are ZNF224, c-SRC, IL-6, CCL2, fibronectin, and miRNAs including let-7b, miR-15, miR-16, miR-18a, and miR-135b. While exosomal miR-135b may promote multiple myeloma bone marrow angiogenesis, its level was significantly lower in plasma of patients than controls. As potential prognostic biomarkers, miR-18a and let-7b were significant predicators of PFS and OS of multiple myeloma patients [181]. EVs could also serve as predictive biomarkers of graft-versus-host disease (GvHD) in multiple myeloma patients. Thus, allograft CD25- and CD46-positive EVs correlated with increased risk of GvHD, while decreased occurrence was associated with CD31- and CD106-positive EVs [182].

12.4.2.6 Lymphoma

Environmental stress such as low pH, heat, and oxidative stress can modulate the composition of EVs released by lymphoma/leukemia T/B cells. For example, under thermal and oxidative stress conditions, exosomes from lymphoma/leukemia cells released NKG2D ligands that functioned as decoys to abrogate NK cytotoxicity dependent on NKG2D receptors [183]. Aggressive B-cell lymphoma cells demonstrated strong exosome release in vitro and in vivo, and the exposed membranes of these exosomes carried CD20 that interacted with rituximab, which could interfere with the efficacy of rituximab in patients [184]. Cancer cells use ATP-binding cassette (ABC) transporters to expel drugs. These transporters are also localized in EV membranes, where they are used to sequester drugs. It was demonstrated that during immunotherapy of aggressive B-cell lymphoma, exosomes used ABCA3 to mediate evasion of tumor cells from humoral immunotherapy. Additionally, EVs could bind complement and thus protect B-cell lymphoma cells from complement-dependent cytolysis [184].

Hodgkin and Reed-Sternberg (HRS) cells released exosomes carrying CD30 that could stimulate innate immune cells such as eosinophil-like cells and primary granulocytes to release IL-8. These CD30-positive exosomes were found predominantly stuck to long actin- and tubulin-based protrusions, which could possibly serve as a network to guide them into the tumor microenvironment [185]. Exosomes from Burkitt lymphoma cell line, DG75, were internalized by B cells to promote their proliferation and T-independent isotype class-switching. Additionally, latent membrane protein transfected DG75 (LMP1-DG75) cell line released exosomes that induced B-cell differentiation into a plasmablast-like phenotype [186].

EVs also serve as biomarkers of lymphoma. The HRS cell marker, CD30, is present in HL EVs and may be associated with disease stage. Thus, lower-stage HL patients harbored more CD30-positve EVs than high-stage patients. Besides, plasma EV miR-21, miR-127, miR-155, and let-7 were indicative of disease presence and thus could serve as therapy response biomarkers and useful in monitoring for residual disease in HL patients [145, 187]. Waldenstrom's macroglobulinemia patients harbor higher serum levels of EVs and their content miR-155 than controls [145]. The miR-155 levels positively correlated with the International Prognostic Scoring System. Because exosomal miRNA content differs at different disease phases, they could serve as biomarkers of Waldenstrom's macroglobulinemia disease progression [188].

12.5 Summary

- Non-Hodgkin lymphoma (509,590) and leukemia (437,033) accounted for 80% of all hematologic malignancies diagnosed globally in 2018.
- In general, hematologic malignancies are characterized by chromosomal aberrations and gene mutations that alter oncogenes and signaling pathways.
- Establishing diagnosis of hematologic malignancies still relies on invasive biopsies that may not be feasible in some patients.
- To overcome invasive sampling procedures for patient management, authenticated biomarkers in blood need to be established for hematologic malignancies.
- While they remain to be validated, the genetic alterations in hematologic malignancies are detectable in circulating cfDNA.

- Extracellular vesicles (EVs) play roles in the functional biology of hematologic malignancies by regulating tumor microenvironment, immunosuppression, and drug resistance. EVs also serve as therapeutic targets and vehicles for drug delivery in hematologic malignancies.
- Noncoding RNAs (miRNAs and lncRNAs) exert important biological effects on hematopoietic and hematologic malignancies.

References

1. Hu W, Yuan B, Flygare J, Lodish HF. Long noncoding RNA-mediated anti-apoptotic activity in murine erythroid terminal differentiation. Genes Dev. 2011;25:2573–8.
2. Alvarez-Dominguez JR, Hu W, Yuan B, et al. Global discovery of erythroid long noncoding RNAs reveals novel regulators of red cell maturation. Blood. 2014;123:570–81.
3. Wagner LA, Christensen CJ, Dunn DM, et al. EGO, a novel, noncoding RNA gene, regulates eosinophil granule protein transcript expression. Blood. 2007;109:5191–8.
4. Ebralidze AK, Guibal FC, Steidl U, et al. PU.1 expression is modulated by the balance of functional sense and antisense RNAs regulated by a shared cis-regulatory element. Genes Dev. 2008;22:2085–92.
5. Sharma S, Findlay GM, Bandukwala HS, et al. Dephosphorylation of the nuclear factor of activated T cells (NFAT) transcription factor is regulated by an RNA-protein scaffold complex. Proc Natl Acad Sci U S A. 2011;108:11381–6.
6. Aoki K, Harashima A, Sano M, et al. A thymus-specific noncoding RNA, thy-ncR1, is a cytoplasmic riboregulator of MFAP4 mRNA in immature T-cell lines. BMC Mol Biol. 2010;11:99.
7. Collier SP, Collins PL, Williams CL, et al. Cutting edge: influence of Tmevpg1, a long intergenic noncoding RNA, on the expression of Ifng by Th1 cells. J Immunol. 2012;189:2084–8.
8. Ranzani V, Rossetti G, Panzeri I, et al. The long intergenic noncoding RNA landscape of human lymphocytes highlights the regulation of T cell differentiation by linc-MAF-4. Nat Immunol. 2015;16:318–25.
9. Yildirim E, Kirby JE, Brown DE, et al. Xist RNA is a potent suppressor of hematologic cancer in mice. Cell. 2013;152:727–42.
10. Bock O, Schlue J, Kreipe H. Reduced expression of H19 in bone marrow cells from chronic myeloproliferative disorders. Leukemia. 2003;17:815–6.
11. Tessema M, Langer F, Bock O, et al. Down-regulation of the IGF-2/H19 locus during normal and malignant hematopoiesis is independent of the imprinting pattern. Int J Oncol. 2005;26:499–507.
12. Takeuchi S, Hofmann WK, Tsukasaki K, et al. Loss of H19 imprinting in adult T-cell leukaemia/lymphoma. Br J Haematol. 2007;137:380–1.
13. Guo G, Kang Q, Zhu X, et al. A long noncoding RNA critically regulates Bcr-Abl-mediated cellular transformation by acting as a competitive endogenous RNA. Oncogene. 2015;34:1768–79.
14. Sun J, Li W, Sun Y, et al. A novel antisense long noncoding RNA within the IGF1R gene locus is imprinted in hematopoietic malignancies. Nucleic Acids Res. 2014;42:9588–601.
15. Zhou Y, Zhong Y, Wang Y, et al. Activation of p53 by MEG3 non-coding RNA. J Biol Chem. 2007;282:24731–42.
16. Benetatos L, Hatzimichael E, Dasoula A, et al. CpG methylation analysis of the MEG3 and SNRPN imprinted genes in acute myeloid leukemia and myelodysplastic syndromes. Leuk Res. 2010;34:148–53.

17. Benetatos L, Dasoula A, Hatzimichael E, et al. Promoter hypermethylation of the MEG3 (DLK1/MEG3) imprinted gene in multiple myeloma. Clin Lymphoma Myeloma. 2008;8:171–5.
18. Khoury H, Suarez-Saiz F, Wu S, Minden MD. An upstream insulator regulates DLK1 imprinting in AML. Blood. 2010;115:2260–3.
19. Garzon R, Volinia S, Papaioannou D, et al. Expression and prognostic impact of lncRNAs in acute myeloid leukemia. Proc Natl Acad Sci U S A. 2014;111:18679–84.
20. Diaz-Beya M, Brunet S, Nomdedeu J, et al. The lincRNA HOTAIRM1, located in the HOXA genomic region, is expressed in acute myeloid leukemia, impacts prognosis in patients in the intermediate-risk cytogenetic category, and is associated with a distinctive microRNA signature. Oncotarget. 2015;6:31613–27.
21. Cho SF, Chang YC, Chang CS, et al. MALAT1 long non-coding RNA is overexpressed in multiple myeloma and may serve as a marker to predict disease progression. BMC Cancer. 2014;14:809.
22. Ronchetti D, Agnelli L, Taiana E, et al. Distinct lncRNA transcriptional fingerprints characterize progressive stages of multiple myeloma. Oncotarget. 2016;7:14814–30.
23. Liu H, Wang H, Wu B, et al. Down-regulation of long non-coding RNA MALAT1 by RNA interference inhibits proliferation and induces apoptosis in multiple myeloma. Clin Exp Pharmacol Physiol. 2017;44:1032–41.
24. Handa H, Kuroda Y, Kimura K, et al. Long non-coding RNA MALAT1 is an inducible stress response gene associated with extramedullary spread and poor prognosis of multiple myeloma. Br J Haematol. 2017;179:449–60.
25. Gao D, Lv AE, Li HP, et al. LncRNA MALAT-1 elevates HMGB1 to promote autophagy resulting in inhibition of tumor cell apoptosis in multiple myeloma. J Cell Biochem. 2017;118:3341–8.
26. Roy M, Liang L, Xiao X, et al. Lycorine downregulates HMGB1 to inhibit autophagy and enhances bortezomib activity in multiple myeloma. Theranostics. 2016;6:2209–24.
27. Li B, Chen P, Qu J, et al. Activation of LTBP3 gene by a long noncoding RNA (lncRNA) MALAT1 transcript in mesenchymal stem cells from multiple myeloma. J Biol Chem. 2014;289:29365–75.
28. Meng YB, He X, Huang YF, et al. Long noncoding RNA CRNDE promotes multiple myeloma cell growth by suppressing miR-451. Oncol Res. 2017;25:1207–14.
29. Haertle L, Maierhofer A, Bock J, et al. Hypermethylation of the non-imprinted maternal MEG3 and paternal MEST alleles is highly variable among normal individuals. PLoS One. 2017;12:e0184030.
30. Zhuang W, Ge X, Yang S, et al. Upregulation of lncRNA MEG3 promotes osteogenic differentiation of mesenchymal stem cells from multiple myeloma patients by targeting BMP4 transcription. Stem Cells. 2015;33:1985–97.
31. Sedlarikova L, Gromesova B, Kubaczkova V, et al. Deregulated expression of long non-coding RNA UCA1 in multiple myeloma. Eur J Haematol. 2017;99:223–33.
32. Yang N, Chen J, Zhang H, et al. LncRNA OIP5-AS1 loss-induced microRNA-410 accumulation regulates cell proliferation and apoptosis by targeting KLF10 via activating PTEN/PI3K/AKT pathway in multiple myeloma. Cell Death Dis. 2017;8:e2975.
33. Hu AX, Huang ZY, Zhang L, Shen J. Potential prognostic long non-coding RNA identification and their validation in predicting survival of patients with multiple myeloma. Tumour Biol. 2017;39:1010428317694563.
34. Shaughnessy JD Jr, Zhan F, Burington BE, et al. A validated gene expression model of high-risk multiple myeloma is defined by deregulated expression of genes mapping to chromosome 1. Blood. 2007;109:2276–84.
35. Ronchetti D, Manzoni M, Agnelli L, et al. lncRNA profiling in early-stage chronic lymphocytic leukemia identifies transcriptional fingerprints with relevance in clinical outcome. Blood Cancer J. 2016;6:e468.

36. Ronchetti D, Agnelli L, Pietrelli A, et al. A compendium of long non-coding RNAs transcriptional fingerprint in multiple myeloma. Sci Rep. 2018;8:6557.
37. Thai TH, Calado DP, Casola S, et al. Regulation of the germinal center response by microRNA-155. Science. 2007;316:604–8.
38. Vigorito E, Perks KL, Abreu-Goodger C, et al. microRNA-155 regulates the generation of immunoglobulin class-switched plasma cells. Immunity. 2007;27:847–59.
39. Dagan LN, Jiang X, Bhatt S, et al. miR-155 regulates HGAL expression and increases lymphoma cell motility. Blood. 2012;119:513–20.
40. Kluiver J, Haralambieva E, de Jong D, et al. Lack of BIC and microRNA miR-155 expression in primary cases of Burkitt lymphoma. Genes Chromosomes Cancer. 2006;45:147–53.
41. Dorsett Y, McBride KM, Jankovic M, et al. MicroRNA-155 suppresses activation-induced cytidine deaminase-mediated Myc-Igh translocation. Immunity. 2008;28:630–8.
42. Muto T, Okazaki IM, Yamada S, et al. Negative regulation of activation-induced cytidine deaminase in B cells. Proc Natl Acad Sci U S A. 2006;103:2752–7.
43. de Yebenes VG, Belver L, Pisano DG, et al. miR-181b negatively regulates activation-induced cytidine deaminase in B cells. J Exp Med. 2008;205:2199–206.
44. Pedersen IM, Otero D, Kao E, et al. Onco-miR-155 targets SHIP1 to promote TNFalpha-dependent growth of B cell lymphomas. EMBO Mol Med. 2009;1:288–95.
45. O'Connell RM, Chaudhuri AA, Rao DS, Baltimore D. Inositol phosphatase SHIP1 is a primary target of miR-155. Proc Natl Acad Sci U S A. 2009;106:7113–8.
46. Yamanaka Y, Tagawa H, Takahashi N, et al. Aberrant overexpression of microRNAs activate AKT signaling via down-regulation of tumor suppressors in natural killer-cell lymphoma/leukemia. Blood. 2009;114:3265–75.
47. Eis PS, Tam W, Sun L, et al. Accumulation of miR-155 and BIC RNA in human B cell lymphomas. Proc Natl Acad Sci U S A. 2005;102:3627–32.
48. Lawrie CH, Soneji S, Marafioti T, et al. MicroRNA expression distinguishes between germinal center B cell-like and activated B cell-like subtypes of diffuse large B cell lymphoma. Int J Cancer. 2007;121:1156–61.
49. Thompson RC, Herscovitch M, Zhao I, et al. NF-kappaB down-regulates expression of the B-lymphoma marker CD10 through a miR-155/PU.1 pathway. J Biol Chem. 2011;286:1675–82.
50. Rai D, Kim SW, McKeller MR, et al. Targeting of SMAD5 links microRNA-155 to the TGF-beta pathway and lymphomagenesis. Proc Natl Acad Sci U S A. 2010;107:3111–6.
51. O'Connell RM, Rao DS, Chaudhuri AA, et al. Sustained expression of microRNA-155 in hematopoietic stem cells causes a myeloproliferative disorder. J Exp Med. 2008;205:585–94.
52. Costinean S, Zanesi N, Pekarsky Y, et al. Pre-B cell proliferation and lymphoblastic leukemia/high-grade lymphoma in E(mu)-miR155 transgenic mice. Proc Natl Acad Sci U S A. 2006;103:7024–9.
53. Costinean S, Sandhu SK, Pedersen IM, et al. Src homology 2 domain-containing inositol-5-phosphatase and CCAAT enhancer-binding protein beta are targeted by miR-155 in B cells of Emicro-MiR-155 transgenic mice. Blood. 2009;114:1374–82.
54. Gottwein E, Mukherjee N, Sachse C, et al. A viral microRNA functions as an orthologue of cellular miR-155. Nature. 2007;450:1096–9.
55. Zhao Y, Xu H, Yao Y, et al. Critical role of the virus-encoded microRNA-155 ortholog in the induction of Marek's disease lymphomas. PLoS Pathog. 2011;7:e1001305.
56. Gatto G, Rossi A, Rossi D, et al. Epstein-Barr virus latent membrane protein 1 trans-activates miR-155 transcription through the NF-kappaB pathway. Nucleic Acids Res. 2008;36:6608–19.
57. Babar IA, Cheng CJ, Booth CJ, et al. Nanoparticle-based therapy in an in vivo microRNA-155 (miR-155)-dependent mouse model of lymphoma. Proc Natl Acad Sci U S A. 2012;109:E1695–704.
58. He L, Thomson JM, Hemann MT, et al. A microRNA polycistron as a potential human oncogene. Nature. 2005;435:828–33.

59. Lenz G, Wright GW, Emre NC, et al. Molecular subtypes of diffuse large B-cell lymphoma arise by distinct genetic pathways. Proc Natl Acad Sci U S A. 2008;105:13520–5.
60. Ventura A, Young AG, Winslow MM, et al. Targeted deletion reveals essential and overlapping functions of the miR-17 through 92 family of miRNA clusters. Cell. 2008;132:875–86.
61. Xiao C, Srinivasan L, Calado DP, et al. Lymphoproliferative disease and autoimmunity in mice with increased miR-17-92 expression in lymphocytes. Nat Immunol. 2008;9:405–14.
62. Tagawa H, Karube K, Tsuzuki S, et al. Synergistic action of the microRNA-17 polycistron and Myc in aggressive cancer development. Cancer Sci. 2007;98:1482–90.
63. O'Donnell KA, Wentzel EA, Zeller KI, et al. c-Myc-regulated microRNAs modulate E2F1 expression. Nature. 2005;435:839–43.
64. Woods K, Thomson JM, Hammond SM. Direct regulation of an oncogenic micro-RNA cluster by E2F transcription factors. J Biol Chem. 2007;282:2130–4.
65. Olive V, Bennett MJ, Walker JC, et al. miR-19 is a key oncogenic component of mir-17-92. Genes Dev. 2009;23:2839–49.
66. Rao E, Jiang C, Ji M, et al. The miRNA-17 approximately 92 cluster mediates chemoresistance and enhances tumor growth in mantle cell lymphoma via PI3K/AKT pathway activation. Leukemia. 2012;26:1064–72.
67. Bagchi A, Mills AA. The quest for the 1p36 tumor suppressor. Cancer Res. 2008;68:2551–6.
68. Lodygin D, Tarasov V, Epanchintsev A, et al. Inactivation of miR-34a by aberrant CpG methylation in multiple types of cancer. Cell Cycle. 2008;7:2591–600.
69. Chim CS, Wong KY, Qi Y, et al. Epigenetic inactivation of the miR-34a in hematological malignancies. Carcinogenesis. 2010;31:745–50.
70. Yamakuchi M, Lowenstein CJ. MiR-34, SIRT1 and p53: the feedback loop. Cell Cycle. 2009;8:712–5.
71. Chang TC, Yu D, Lee YS, et al. Widespread microRNA repression by Myc contributes to tumorigenesis. Nat Genet. 2008;40:43–50.
72. Craig VJ, Tzankov A, Flori M, et al. Systemic microRNA-34a delivery induces apoptosis and abrogates growth of diffuse large B-cell lymphoma in vivo. Leukemia. 2012;26:2421–4.
73. Craig VJ, Cogliatti SB, Imig J, et al. Myc-mediated repression of microRNA-34a promotes high-grade transformation of B-cell lymphoma by dysregulation of FoxP1. Blood. 2011;117:6227–36.
74. Sonoki T, Iwanaga E, Mitsuya H, Asou N. Insertion of microRNA-125b-1, a human homologue of lin-4, into a rearranged immunoglobulin heavy chain gene locus in a patient with precursor B-cell acute lymphoblastic leukemia. Leukemia. 2005;19:2009–10.
75. Bousquet M, Quelen C, Rosati R, et al. Myeloid cell differentiation arrest by miR-125b-1 in myelodysplastic syndrome and acute myeloid leukemia with the t(2;11)(p21;q23) translocation. J Exp Med. 2008;205:2499–506.
76. Bousquet M, Harris MH, Zhou B, Lodish HF. MicroRNA miR-125b causes leukemia. Proc Natl Acad Sci U S A. 2010;107:21558–63.
77. Ooi AG, Sahoo D, Adorno M, et al. MicroRNA-125b expands hematopoietic stem cells and enriches for the lymphoid-balanced and lymphoid-biased subsets. Proc Natl Acad Sci U S A. 2010;107:21505–10.
78. Malumbres R, Sarosiek KA, Cubedo E, et al. Differentiation stage-specific expression of microRNAs in B lymphocytes and diffuse large B-cell lymphomas. Blood. 2009;113:3754–64.
79. Enomoto Y, Kitaura J, Hatakeyama K, et al. Emu/miR-125b transgenic mice develop lethal B-cell malignancies. Leukemia. 2011;25:1849–56.
80. Kim SW, Ramasamy K, Bouamar H, et al. MicroRNAs miR-125a and miR-125b constitutively activate the NF-kappaB pathway by targeting the tumor necrosis factor alpha-induced protein 3 (TNFAIP3, A20). Proc Natl Acad Sci U S A. 2012;109:7865–70.
81. Navarro A, Gaya A, Martinez A, et al. MicroRNA expression profiling in classic Hodgkin lymphoma. Blood. 2008;111:2825–32.
82. Wang X, Li C, Ju S, et al. Myeloma cell adhesion to bone marrow stromal cells confers drug resistance by microRNA-21 up-regulation. Leuk Lymphoma. 2011;52:1991–8.

83. Medina PP, Nolde M, Slack FJ. OncomiR addiction in an in vivo model of microRNA-21-induced pre-B-cell lymphoma. Nature. 2010;467:86–90.
84. de Yebenes VG, Bartolome-Izquierdo N, Nogales-Cadenas R, et al. miR-217 is an oncogene that enhances the germinal center reaction. Blood. 2014;124:229–39.
85. Nie K, Gomez M, Landgraf P, et al. MicroRNA-mediated down-regulation of PRDM1/Blimp-1 in Hodgkin/Reed-Sternberg cells: a potential pathogenetic lesion in Hodgkin lymphomas. Am J Pathol. 2008;173:242–52.
86. Lin J, Lwin T, Zhao JJ, et al. Follicular dendritic cell-induced microRNA-mediated upregulation of PRDM1 and downregulation of BCL-6 in non-Hodgkin's B-cell lymphomas. Leukemia. 2011;25:145–52.
87. Leucci E, Zriwil A, Gregersen LH, et al. Inhibition of miR-9 de-represses HuR and DICER1 and impairs Hodgkin lymphoma tumour outgrowth in vivo. Oncogene. 2012;31:5081–9.
88. Melzner I, Weniger MA, Menz CK, Moller P. Absence of the JAK2 V617F activating mutation in classical Hodgkin lymphoma and primary mediastinal B-cell lymphoma. Leukemia. 2006;20:157–8.
89. Navarro A, Diaz T, Martinez A, et al. Regulation of JAK2 by miR-135a: prognostic impact in classic Hodgkin lymphoma. Blood. 2009;114:2945–51.
90. Bezman NA, Chakraborty T, Bender T, Lanier LL. miR-150 regulates the development of NK and iNKT cells. J Exp Med. 2011;208:2717–31.
91. Ghisi M, Corradin A, Basso K, et al. Modulation of microRNA expression in human T-cell development: targeting of NOTCH3 by miR-150. Blood. 2011;117:7053–62.
92. Watanabe A, Tagawa H, Yamashita J, et al. The role of microRNA-150 as a tumor suppressor in malignant lymphoma. Leukemia. 2011;25:1324–34.
93. Calin GA, Dumitru CD, Shimizu M, et al. Frequent deletions and down-regulation of microRNA genes miR15 and miR16 at 13q14 in chronic lymphocytic leukemia. Proc Natl Acad Sci U S A. 2002;99:15524–9.
94. Cimmino A, Calin GA, Fabbri M, et al. miR-15 and miR-16 induce apoptosis by targeting BCL2. Proc Natl Acad Sci U S A. 2005;102:13944–9.
95. Fabbri M, Bottoni A, Shimizu M, et al. Association of a microRNA/TP53 feedback circuitry with pathogenesis and outcome of B-cell chronic lymphocytic leukemia. JAMA. 2011;305:59–67.
96. Raveche ES, Salerno E, Scaglione BJ, et al. Abnormal microRNA-16 locus with synteny to human 13q14 linked to CLL in NZB mice. Blood. 2007;109:5079–86.
97. Calin GA, Ferracin M, Cimmino A, et al. A MicroRNA signature associated with prognosis and progression in chronic lymphocytic leukemia. N Engl J Med. 2005;353:1793–801.
98. Klein U, Lia M, Crespo M, et al. The DLEU2/miR-15a/16-1 cluster controls B cell proliferation and its deletion leads to chronic lymphocytic leukemia. Cancer Cell. 2010;17:28–40.
99. Lia M, Carette A, Tang H, et al. Functional dissection of the chromosome 13q14 tumor-suppressor locus using transgenic mouse lines. Blood. 2012;119:2981–90.
100. Fulci V, Chiaretti S, Goldoni M, et al. Quantitative technologies establish a novel microRNA profile of chronic lymphocytic leukemia. Blood. 2007;109:4944–51.
101. Ouillette P, Erba H, Kujawski L, et al. Integrated genomic profiling of chronic lymphocytic leukemia identifies subtypes of deletion 13q14. Cancer Res. 2008;68:1012–21.
102. Wang M, Tan LP, Dijkstra MK, et al. miRNA analysis in B-cell chronic lymphocytic leukaemia: proliferation centres characterized by low miR-150 and high BIC/miR-155 expression. J Pathol. 2008;215:13–20.
103. Dejean E, Renalier MH, Foisseau M, et al. Hypoxia-microRNA-16 downregulation induces VEGF expression in anaplastic lymphoma kinase (ALK)-positive anaplastic large-cell lymphomas. Leukemia. 2011;25:1882–90.
104. Chen RW, Bemis LT, Amato CM, et al. Truncation in CCND1 mRNA alters miR-16-1 regulation in mantle cell lymphoma. Blood. 2008;112:822–9.

105. Zhang X, Chen X, Lin J, et al. Myc represses miR-15a/miR-16-1 expression through recruitment of HDAC3 in mantle cell and other non-Hodgkin B-cell lymphomas. Oncogene. 2012;31:3002–8.
106. Vasioukhin V, Anker P, Maurice P, et al. Point mutations of the N-ras gene in the blood plasma DNA of patients with myelodysplastic syndrome or acute myelogenous leukaemia. Br J Haematol. 1994;86:774–9.
107. Iriyama C, Tomita A, Hoshino H, et al. Using peripheral blood circulating DNAs to detect CpG global methylation status and genetic mutations in patients with myelodysplastic syndrome. Biochem Biophys Res Commun. 2012;419:662–9.
108. Suzuki Y, Tomita A, Nakamura F, et al. Peripheral blood cell-free DNA is an alternative tumor DNA source reflecting disease status in myelodysplastic syndromes. Cancer Sci. 2016;107:1329–37.
109. Albitar F, Ma W, Diep K, et al. Deep sequencing of cell-free peripheral blood DNA as a reliable method for confirming the diagnosis of myelodysplastic syndrome. Genet Test Mol Biomarkers. 2016;20:341–5.
110. Yeh P, Dickinson M, Ftouni S, et al. Molecular disease monitoring using circulating tumor DNA in myelodysplastic syndromes. Blood. 2017;129:1685–90.
111. Rogers A, Joe Y, Manshouri T, et al. Relative increase in leukemia-specific DNA in peripheral blood plasma from patients with acute myeloid leukemia and myelodysplasia. Blood. 2004;103:2799–801.
112. Quan J, Gao YJ, Yang ZL, et al. Quantitative detection of circulating nucleophosmin mutations DNA in the plasma of patients with acute myeloid leukemia. Int J Med Sci. 2015;12:17–22.
113. Schwarz AK, Stanulla M, Cario G, et al. Quantification of free total plasma DNA and minimal residual disease detection in the plasma of children with acute lymphoblastic leukemia. Ann Hematol. 2009;88:897–905.
114. Frickhofen N, Muller E, Sandherr M, et al. Rearranged Ig heavy chain DNA is detectable in cell-free blood samples of patients with B-cell neoplasia. Blood. 1997;90:4953–60.
115. Albitar A, Ma W, DeDios I, et al. Using high-sensitivity sequencing for the detection of mutations in BTK and PLCgamma2 genes in cellular and cell-free DNA and correlation with progression in patients treated with BTK inhibitors. Oncotarget. 2017;8:17936–44.
116. Hohaus S, Giachelia M, Massini G, et al. Cell-free circulating DNA in Hodgkin's and non-Hodgkin's lymphomas. Ann Oncol. 2009;20:1408–13.
117. Primerano S, Burnelli R, Carraro E, et al. Kinetics of circulating plasma cell-free DNA in Paediatric classical Hodgkin lymphoma. J Cancer. 2016;7:364–6.
118. Mussolin L, Burnelli R, Pillon M, et al. Plasma cell-free DNA in paediatric lymphomas. J Cancer. 2013;4:323–9.
119. Zhong L, Huang WF. Better detection of Ig heavy chain and TCRgamma gene rearrangement in plasma cell-free DNA from patients with non-Hodgkin lymphoma. Neoplasma. 2010;57:507–11.
120. Armand P, Oki Y, Neuberg DS, et al. Detection of circulating tumour DNA in patients with aggressive B-cell non-Hodgkin lymphoma. Br J Haematol. 2013;163:123–6.
121. Hosny G, Farahat N, Hainaut P. TP53 mutations in circulating free DNA from Egyptian patients with non-Hodgkin's lymphoma. Cancer Lett. 2009;275:234–9.
122. Bohers E, Viailly PJ, Dubois S, et al. Somatic mutations of cell-free circulating DNA detected by next-generation sequencing reflect the genetic changes in both germinal center B-cell-like and activated B-cell-like diffuse large B-cell lymphomas at the time of diagnosis. Haematologica. 2015;100:e280–4.
123. Camus V, Sarafan-Vasseur N, Bohers E, et al. Digital PCR for quantification of recurrent and potentially actionable somatic mutations in circulating free DNA from patients with diffuse large B-cell lymphoma. Leuk Lymphoma. 2016;57:2171–9.
124. Camus V, Stamatoullas A, Mareschal S, et al. Detection and prognostic value of recurrent exportin 1 mutations in tumor and cell-free circulating DNA of patients with classical Hodgkin lymphoma. Haematologica. 2016;101:1094–101.

125. Sata H, Shibayama H, Maeda I, et al. Quantitative polymerase chain reaction analysis with allele-specific oligonucleotide primers for individual IgH VDJ regions to evaluate tumor burden in myeloma patients. Exp Hematol. 2015;43:374–81. e372
126. Oberle A, Brandt A, Voigtlaender M, et al. Monitoring multiple myeloma by next-generation sequencing of V(D)J rearrangements from circulating myeloma cells and cell-free myeloma DNA. Haematologica. 2017;102:1105–11.
127. Mithraprabhu S, Khong T, Ramachandran M, et al. Circulating tumour DNA analysis demonstrates spatial mutational heterogeneity that coincides with disease relapse in myeloma. Leukemia. 2017;31:1695–705.
128. Huan J, Hornick NI, Shurtleff MJ, et al. RNA trafficking by acute myelogenous leukemia exosomes. Cancer Res. 2013;73:918–29.
129. Hong CS, Muller L, Whiteside TL, Boyiadzis M. Plasma exosomes as markers of therapeutic response in patients with acute myeloid leukemia. Front Immunol. 2014;5:160.
130. Ohyashiki JH, Umezu T, Ohyashiki K. Exosomes promote bone marrow angiogenesis in hematologic neoplasia: the role of hypoxia. Curr Opin Hematol. 2016;23:268–73.
131. Szczepanski MJ, Szajnik M, Welsh A, et al. Blast-derived microvesicles in sera from patients with acute myeloid leukemia suppress natural killer cell function via membrane-associated transforming growth factor-beta1. Haematologica. 2011;96:1302–9.
132. Hong CS, Funk S, Muller L, et al. Isolation of biologically active and morphologically intact exosomes from plasma of patients with cancer. J Extracell Vesicles. 2016;5:29289.
133. Boyiadzis M, Whiteside TL. Plasma-derived exosomes in acute myeloid leukemia for detection of minimal residual disease: are we ready? Expert Rev Mol Diagn. 2016;16:623–9.
134. Wang Y, Cheng Q, Liu J, Dong M. Leukemia stem cell-released microvesicles promote the survival and migration of myeloid leukemia cells and these effects can be inhibited by MicroRNA34a overexpression. Stem Cells Int. 2016;2016:9313425.
135. Hornick NI, Doron B, Abdelhamed S, et al. AML suppresses hematopoiesis by releasing exosomes that contain microRNAs targeting c-MYB. Sci Signal. 2016;9:–ra88.
136. Huan J, Hornick NI, Goloviznina NA, et al. Coordinate regulation of residual bone marrow function by paracrine trafficking of AML exosomes. Leukemia. 2015;29:2285–95.
137. Razmkhah F, Soleimani M, Mehrabani D, et al. Leukemia microvesicles affect healthy hematopoietic stem cells. Tumour Biol. 2017;39:1010428317692234.
138. Gu H, Chen C, Hao X, et al. Sorting protein VPS33B regulates exosomal autocrine signaling to mediate hematopoiesis and leukemogenesis. J Clin Invest. 2016;126:4537–53.
139. Horiguchi H, Kobune M, Kikuchi S, et al. Extracellular vesicle miR-7977 is involved in hematopoietic dysfunction of mesenchymal stromal cells via poly(rC) binding protein 1 reduction in myeloid neoplasms. Haematologica. 2016;101:437–47.
140. Muntion S, Ramos TL, Diez-Campelo M, et al. Microvesicles from mesenchymal stromal cells are involved in HPC-microenvironment crosstalk in myelodysplastic patients. PLoS One. 2016;11:e0146722.
141. Viola S, Traer E, Huan J, et al. Alterations in acute myeloid leukaemia bone marrow stromal cell exosome content coincide with gains in tyrosine kinase inhibitor resistance. Br J Haematol. 2016;172:983–6.
142. Wojtuszkiewicz A, Schuurhuis GJ, Kessler FL, et al. Exosomes secreted by apoptosis-resistant acute myeloid leukemia (AML) Blasts Harbor regulatory network proteins potentially involved in antagonism of apoptosis. Mol Cell Proteomics. 2016;15:1281–98.
143. Hansen HP, Trad A, Dams M, et al. CD30 on extracellular vesicles from malignant Hodgkin cells supports damaging of CD30 ligand-expressing bystander cells with Brentuximab-Vedotin, in vitro. Oncotarget. 2016;7:30523–35.
144. Johnson SM, Dempsey C, Chadwick A, et al. Metabolic reprogramming of bone marrow stromal cells by leukemic extracellular vesicles in acute lymphoblastic leukemia. Blood. 2016;128:453–6.

145. Caivano A, La Rocca F, Simeon V, et al. MicroRNA-155 in serum-derived extracellular vesicles as a potential biomarker for hematologic malignancies – a short report. Cell Oncol (Dordr). 2017;40:97–103.
146. Corrado C, Raimondo S, Saieva L, et al. Exosome-mediated crosstalk between chronic myelogenous leukemia cells and human bone marrow stromal cells triggers an interleukin 8-dependent survival of leukemia cells. Cancer Lett. 2014;348:71–6.
147. Cai J, Han Y, Ren H, et al. Extracellular vesicle-mediated transfer of donor genomic DNA to recipient cells is a novel mechanism for genetic influence between cells. J Mol Cell Biol. 2013;5:227–38.
148. Cai J, Wu G, Tan X, et al. Transferred BCR/ABL DNA from K562 extracellular vesicles causes chronic myeloid leukemia in immunodeficient mice. PLoS One. 2014;9:e105200.
149. Marinaccio C, Ingravallo G, Gaudio F, et al. Microvascular density, CD68 and tryptase expression in human diffuse large B-cell lymphoma. Leuk Res. 2014;38:1374–7.
150. Taverna S, Flugy A, Saieva L, et al. Role of exosomes released by chronic myelogenous leukemia cells in angiogenesis. Int J Cancer. 2012;130:2033–43.
151. Corrado C, Flugy AM, Taverna S, et al. Carboxyamidotriazole-orotate inhibits the growth of imatinib-resistant chronic myeloid leukaemia cells and modulates exosomes-stimulated angiogenesis. PLoS One. 2012;7:e42310.
152. Mineo M, Garfield SH, Taverna S, et al. Exosomes released by K562 chronic myeloid leukemia cells promote angiogenesis in a Src-dependent fashion. Angiogenesis. 2012;15:33–45.
153. Taverna S, Amodeo V, Saieva L, et al. Exosomal shuttling of miR-126 in endothelial cells modulates adhesive and migratory abilities of chronic myelogenous leukemia cells. Mol Cancer. 2014;13:169.
154. Umezu T, Ohyashiki K, Kuroda M, Ohyashiki JH. Leukemia cell to endothelial cell communication via exosomal miRNAs. Oncogene. 2013;32:2747–55.
155. Tadokoro H, Umezu T, Ohyashiki K, et al. Exosomes derived from hypoxic leukemia cells enhance tube formation in endothelial cells. J Biol Chem. 2013;288:34343–51.
156. Umezu T, Shibata Y. Different behavioral effect dose-response profiles in mice exposed to two-carbon chlorinated hydrocarbons: influence of structural and physical properties. Toxicol Appl Pharmacol. 2014;279:103–12.
157. Milani G, Lana T, Bresolin S, et al. Expression profiling of circulating microvesicles reveals intercellular transmission of oncogenic pathways. Mol Cancer Res. 2017;15:683–95.
158. Zhu X, You Y, Li Q, et al. BCR-ABL1-positive microvesicles transform normal hematopoietic transplants through genomic instability: implications for donor cell leukemia. Leukemia. 2014;28:1666–75.
159. Gutkin A, Uziel O, Beery E, et al. Tumor cells derived exosomes contain hTERT mRNA and transform nonmalignant fibroblasts into telomerase positive cells. Oncotarget. 2016;7:59173–88.
160. Feng DQ, Huang B, Li J, et al. Selective miRNA expression profile in chronic myeloid leukemia K562 cell-derived exosomes. Asian Pac J Cancer Prev. 2013;14:7501–8.
161. Ohyashiki K, Umezu T, Katagiri S, et al. Downregulation of plasma miR-215 in chronic myeloid leukemia patients with successful discontinuation of Imatinib. Int J Mol Sci. 2016;17:570.
162. Caivano A, Laurenzana I, De Luca L, et al. High serum levels of extracellular vesicles expressing malignancy-related markers are released in patients with various types of hematological neoplastic disorders. Tumour Biol. 2015;36:9739–52.
163. Fei F, Joo EJ, Tarighat SS, et al. B-cell precursor acute lymphoblastic leukemia and stromal cells communicate through Galectin-3. Oncotarget. 2015;6:11378–94.
164. El-Saghir J, Nassar F, Tawil N, El-Sabban M. ATL-derived exosomes modulate mesenchymal stem cells: potential role in leukemia progression. Retrovirology. 2016;13:73.

165. Farahani M, Rubbi C, Liu L, et al. CLL exosomes modulate the transcriptome and behaviour of recipient stromal cells and are selectively enriched in miR-202-3p. PLoS One. 2015;10:e0141429.
166. Paggetti J, Haderk F, Seiffert M, et al. Exosomes released by chronic lymphocytic leukemia cells induce the transition of stromal cells into cancer-associated fibroblasts. Blood. 2015;126:1106–17.
167. Ferrajoli A, Shanafelt TD, Ivan C, et al. Prognostic value of miR-155 in individuals with monoclonal B-cell lymphocytosis and patients with B chronic lymphocytic leukemia. Blood. 2013;122:1891–9.
168. Reiners KS, Topolar D, Henke A, et al. Soluble ligands for NK cell receptors promote evasion of chronic lymphocytic leukemia cells from NK cell anti-tumor activity. Blood. 2013;121:3658–65.
169. De Luca L, D'Arena G, Simeon V, et al. Characterization and prognostic relevance of circulating microvesicles in chronic lymphocytic leukemia. Leuk Lymphoma. 2017;58:1424–32.
170. Boysen J, Nelson M, Magzoub G, et al. Dynamics of microvesicle generation in B-cell chronic lymphocytic leukemia: implication in disease progression. Leukemia. 2017;31:350–60.
171. Yeh YY, Ozer HG, Lehman AM, et al. Characterization of CLL exosomes reveals a distinct microRNA signature and enhanced secretion by activation of BCR signaling. Blood. 2015;125:3297–305.
172. Roccaro AM, Sacco A, Maiso P, et al. BM mesenchymal stromal cell-derived exosomes facilitate multiple myeloma progression. J Clin Invest. 2013;123:1542–55.
173. Liu Y, Zhu XJ, Zeng C, et al. Microvesicles secreted from human multiple myeloma cells promote angiogenesis. Acta Pharmacol Sin. 2014;35:230–8.
174. Wang J, Hendrix A, Hernot S, et al. Bone marrow stromal cell-derived exosomes as communicators in drug resistance in multiple myeloma cells. Blood. 2014;124:555–66.
175. Arendt BK, Walters DK, Wu X, et al. Multiple myeloma dell-derived microvesicles are enriched in CD147 expression and enhance tumor cell proliferation. Oncotarget. 2014;5:5686–99.
176. Raimondi L, De Luca A, Amodio N, et al. Involvement of multiple myeloma cell-derived exosomes in osteoclast differentiation. Oncotarget. 2015;6:13772–89.
177. Vardaki I, Sanchez C, Fonseca P, et al. Caspase-3-dependent cleavage of Bcl-xL in the stroma exosomes is required for their uptake by hematological malignant cells. Blood. 2016;128:2655–65.
178. Purushothaman A, Bandari SK, Liu J, et al. Fibronectin on the surface of myeloma cell-derived exosomes mediates exosome-cell interactions. J Biol Chem. 2016;291:1652–63.
179. Wang J, De Veirman K, Faict S, et al. Multiple myeloma exosomes establish a favourable bone marrow microenvironment with enhanced angiogenesis and immunosuppression. J Pathol. 2016;239:162–73.
180. Chillemi A, Quarona V, Antonioli L, et al. Roles and modalities of ectonucleotidases in remodeling the multiple myeloma niche. Front Immunol. 2017;8:305.
181. Manier S, Liu CJ, Avet-Loiseau H, et al. Prognostic role of circulating exosomal miRNAs in multiple myeloma. Blood. 2017;129:2429–36.
182. Lia G, Brunello L, Bruno S, et al. Extracellular vesicles as potential biomarkers of acute graft-vs-host disease. Leukemia. 2018;32:765–73.
183. Hedlund M, Nagaeva O, Kargl D, et al. Thermal- and oxidative stress causes enhanced release of NKG2D ligand-bearing immunosuppressive exosomes in leukemia/lymphoma T and B cells. PLoS One. 2011;6:e16899.
184. Aung T, Chapuy B, Vogel D, et al. Exosomal evasion of humoral immunotherapy in aggressive B-cell lymphoma modulated by ATP-binding cassette transporter A3. Proc Natl Acad Sci U S A. 2011;108:15336–41.

185. Hansen HP, Engels HM, Dams M, et al. Protrusion-guided extracellular vesicles mediate CD30 trans-signalling in the microenvironment of Hodgkin's lymphoma. J Pathol. 2014;232:405–14.
186. Gutzeit C, Nagy N, Gentile M, et al. Exosomes derived from Burkitt's lymphoma cell lines induce proliferation, differentiation, and class-switch recombination in B cells. J Immunol. 2014;192:5852–62.
187. van Eijndhoven MA, Zijlstra JM, Groenewegen NJ, et al. Plasma vesicle miRNAs for therapy response monitoring in Hodgkin lymphoma patients. JCI Insight. 2016;1:e89631.
188. Bouyssou JM, Liu CJ, Bustoros M, et al. Profiling of circulating exosomal miRNAs in patients with Waldenstrom Macroglobulinemia. PLoS One. 2018;13:e0204589.

Chapter 13
Cancer Biomarkers in Interstitial Fluids

13.1 Introduction

Despite its complexity, tumor interstitial fluid is a rich source of cancer-specific biomarkers that can be explored and leveraged in easily accessible body fluids such as blood, saliva, sputum, stool, and urine. The interstitium or commonly referred to as interstitial or extracellular space is the connective tissue components interposed between the vasculature (blood and lymphatic) and cells. It is the supporting tissue for cells within which intercellular communication also occurs. The two components of this space are the structural molecules referred to as the extracellular matrix (ECM) and the interstitial fluid (IF). The ECM or ground substance is made of proteoglycans, glycoproteins, and fibrous elements. The IF serves as a medium for exchange of nutrients and waste products between capillaries and cells and also contains high concentration of substances that are locally produced or preferentially transported to the tissue via the circulation. The cells in the interstitial space are either tissue-specific such as parenchymal cells or non-tissue-specific (or shared) cells such as immune cells and fibroblasts.

The tumor interstitium, preferably referred to as tumor microenvironment, plays an important role in tumor growth, invasion, and metastasis. This medium contains numerous soluble and membrane-enclosed signaling molecules used in multidimensional communication among cells in the tumor microenvironment. The tumor interstitial fluid (TIF) is rich in secreted biomolecules (the secretome) from tumor and reactive stromal cells. These biomolecules eventually percolate into the lymphatic and hence systemic circulation, as well as organ- or tissue-associated proximal fluids such as saliva or urine.

Unlike the interstitial space of normal cells, that of the cancer cell is "reactive." It contains increased numbers of activated endothelial cells, fibroblasts, and inflammatory cells with altered phenotypes. Macrophages in the tumor microenvironment tend to be pro-tumoral M2-activated cells. Other reactive cells that impact on tumor

G. D. Dakubo, *Cancer Biomarkers in Body Fluids*,
https://doi.org/10.1007/978-3-030-24725-6_13

behaviors are regulatory T cells (Tregs), tumor-infiltrating cytotoxic T cells, myeloid-derived suppressor cells (MDSCs), and cancer-associated fibroblasts (CAFs).

The complexity of plasma proteins and the dilution of low-abundant disease proteins (1–10 pg/ml or lower) are obstacles to accurate biomarker discovery in blood. Because the concentration of disease biomarkers in local IF or tumor microenvironment is high (1000–5000 times higher than in blood), TIF analysis offers the advantage of enabling accurate biomarker discovery. Thus, TIF exploration is a popular strategy for cancer biomarker (especially proteomic) discovery.

13.2 The Tumor Microenvironment

The tumor interstitial compartment or microenvironment is everything interposed between the plasma membrane of the cancer cell and the vascular wall of newly formed vessels [1]. This microenvironment supports cancer cell growth and progression through networks of interactions with multiple factors produced by cells in this compartment, as well as those brought in by the circulation. Unlike the microenvironment of normal tissues, that of the tumor is very "reactive and complex."

The interstitium of both normal and tumor tissues consists of collagen network, gel phase of glycosaminoglycans (GAGs), salt solution, and plasma proteins, in which numerous cells suspend. Compared to the normal tissue microenvironment, the tumor interstitium has increased the number of activated inflammatory cells, endothelial cells, fibroblasts, and several signaling molecules, all of which function to enhance tumor growth.

The effector immune cells in the tumor microenvironment include tumor-associated macrophages (TAMs), tumor-infiltrating lymphocytes (TILs), and myeloid-derived suppressor cells (MDSCs). Classical macrophage activation, as occurs during immune defense against microbes, is induced primarily by TH_1 cytokine (IFNγ), but could also be through microbial structures (pathogen- or microbe-associated molecular patterns – PAMPs or MAMPs) such as lipopolysaccharide (LPS), or other cytokines such as TNF-α and GM-CSF. This type of macrophage activation in the tumor microenvironment exerts antitumoral effects. However, other cytokines and factors in the tumor microenvironment induce rather an alternative macrophage activation (M2) that supports tumorigenesis. These factors include TH2 cytokines (IL-4 and IL-13) and macrophage colony-stimulating factor (M-CSF) that are produced by tumor and stromal cells. TILs can kill tumor cells directly through their recognition, and production of perforins that make holes in the tumor plasma membrane, followed by secretion of granzymes into the cancer cell to induce apoptosis. The functions of TILs are augmented by CD4+ helper T cells through production of IL-2 and IFNγ. Thus, increased numbers of these adaptive immune cells in the tumor microenvironment are associated with good prognosis. On the contrary, MDSCs perform pro-tumoral functions by suppressing the functions of CD8+ T cells through expression of arginase 1 (ARG1) and nitric oxide synthase 2 (NOS2) as well as inducing alternative macrophage activation.

M2 cells can activate fibroblasts to become cancer-associated fibroblasts (CAFs) that are involved in ECM remodeling resembling wound healing, except this process is dysregulated in the tumor interstitium. CAFs produce excess collagen, proteoglycans, and GAGs. Cancer cells, fibroblasts, inflammatory cells, and endothelial cells secrete angiogenic factors such as VEGF-A that play an important role in new blood vessel formation. Several other growth factors are found in the reactive tumor microenvironment.

13.3 Tumor Interstitial Fluid Formation

The physiologic role of the circulatory system is to distribute oxygen and nutrients to cells and to remove carbon dioxide and cellular waste products. These functions occur at the level of the microcirculation. The tissue interstitial fluid formed at the capillary bed is reabsorbed mainly via the lymphatics and returned to the blood circulation via the superior and inferior vena cava. Starling in 1896 initially conceived the physiologic principles governing fluid exit from the microcirculation into the interstitial space and subsequent reabsorption [2]. Three critical factors were considered by Starling: vascular wall permeability, differences in capillary and interstitial hydrostatic pressures, and differences in capillary and interstitial colloid (oncotic) osmotic pressures. These variables were used to formulate the Starling equation:

$$J_v = L_p S\left[\left(P_c - P_i\right) - \sigma\left(\pi_p - \pi_i\right)\right]$$

J_v = transendothelial solvent filtration volume per second (ml min^{-1})
$(P_c - P_i) - \sigma(\pi_p - \pi_i)$ = net driving force (mmHg)
P_c = capillary hydrostatic pressure (mmHg)
P_i = interstitial hydrostatic pressure (mmHg)
π_p = plasma protein oncotic pressure (mmHg)
π_i = interstitial protein oncotic pressure (mmHg)
σ = Staverman's osmotic reflection coefficient of vessel wall (0, when membrane is fully permeable to molecules, and 1 when impermeable)
L_p = hydraulic conductivity of the membrane (cm × min^{-1} × mmHg^{-1})
S = capillary surface area (cm^2)

Modifications were subsequently made to the Starling equation. Starling had considered only colloid osmotic pressure between the capillary lumen and the interstitial space. The Starling forces based on the initial equation favored fluid filtration at the arteriolar end and reabsorption at the venular end of the microcirculation. However, these continuous capillaries filter along their entire lengths, with return of filtered fluid back into the blood circulation mostly via the lymphatics. It was later uncovered that the subendothelial glycocalyx rather than interstitial fluid colloid osmotic pressure influenced fluid filtration. This "no reabsorption rule" is the glycocalyx or Michel-Weinbaum model. Thus, the revised Starling equation [3] is:

$$J_v = L_p S\left[\left(P_c - P_i\right) - \sigma\left(\pi_p - \pi_g\right)\right],$$

where π_i is replaced with π_g (glycocalyx oncotic pressure).

The disordered tumor microenvironment and abnormal new blood and lymphatic vessels lead to increased TIF pressure and volume. The P_i of solid tumors is high compared to normal tissues. For example, while normal skin and muscle tissue P_i ranges from – 2 to 0 mmHg [4], the P_i in tumor tissues is in the range of 10–40 mmHg, and even a P_i of 99 mmHg has been recorded in a pancreatic adenocarcinoma model [5]. This high TIF pressure has been a hindrance to delivery of therapeutics to solid tumors.

The disordered intratumoral vasculature summarized here underlies the increased TIF pressure:

- The endothelial cells of tumor blood vessels are irregularly shaped, are disordered, and even overlap, with loose interconnections between them that leave openings of about 2 um between them.
- Dysfunctional pericytes during neovascularization lead to ECM deposition in perivascular regions causing defective basement membrane formation.
- Production of VEGF and vasoactive factors such as bradykinin, nitric oxide, and peroxynitrite derivatives causes endothelial cell dilatation and increased permeability.
- Tumor neovessels are architecturally tortuous, lacking normal arteriolar and venular structures with high arteriovenous anastomoses, further enhancing their leakiness.
- Normal-functioning lymphatics are located at the periphery of solid tumors. Intratumoral lymphatics are compressed, collapsed, and hence dysfunctional. Thus, TIF pressure is highest in the center of the tumor and decreases toward the periphery.

Thus, leakage of proteins and water into the interstitial space will cause high L_p and low σ and hence increased P_i. Decreased lymphatic drainage in the tumor will lead to increased P_i. Moreover, intratumoral blood vessel compression will squeeze out fluid to increase P_i. Finally, direct effects of VEGF, TGFβ, and PDGF in tumor microenvironment cause elevation in the P_i.

13.4 Interstitial Fluid Extraction Methods

The teams of Gullino and Sylven pioneered studies of TIF [1, 6]. The methodologies for obtaining TIF were different between the groups, and those of Gullino's group were more reminiscent of the in vivo pathophysiologic processes. Thus, Gullino's method could more accurately determine TIF composition, interstitial fluid pressure, tumor metabolism, pH, and pharmacokinetics of drugs. Several refined methodologies for obtaining TIF without intracellular contamination have since been developed [7, 8].

From a practical standpoint, two methods or ex vivo approaches appear appropriate for obtaining TIF from resected tissue samples. These are tissue elution and centrifugation, both of which have been validated in a number of studies. There are several in vivo methods including catheter insertion techniques and capsule implantation that enable acquisition of TIF for pathophysiologic, pharmacokinetics, pharmacodynamics, and possibly metabolomic studies. Because of their invasive nature, these in vivo techniques are mostly used in model animal studies.

Obtaining IF for biomarker exploration, mostly proteomic analysis, faces numerous technical challenges. The tumor microenvironment is very different from normal tissue microenvironment by being vascular, cellular, and with abnormal blood and lymphatic vessels. Cautionary measures must be taken to minimize IF contamination with blood or intracellular content released by cell lysis, damage, or death.

13.4.1 Ex Vivo Approaches

These methods include tissue elution and centrifugation techniques. They are the primary approaches mostly used in cancer biomarker exploration from resected tissues.

13.4.1.1 Tissue Elution Technique

This technique was developed by the Copenhagen group [9]. It is a passive process for extraction of IFs from surgically resected small tissue specimens using physiologic solutions such as phosphate-buffered solution (PBS). A comparative study of various physiologic solutions did not find significant differences in protein composition between the five solutions studied including PBS. However, components within the four other solutions, namely, DMEM, University of Wisconsin, Celsior solution S, and histidine-tryptophan-ketoglutarate, could confound downstream LC-MS/MS proteomic analysis [10].

In the initial procedural development, about 0.25 g of tissue biopsies were cut into 1–3 mm^3 little pieces, washed in 5 ml PBS, and placed in 10 ml conical plastic tubes with 0.8 ul PBS. The samples were then incubated at 37 °C in humidified CO_2 chamber for various time periods from 0 to 24 h. The samples were centrifuged at 170 g for 20 min, and the supernatant was transferred using a Pasteur pipette into another tube. To concentrate biomarkers, a final centrifugation at 2800 g for 20 min at 4 °C was performed. The supernatant with concentrated proteins up to 4 ug/ml was collected and stored at – 80 °C for later analysis.

This method of TIF extraction faces obvious challenges. Cutting through such vascularized tumor tissue may lead to release of both intracellular and intravascular components into the TIF. Also because the eluent is recovered with PBS, IF biomarkers will certainly be diluted and thus require further concentration methods such as lyophilization, ultrafiltration, and centrifugation. This method has however been validated for efficient collection of TIF.

13.4.1.2 Tissue Centrifugation Technique

This method was originally developed for collecting IF from collagen-rich and cell-poor tissues such as cornea and tendons, as well as from experimental tumor models. However, by applying the appropriate centrifugation forces, it has been adapted to efficiently collect IF from human-resected tissues.

In this procedure, flushing with saline buffer cleans the excised tissue, which is then sectioned and gently blotted with tissue paper to remove excess saline. The tissue is then centrifuged at appropriate gravitational force based on tissue type. The G-forces should be low to minimize damage to cells and tissues. A G-force $\leq$424 appears not to be associated with dilution of extracellular fluid and is representative of TIF. Human ovarian cancer IF was successfully isolated by centrifugation through a nylon mesh at 106 g for 10 min [8].

There are equally challenges with this method in obtaining uncontaminated TIF. Because the resected tumors are sectioned, this suffers similar possible contamination issues as in the elution method. Another critical issue is determining the optimal G-force for the tissue in question. This has to be empirically determined for each tissue type. High G-forces may lead to cell and tissue damage and thus contamination of TIF with intracellular content. Also observed is the low yield of TIF, especially with hard tissues, which are reminiscent of solid tumors. This method, however, has been successfully employed in the discovery of biomarkers in TIF.

13.4.2 In Vivo Approaches

These approaches are developed mostly for studying physiologic and pathologic features of IFs of mostly animal models because of their invasive nature. Nonetheless, some techniques such as microdialysis, because of its low invasiveness, have been used to obtain TIF from humans for proteomic studies.

13.4.2.1 Catheter Insertion Techniques

Originally developed for fluid sampling from the brain, microdialysis has been adapted for sampling TIFs. While extensively used to obtain TIF, most have focused on pharmacological studies. In this procedure, a microcatheter or probe with a semi-permeable membrane at the tip is inserted into the tissue. The method relies on passive movement of fluid across the semipermeable membrane implanted in the extracellular space. This method of IF recovery is more suitable for low molecular weight substances such as metabolites, for which it was developed. Although the recovery is low, microdialysis has been used to successfully study IF proteome. The major disadvantage is the low recovery (~1%) of macromolecules.

Capillary ultrafiltration is a technique used for purification of chemicals. It has been adapted for recovery of TIF for analysis. This method involves in vivo placement of a capillary probe with application of negative pressure to the probe to facilitate IF extraction. While the method is optimal for recovery of small molecules, selective pressures at the tissue-membrane interface restrict macromolecular passage. Thus, for proteomic studies, membranes with high molecular weight cutoffs (e.g., 400 kDa) that allow passage of proteins and peptides have been employed for IF recovery. This method has also been successfully used to study TIF of mouse models [11].

Wicked-in-needle technique is another method employed for the study of TIF in animal models. It is also mostly applied to measure osmotic pressure and IF pressure. In this procedure, a nylon wick soaked in buffered saline solution is inserted into established tumors or simultaneously with tumor transplantation into mice. The main drawbacks are tissue damage with associated inflammation from the invasive procedure and contamination of TIF from intracellular components as a result of cell or tissue damage from the procedure.

Developed by Sylven and Bois, glass capillary method is based on the tenet that tumor periphery is rich in edema-like IF that could easily be collected via glass capillary insertion [6]. However, because of the presence of normal tissue and other elements of tumor margins, the collected fluid is not a true reflection of TIF. Contamination of the TIF can also occur from damage to cells caused by the procedure.

13.4.2.2 Capsular Implantation

Guyton et al. developed the implanted capsule method for the study of IF pressure [12]. This approach helped disprove the previous (until 1960) notion that the IF pressure was positive. Gullino subsequently improved upon this procedure by creating a capsule that enabled both IF pressure measurement and extraction of TIF. The Gullino capsule consists of a 1–2 mm ring with the upper and lower ends covered with a Millipore membrane. It has a small cavity inside that is connected externally to enable fluid collection via a catheter as well as IF pressure measurement. The capsule is placed and left in situ to grow with the tumor. This enables longitudinal study of TIF or microenvironment with tumor progression. The drawbacks of this approach are the inflammatory response to a foreign object and wound healing process following implantation, all of which will be associated with different biomolecular secretions into TIF, but which are not reflective of the carcinogenic process.

13.5 Tumor Interstitial Fluid Composition

The TIF is the fluid phase of the interstitium that percolates the tumor and tumor stromal cells (TAM, CAF, other immune cells, mesenchymal cells, and adipocytes), as well as the gel phase ECM composed of GAGs, proteoglycans, and collagen. TIF composition is therefore important to the pathophysiologic functions of these reactive cells. The composition of TIF has been extensively studied, being pioneered by Gullino's group who analyzed the composition of TIF in transplanted rat models [13].

The TIF differs in pH, dissolved gases, macromolecules, and extracellular vesicles when compared to plasma and subcutaneous IF. The pH of TIF is in the order of 0.2–0.4 units lower than plasma, but this appears to depend on tumor size, because it has been demonstrated to decrease from about 7.3 to 6.2 with increasing tumor size up to 50 g [14]. Dissolved CO_2 is about 1 mm higher leading to increased PCO_2, which is 16–39 mmHg higher than plasma. TIF PO_2 is, however, lower. While TIF protein is relatively high, leading to increased colloid osmotic pressure, it is lower than plasma, being about 80% that of plasma proteins. Fibrinogen is completely absent in TIF. However, TIF protein is significantly higher than subcutaneous tissue IF. Free amino acids are higher in TIF than plasma. There is low hyaluronic acid in TIF due to increased hyaluronidase activity. TIF is rich in extracellular vesicles, particularly exosomes, and bioactive substances called matrikines. Matrikines are peptide derivatives from partial proteolysis of extracellular proteins and GAGs. They are biologically active molecules that can regulate cellular functions and extracellular matrix degradation [15, 16].

The increased TIF osmolality, primarily due to albumin, has been linked to a number of biologic activities in the tumor microenvironment. The elevated osmotic pressure acts as a potent pro-inflammatory stimulus [17]. Macrophages respond to the hyperosmolar environment by producing pro-inflammatory molecules such as TNF, IL-1, IL-6, and IL-8 [18]. Additionally, the increased osmolality activates NF-κB, which promotes tumor growth [19, 20].

13.6 The Secretome

The ideal diagnostic or screening biomarker should be accurately measureable in blood or other noninvasively procured proximal fluid such as saliva, sputum, or urine. Cancer biomarkers in circulation are released by the cancer cell either via secretion or other means and have to percolate into the microcirculation or proximal fluid. Due to the sheer volume of blood and other proximal fluids, biomarkers in these media are very dilute, thus requiring concentration, amplification, and sensitive technologies for their measurement. Thus, cancer biomarker discovery in these body fluids is less attractive. Obviously, the highest concentration of cancer biomarkers is in the cancer cell, making pure cancer cell analysis the ideal for biomarker discovery. However, if such intracellular biomarker is not secreted, it is unlikely to be present in circulation and proximal fluids to be used as a screening or diagnostic biomarker. Therefore, searching for screening biomarkers has focused on samples close to the disease site. To this end, the TIF is considered the ideal sample for discovery of secreted biomarkers (the secretome) by cancer cells.

The secretome has been studied using cell culture systems and TIFs. While secreted molecules into cell culture media have provided important biomarker targets, it is unlikely to capture all relevant biomarkers because of the lack of tumor microenvironmental interactions. Another challenge is the inability to differentiate between secreted biomarkers and those released into the medium due to cell death. Analysis for cell death prior to harvesting the supernatant for study should help minimize this confounding variable. Notwithstanding, secretome studies of in vivo or ex vivo TIF also face challenges. The TIF is a complex medium reflective of all available biomolecules from cancer and stromal cells, as well as those from the circulation. Secondly, methodological issues with TIF collection may not be optimal leading to contamination with intracellular or vascular contents. Despite these confounding factors, secretome studies using TIF and cell culture systems should enable discovery of authentic cancer biomarkers for translation.

13.7 Cancer Biomarkers in Interstitial Fluids

A number of TIF biomarkers have been identified, with some validated and translated successfully using blood (Table 13.1).

13.7.1 Head and Neck Cancer Biomarkers in Interstitial Fluids

Stone et al. used ultrafiltration catheter to collect IF from head and neck squamous cell carcinoma (HNSCC) patients for proteomic studies [21]. The sample was immune depleted of high abundance serum proteins before trypsinization. The peptides were fractionated in three dimensions before MS analysis that identified 525 proteins constituting the first catalog of HNSCC IF proteome. The following

Table 13.1 Tumor interstitial fluid (TIF) biomarkers

Cancer	TIF biomarkers
Breast	CD276, CRABP2, CLIC1, TCPT, S100A9, EF1β, PRDX2, PD-ECGF, PDI, UCTH5, GDI1, YWHA2, HNRNPD, calreticulin, calumenin
Head and neck	MMP8, MMP9, neurotrypsin, trypsin1, fascin
Lung	Perixiredoxin, PRDX1
Liver	SPARC, THBS2, S100A2, AFP, SERBB, S100A9
Colorectal	Desmocollin, fibrinogen chain
Renal	ENO2, NNMT, TSP1
Ovarian	PRDX1, WDR1, S100A8, STIP1, LAP3, TPI1, UCHL1, BNDF, transferrin

evidences confirmed minimal contamination of the HNSCC IF from cell lysis: (i) the fluid was enriched for "extracellular" proteins by Gene Ontology annotation, (ii) proteins in the HNSCC IF were distinct from proteins in other body fluids, (iii) the IF proteins had higher overlap with human salivary proteome (76%) than plasma proteome (46%), and (iv) many of the HNSCC IF proteins had overlap with proteins identified as HNSCC biomarkers in other body fluids. The use of microdialysis to extract interstitial fluid from oral squamous cell carcinoma (OSCC) enabled identification of 217 proteins. Among them, proteases were most abundant [22]. The authors concluded that this methodology that is commonly applied in collection of brain interstitial fluid could be broadly adopted for biomarker mining. Gel-based MS proteomics of HNC IF and normal IF (NIF) uncovered 189 peptides corresponding to 75 proteins [23]. The most elevated protein, fascin, was confirmed in cancer tissues and cell culture supernatant by immunoblot and immunohistochemistry. The diagnostic accuracy of serum fascin levels with AUROCC of 0.808 was superior to the 0.501 achieved for squamous cell carcinoma antigen (SCCA) in this cohort. Elevated fascin levels also correlated with lymph node metastasis.

13.7.2 Lung Cancer Biomarkers in Interstitial Fluids

Li et al. used the centrifugation method to obtain TIF from 20 NSCLC patients for study [24]. Peroxiredoxin was uncovered to be significantly elevated in TIF compared to IF from benign lung pathologies. The increased peroxiredoxin levels in TIF were associated with apoptosis resistance, as well as clinicopathologic variables such as age, lymph node involvement, and TNM classification.

IF pressure is in general high in solid tumors and this influences many pathophysiologic aspects of tumors. Prospective measurements of TIF pressure in 211 lung cancer patients revealed a mean pressure of 8.5 mmHg [25]. The increased tumor ITP significantly correlated with tumor size, TNM, vessel and pleural invasion, Ki-67 index, and maximum standardized uptake value (SUV_{max}). Compared to high, low TIF pressure was associated with better recurrence-free survival (RFS), and this was an independent prognostic factor for adenocarcinoma.

13.7.3 Breast Cancer Biomarkers in Interstitial Fluids

Potential breast cancer IF biomarkers have been uncovered for subsequent translational studies [9, 26]. A group from Copenhagen University, Denmark, has performed proteomic analysis on IF from 69 breast cancer patients. The TIF and NIF were prospectively collected over 6 years. While topologically TIF and NIF proteins were identical, the levels of NIF proteins were lower than their TIF counterparts. This finding could be due to the differential sources and mode of release of IF between normal and cancerous breast tissues. In the normal breast (especially postmenopausal), more proteins are from connective than glandular tissue, and the opposite is true for cancerous breast tissue. Because all breast cancer IFs irrespective of histopathological subtype shared a significant proportion of all identified proteins, a phased discovery approach was employed for analysis rather than simple sample comparison [26]. In phase 1, 110 of the 623 identified proteins in breast cancer IFs were observed to have increased by a factor of 2 or more when compared to corresponding NIF in one patient. In phase 2, breast cancer IF and NIF from 68 and 28 patients, respectively, were comparatively studied using computer-assisted analysis of the 2D gels. This approach uncovered 26 unique proteins that were present at elevated levels in >90% of breast cancer IFs compared to NIFs. The third phase of the discovery process was validation of the 26 proteins using a commercially available breast cancer tissue microarray, Pantomics BRC1503. This analysis confirmed the upregulation of nine proteins, namely, calreticulin, CRABP-II, CLIC1, EF-1β, galectin-1, PRDX2, PD-ECGF, PDI, and UCTH5. The breast cancer IF proteins are unique in some respect. First, only a few of the 26 proteins (calreticulin, lactate dehydrogenase, GSTP1, thioredoxin, PDI, TPI, EF-1β, and galectin) have been shown to be dysregulated in breast cancer, with the vast majority being novel. Second, none of the 26 elevated breast cancer IF proteins have been demonstrated to be upregulated in breast cancer cells, which may be due to the lack of interaction between cultured cells and stromal cells, as occurs in vivo. Additionally, the cell culture process could affect protein profile. In another analysis, of 93 elevated proteins in breast cancer IF, CD276 was validated by immunohistochemistry as breast cancer biomarker [27]. Similarly, of 1324 non-redundant proteins uncovered in breast cancer IF, GDI-1, HNRNPD, and YWHAZ were validated by Western blot as breast cancer biomarkers [28].

Tchafa et al. investigated the role of IF flow on signaling in ERBB2-positive breast cancer cells. Invasion of these cells was induced by IF flow through activation of the PI3K pathway [29]. In ERBB2-expressing cells that had undergone EMT, IF flow-induced invasion required CXCR4 chemokine receptor, a gradient of its ligand, CXCL12, as well as activity of p100α and β. In breast cancer cells expressing wild-type ERBB2, IF flow-mediated invasion required only p100α activation but not CXCR4.

miRNA profiling of matched TIF and NIF samples from women with breast cancer uncovered 266 miRNAs that were elevated in TIF compared to NIF [30]. Sixty-one of these miRNAs were also present in >75% of serum samples, and seven were associated with poor survival.

13.7.4 Hepatocellular Carcinoma Biomarkers in Interstitial Fluids

A proof of concept study of biomarker discovery in hepatocellular carcinoma (HCC) IF was conducted using mouse liver [31]. Ex vivo incubation of tissue in PBS was used for TIF extraction followed by reverse-phase HPLC-MS/MS proteomic analysis. Lack of intracellular protein contamination of TIF was confirmed by the absence of organellar proteins indicated by nuclear lamin B, mitochondrial cytochrome C, and plasma membrane flotillin. Linear trap quadrupole (LTQ) analysis and database search led to identification of 1450 proteins in mouse liver TIF. Potential blood-based HCC biomarkers were putatively uncovered after comparing proteins from mouse liver tissue (7090), liver TIF (1450), hepatocyte (1125), and plasma (4721). Further analysis of paired liver TIF and NIF from a patient with HCC supported this biomarker discovery process. Analysis of HCC IF and NIF identified 72 proteins of interest, of which sERBB3 was validated by Western blot [32]. Soluble ERBB3 and AFP were examined in serum samples from HCC patients and controls that consisted of chronic hepatitis and cirrhotic patients.

Sun et al. used iTRAQ to analyze HCC IF and matched NIF that enabled identification of 241 elevated and 288 decreased proteins in TIF [33]. S100A9 was remarkably elevated in TIF (ratio of 19) and was validated in serum samples using ELISA. There were significantly elevated levels in sera from HCC patients compared to those with cirrhosis, and this achieved a sensitivity, specificity, and AUROCC of 91%, 66%, and 0.83, respectively, in separating between the two groups of patients. Zhang et al. used iTRAQ to analyze 16 HCC IFs and paired NIFs [34]. Of the 3357 quantified proteins, 232 were significantly elevated and 257 were decreased in TIF. Two of the elevated proteins, SPARC and THBS2, were validated in serum samples using ELISA and were equally significantly increased in HCC patients than healthy controls. The combined serum biomarkers achieved a sensitivity of 86%, specificity of 100%, and AUROCC of 0.97 in distinguishing HCC patients and a sensitivity of 80%, specificity of 93%, and AUROCC of 0.95 in differentiating AFP-negative HCC patients from healthy controls. For patients with benign liver diseases, the sensitivity was 80%, and specificity was 94%, with AUROCC of 0.93. Serum level of THBS2 was an independent HCC prognostic biomarker.

13.7.5 Colorectal Cancer Biomarkers in Interstitial Fluids

In a colorectal cancer (CRC) explant eluate to obtain TIF and NIF for proteomic analysis, 32 differential protein levels were uncovered, with desmocollin and fibrinogen γ-chain identified as potential biomarkers [35]. Analysis of TIF and NIF from mouse CRC model enabled identification of 2172 proteins with 1958 having human homologs [36]. Of 52 suggested candidates, MCM4 and S100A9 were verified by immunohistochemistry in mouse tissues, while serum samples from CRC and adenoma patients were analyzed using ELISA targeting CHI3L1 and CEA. Small hyaluronan oligosaccharide concentration up to 6 ug/ml was detected in some CRC IF but not NIF [37]. In a cohort of 72 CRC patients, increased small hyaluronan oligosaccharide concentration in TIF was associated with lymphatic invasion and lymph node metastasis.

iTRAQ proteomic analysis of TIF from inflammation-related CRC mouse model (AOM-DSS) was conducted [38]. A total of 144 proteins, including 45 that increased and 17 that decreased, demonstrated changes with tumor progression. Twelve of the elevated TIF proteins were examined using multiple reaction monitoring (MRM) in serum samples. Significantly increased in CRC compared to control mice were leucine-rich α-2-glycoprotein 1 (LRG1), tubulin β-5 chain (TUBB5), and Ig J chain (IGJ). Verification in clinical samples using MRM confirmed elevated LRG1 and TUBB5 as potential CRC serum biomarkers. Xie et al. also used iTRAQ to analyze TIF from ApcMin/+ CRC mouse model, which enabled identification of 46 elevated proteins, of which 6 serine proteases, chymotrypsin-like elastase 1 (CELA1), chymotrypsin-like elastase 2A (CEL2A), chymopasin, chymotrypsinogen B (CTRB1), trypsin 2 (TRY2), and trypsin 4 (TRY4), were verified using MRM [39]. In serum samples from human CRC patients, CELA1, CEL2A, CTRL/chymopasin, and TRY2 were significantly elevated. A panel of CELA1 and CTRL achieved a diagnostic sensitivity of 90% and specificity of 80% for CRC detection.

13.7.6 Epithelial Ovarian Cancer Biomarkers in Interstitial Fluids

Not surprisingly because of the lack of proximal fluid, except ascites that develops after overt malignancy, there has been keen interest in biomarker exploration in ovarian cancer IF that could be developed as blood-based screening [8, 40, 41]. Differential protein levels between human ovarian cancer IF and NIF were uncovered using comprehensive 2D electrophoresis comparative study [40]. The identified proteins included stress-induced phosphoprotein 1 (STIP1), type I keratin 16, LAP3, MACF1, BDNF isoform b preproprotein (BDNF1), and TPI1. Immunohistochemistry was used to confirm the overexpression of STIP1 in ovarian cancer compared to normal ovarian tissue. Moreover, the secretion of STIP1 and subsequent significantly elevated circulating levels of STIP1 in ovarian cancer patients compared to age-matched normal controls were demonstrated. In another study, LC-MS/MS was used to analyze paired TIF and ascitic fluid from four papillary serous epithelial ovarian cancer (EOC) patients [41]. A total of 569 proteins identified were common to all ovarian cancer IF samples. This contrasted with only 171 proteins commonly identified in the corresponding ascetic fluid. The level of peroxiredoxin 1 (PRDX1) was higher in ovarian cancer IF than ascites and was much significantly elevated in 20 EOC patients with a mean level of 20.0 ng/ml compared to 4.19 ng/ml in 16 individuals with normal or benign ovarian tumors. Haslene-Hox et al. used a centrifugation technique to collect ovarian cancer IF and verified to be interstitial fluid with negligible contamination from cell lysis [8]. LC-MS/MS was used to uncover 769 proteins that were sixfold elevated in ovarian cancer IF compared to plasma. The ovarian cancer IF proteins were compared to two protein datasets, the proteomes of ascites derived from ovarian cancer patients and ovarian cancer cell lines, and as many as 454 of the ovarian cancer IF proteins were absent in the two datasets. Thus, the EOC IF is highly concentrated with secreted proteins that should facilitate discovery of clinically relevant biomarkers.

Analysis of ovarian cancer IF and NIF identified 58 proteins of interest [42]. Validation by immunohistochemistry identified S100A8 as ovarian cancer biomarker. Six proteins including CEACAM5, FREM2, MUC5AC, TFF3, PYCARD, and WDR1 among several identified in ovarian cancer IF were validated by Western blot, selected reaction monitoring (SRM) and MRM, and WDR1 identified as candidate ovarian cancer biomarker [43].

13.7.7 Uterine Leiomyoma Biomarkers in Interstitial Fluids

2D gel electrophoresis and MS analysis of leiomyoma and normal myometrial IFs uncovered differential levels of seven proteins. Desmin, α-1-antitrypsin, and peroxiredoxin levels were high, while α-actin 1, prelamin-A/C, transgelin, and HSP70 kDa protein 1A/B levels were low in leiomyoma IF compared to NIF. Immunohistochemistry was used to validate desmin and α-1-antitrypsin.

13.7.8 Urinary Bladder Cancer Biomarkers in Interstitial Fluids

A number of urinary bladder cancer biomarkers in urine are clinically available. However, there is continuous pursuit to discover novel urinary bladder cancer biomarkers in TIF that could leak into urine. Thus, 2D PAGE and cytokine arrays have been used to analyze urinary bladder cancer IF [44]. Extracted urinary bladder cancer IF was devoid of intracellular components indicative of lack of contamination from cell lysis. The observed protein profile of urinary bladder cancer IF and matched urinary samples from the same patients were remarkably different in composition, though major serum proteins were identical. It appears that not all urinary bladder cancer IF proteins leak into urine, because Western blot analysis of urine from transitional cell carcinoma patient using antibodies against major TIF proteins revealed that while some proteins including CuZn SOD, cathepsin D, and calreticulin were present in urine, others such as annexin 2, prostaglandin dehydrogenase, α-enolase, 14-3-3σ, protein disulfide isomerase, maspin, triosephosphate isomerase, and HSP27 were not. This same group had previously uncovered 15-prostaglandin dehydrogenase (15-PGDH) expressed by low-grade urinary bladder cancer to be present in tumor microenvironment [45].

13.7.9 Renal Cell Carcinoma Biomarkers in Interstitial Fluids

MS-based proteomic workflow and peptide-centric analysis uncovered differential protein levels between renal cell carcinoma (RCC) IF and IF from matched normal adjacent kidney samples [46]. After depletion of top 14 abundant serum proteins,

138 proteins were identified to demonstrate differential levels between clear cell RCC (ccRCC) IF and matched NIF. The significantly elevated proteins in ccRCC IF include nicotinamide n-methyltransferase (NNMT), thrombospondin-1 (TSP-1), enolase 2 (ENO2) annexin A4, ferritin, CD14, galectin-1, and thyroxine-binding globulin (TBG). Western blot analysis and selected reaction monitoring (SRM) were used to confirm the elevated levels of these proteins in ccRCC IF. ELISA analysis of serum samples uncovered elevated ENO2 and TSP1 in ccRCC patient samples compared to normal controls. Indeed TSP1 levels were 14-fold higher in sera from ccRCC patients than normal controls by both ELISA and SRM analysis.

13.8 Summary

- The structures interposed between cells and vessels form the interstitial space or interstitium.
- The interstitium is composed of the interstitial fluid that contains the structural elements.
- The dynamic range and high-abundant proteins in circulation tend to make biomarker exploration in plasma difficult.
- The secretome is enriched with biomarkers that can be accurately assayed, validated, and leveraged in other body fluids for noninvasive clinical utility.
- TIF can be extracted from resected tissues using elution and centrifugation methods.
- In vivo techniques including catheter insertion and capsule implantation are used in model animal studies.
- Interstitial fluid biomarkers of some tumors have been discovered and validated in blood.

References

1. Gullino PM, Clark SH, Grantham FH. The interstitial fluid of solid tumors. Cancer Res. 1964;24:780–94.
2. Starling EH. On the absorption of fluids from the connective tissue spaces. J Physiol. 1896;19:312–26.
3. Levick JR, Michel CC. Microvascular fluid exchange and the revised Starling principle. Cardiovasc Res. 2010;87:198–210.
4. Wiig H. Evaluation of methodologies for measurement of interstitial fluid pressure (Pi): physiological implications of recent Pi data. Crit Rev Biomed Eng. 1990;18:27–54.
5. Provenzano PP, Cuevas C, Chang AE, et al. Enzymatic targeting of the stroma ablates physical barriers to treatment of pancreatic ductal adenocarcinoma. Cancer Cell. 2012;21:418–29.
6. Sylven B, Bois I. Protein content and enzymatic assays of interstitial fluid from some normal tissues and transplanted mouse tumors. Cancer Res. 1960;20:831–6.
7. Gromov P, Gromova I, Olsen CJ, et al. Tumor interstitial fluid – a treasure trove of cancer biomarkers. Biochim Biophys Acta. 2013;1834:2259–70.

8. Haslene-Hox H, Oveland E, Berg KC, et al. A new method for isolation of interstitial fluid from human solid tumors applied to proteomic analysis of ovarian carcinoma tissue. PLoS One. 2011;6:e19217.
9. Celis JE, Gromov P, Cabezon T, et al. Proteomic characterization of the interstitial fluid perfusing the breast tumor microenvironment: a novel resource for biomarker and therapeutic target discovery. Mol Cell Proteomics. 2004;3:327–44.
10. Teng PN, Rungruang BJ, Hood BL, et al. Assessment of buffer systems for harvesting proteins from tissue interstitial fluid for proteomic analysis. J Proteome Res. 2010;9:4161–9.
11. Huang CM, Ananthaswamy HN, Barnes S, et al. Mass spectrometric proteomics profiles of in vivo tumor secretomes: capillary ultrafiltration sampling of regressive tumor masses. Proteomics. 2006;6:6107–16.
12. Guyton CGH, Taylor A. Interstitial fluid pressure. Physiol Rev. 1971;5:527–63.
13. Duyverman AM, Kohno M, Roberge S, et al. An isolated tumor perfusion model in mice. Nat Protoc. 2012;7:749–55.
14. Jain RK, Shah SA, Finney PL. Continuous noninvasive monitoring of pH and temperature in rat Walker 256 carcinoma during normoglycemia and hyperglycemia. J Natl Cancer Inst. 1984;73:429–36.
15. Baronzio G, Schwartz L, Kiselevsky M, et al. Tumor interstitial fluid as modulator of cancer inflammation, thrombosis, immunity and angiogenesis. Anticancer Res. 2012;32:405–14.
16. Maquart FX, Bellon G, Pasco S, Monboisse JC. Matrikines in the regulation of extracellular matrix degradation. Biochimie. 2005;87:353–60.
17. Brocker C, Thompson DC, Vasiliou V. The role of hyperosmotic stress in inflammation and disease. Biomol Concepts. 2012;3:345–64.
18. Schwartz L, Guais A, Pooya M, Abolhassani M. Is inflammation a consequence of extracellular hyperosmolarity? J Inflamm (London). 2009;6:21.
19. Nemeth ZH, Deitch EA, Szabo C, Hasko G. Hyperosmotic stress induces nuclear factor-kappaB activation and interleukin-8 production in human intestinal epithelial cells. Am J Pathol. 2002;161:987–96.
20. Gupta SC, Kim JH, Kannappan R, et al. Role of nuclear factor kappaB-mediated inflammatory pathways in cancer-related symptoms and their regulation by nutritional agents. Exp Biol Med (Maywood). 2011;236:658–71.
21. Stone MD, Odland RM, McGowan T, et al. Novel in situ collection of tumor interstitial fluid from a head and neck squamous carcinoma reveals a unique proteome with diagnostic potential. Clin Proteomics. 2010;6:75–82.
22. Hardt M, Lam DK, Dolan JC, Schmidt BL. Surveying proteolytic processes in human cancer microenvironments by microdialysis and activity-based mass spectrometry. Proteomics Clin Appl. 2011;5:636–43.
23. Lee LY, Chen YJ, Lu YC, et al. Fascin is a circulating tumor marker for head and neck cancer as determined by a proteomic analysis of interstitial fluid from the tumor microenvironment. Clin Chem Lab Med. 2015;53:1631–41.
24. Li S, Wang R, Zhang M, et al. Proteomic analysis of non-small cell lung cancer tissue interstitial fluids. World J Surg Oncol. 2013;11:173.
25. Mori T, Koga T, Shibata H, et al. Interstitial fluid pressure correlates clinicopathological factors of lung Cancer. Ann Thorac Cardiovasc Surg. 2015;21:201–8.
26. Gromov P, Gromova I, Bunkenborg J, et al. Up-regulated proteins in the fluid bathing the tumour cell microenvironment as potential serological markers for early detection of cancer of the breast. Mol Oncol. 2010;4:65–89.
27. Turtoi A, Dumont B, Greffe Y, et al. Novel comprehensive approach for accessible biomarker identification and absolute quantification from precious human tissues. J Proteome Res. 2011;10:3160–82.
28. Raso C, Cosentino C, Gaspari M, et al. Characterization of breast cancer interstitial fluids by TmT labeling, LTQ-Orbitrap Velos mass spectrometry, and pathway analysis. J Proteome Res. 2012;11:3199–210.

29. Tchafa AM, Ta M, Reginato MJ, Shieh AC. EMT transition alters interstitial fluid flow-induced signaling in ERBB2-positive breast Cancer cells. Mol Cancer Res. 2015;13:755–64.
30. Halvorsen AR, Helland A, Gromov P, et al. Profiling of microRNAs in tumor interstitial fluid of breast tumors – a novel resource to identify biomarkers for prognostic classification and detection of cancer. Mol Oncol. 2017;11:220–34.
31. Sun W, Ma J, Wu S, et al. Characterization of the liver tissue interstitial fluid (TIF) proteome indicates potential for application in liver disease biomarker discovery. J Proteome Res. 2010;9:1020–31.
32. Hsieh SY, He JR, Yu MC, et al. Secreted ERBB3 isoforms are serum markers for early hepatoma in patients with chronic hepatitis and cirrhosis. J Proteome Res. 2011;10:4715–24.
33. Sun W, Xing B, Guo L, et al. Quantitative proteomics analysis of tissue interstitial fluid for identification of novel serum candidate diagnostic marker for hepatocellular carcinoma. Sci Rep. 2016;6:26499.
34. Zhang J, Hao N, Liu W, et al. In-depth proteomic analysis of tissue interstitial fluid for hepatocellular carcinoma serum biomarker discovery. Br J Cancer. 2017;117:1676–84.
35. Shi HJ, Stubbs R, Hood K. Characterization of de novo synthesized proteins released from human colorectal tumour explants. Electrophoresis. 2009;30:2442–53.
36. Fijneman RJ, de Wit M, Pourghiasian M, et al. Proximal fluid proteome profiling of mouse colon tumors reveals biomarkers for early diagnosis of human colorectal cancer. Clin Cancer Res. 2012;18:2613–24.
37. Schmaus A, Klusmeier S, Rothley M, et al. Accumulation of small hyaluronan oligosaccharides in tumour interstitial fluid correlates with lymphatic invasion and lymph node metastasis. Br J Cancer. 2014;111:559–67.
38. Wang Y, Shan Q, Hou G, et al. Discovery of potential colorectal cancer serum biomarkers through quantitative proteomics on the colonic tissue interstitial fluids from the AOM-DSS mouse model. J Proteome. 2016;132:31–40.
39. Xie Y, Chen L, Lv X, et al. The levels of serine proteases in colon tissue interstitial fluid and serum serve as an indicator of colorectal cancer progression. Oncotarget. 2016;7:32592–606.
40. Wang TH, Chao A, Tsai CL, et al. Stress-induced phosphoprotein 1 as a secreted biomarker for human ovarian cancer promotes cancer cell proliferation. Mol Cell Proteomics. 2010;9:1873–84.
41. Hoskins ER, Hood BL, Sun M, et al. Proteomic analysis of ovarian cancer proximal fluids: validation of elevated peroxiredoxin 1 in patient peripheral circulation. PLoS One. 2011;6:e25056.
42. Cortesi L, Rossi E, Della Casa L, et al. Protein expression patterns associated with advanced stage ovarian cancer. Electrophoresis. 2011;32:1992–2003.
43. Haslene-Hox H, Oveland E, Woie K, et al. Increased WD-repeat containing protein 1 in interstitial fluid from ovarian carcinomas shown by comparative proteomic analysis of malignant and healthy gynecological tissue. Biochim Biophys Acta. 2013;1834:2347–59.
44. Celis JE, Gromova I, Moreira JM, et al. Impact of proteomics on bladder cancer research. Pharmacogenomics. 2004;5:381–94.
45. Celis JE, Ostergaard M, Basse B, et al. Loss of adipocyte-type fatty acid binding protein and other protein biomarkers is associated with progression of human bladder transitional cell carcinomas. Cancer Res. 1996;56:4782–90.
46. Teng PN, Hood BL, Sun M, et al. Differential proteomic analysis of renal cell carcinoma tissue interstitial fluid. J Proteome Res. 2011;10:1333–42.

Chapter 14
Body Fluid Microbiome as Cancer Biomarkers

14.1 Introduction

While composed of 10 times more cells than the human body, 1000 more genes than in the human genome, and forms 1–3% of the human body mass, the importance of this neglected "organ" of the human body composition is being realized. That a single gene or multiple gene alterations cause cancer is well established. Moreover, though they faced some difficulties before acceptance, some tissue-specific microbial infections such as *Helicobacter pylori* and human papilloma virus (HPV) are etiologic agents of cancer. This Koch's postulate-based infectious causes of cancer are well established, and advances are made in disease prevention and management. But that global microbial alterations, for example, changes in gut microbial population diversity or density, could cause distant cancers such as those of the breast or prostate came as a surprise. Established also is that many cancers are not caused by simple single gene mutations but rather a complex interplay of gene-environment interaction. Again, many environmental etiologic influences on cancer such as occupational and lifestyle exposures, specific infectious agents, as well as lifestyle and genetic causes of increased body mass index are well affirmed. However, the influence of a component of the environment that resides within and on us, our "ancillary organ," the microbiome has before now been forgotten.

Thanks to technological developments, next-generation sequencing, and advanced computational and bioinformatic efforts, the entire human microbial community of bacteria, archaea, fungi, protists, and viruses has been deciphered. Disturbances in this community that impinge on signaling pathways such as those involved in nutrition, metabolism, hormonal changes, metabolite detoxification, as well as immune functions and inflammation contribute to carcinogenesis. The interaction of altered microbiome, metabolism, inflammation, and tumor microenvironment in cancer initiation and sustenance requires illumination. Current efforts at unraveling the effects of taxonomic alterations of the microbiome on human health and disease have been championed by the NIH-funded Human Microbiome Project

G. D. Dakubo, *Cancer Biomarkers in Body Fluids*,
https://doi.org/10.1007/978-3-030-24725-6_14

(HMP) and the European Metagenomics of the Human Intestinal Tract (MetaHIT) projects. The emerging mechanistic roles of altered human microbiome or microbial dysbiosis in cancer are the subject of this chapter.

14.2 The Human Microbiome

The entirety of microorganisms or microbiota including archaea, bacteria, viruses, and eukaryotes (yeast and fungi) and their collective genomes constitute the human microbiome. This microbiota, which is greater than 10^{14} per body, is about tenfold greater than the cellular composition of the human body. The microbiome community exists in symbiotic or commensal relationship with the host. They are involved in the breakdown of food (e.g., carbohydrates), synthesis of vitamin, immune competency, and production of anti-inflammatory substances. These microbes occupy various anatomic niches including the skin, eyes, ears, nose, upper aerodigestive tract, gastrointestinal tract, and urogenital tract. Bacterial species differences occur at these anatomic locations. For example, there are approximately 1000, 400, and 120 species in the gastrointestinal tract, oral cavity, and skin, respectively. Metagenomic characterization of the microbiome indicates variable composition at these anatomic sites, with the vast majority (>90%) being luminal bacteria of the gastrointestinal tract.

These microbes are conserved at the higher taxonomic level but show great diversity or variation at the genus and species levels among individuals. Both genetics and environmental factors influence the composition of microbes of an individual. Thus, the host microbiota varies in response to numerous factors including diet, household environment, medication use, and stress level, as well as over their lifespan. Additionally, genome-wide association study (GWAS) of mouse cell line identified a number of quantitative trait loci associated with the relative abundance of specific microbial taxa, suggesting individual quantitative trait loci (QTLs) influence their microbial composition.

14.3 The Human Microbiome Projects

In order to achieve a comprehensive understanding of the role of the human microbiome in health and disease, the Human Microbiome Project (HMP) and Metagenomics of the Human Intestinal Tract (MetaHIT) project were established with specific goals.

In 2008, the HMP was established with the primary mission of gathering resources to enable comprehensive characterization of the human microbiota. This interdisciplinary effort, funded by the NIH common fund, involves several investigators and sequencing centers such as the J. Craig Venter Institute, the Broad Institute, the Baylor College of Medicine, Washington University, and Data Analysis and Coordinating Center (DACC). The specific aim was to attempt to unravel the role of the microbiome on human health and disease. This ambition was based on metagenomics technologies that obviate the need for cell culture to characterize individual organisms. The metagenomics approach also enabled sampling and analysis of microbes from their natural physiologic states. Thus, characterization of the diverse microbes in their specific communities on and in the human body should uncover the norm and how deviations impact human health and disease. The HMP has currently characterized microbes in different parts of the human body including the skin, nasal passages, oral cavity, gastrointestinal tract, and urogenital tract with five specific aims:

- To develop a reference set of 3000 isolated microbial genome sequences
- To use 16S rRNA and whole genome sequencing metagenomics to estimate the complexity of the microbial community at each of the selected body site and to address the question of whether there is a "core" microbiome at each site
- To demonstrate the connection between changes in the human microbiome and disease
- To develop new tools and technologies for computational analysis of the genomes, through establishment of Data Analysis and Coordinating Center (DACC), as well as resource repositories
- To examine the ethical, legal, and social implications (ELSI) needed to be considered in the study and use of metagenomic analysis of the human microbiome

Funded by the European Commission, MetaHIT is a project aimed at establishing associations between genes of the human gastrointestinal tract microbiota with health and disease. The consortium includes industry and academic partners from eight European countries and is charged with the responsibility of finding the influence of the gut microbiota and two diseases, irritable bowel syndrome (IBS), and obesity, which are plaguing Europe and the rest of the world. The primary objective will be achieved through completion of the following specific aims:

- To establish an extensive reference catalog of human intestinal microbial genes
- To develop bioinformatics tools to store, organize, and interpret the information generated
- To develop tools for determining which genes within the reference catalog are present in different individuals and their frequencies
- To determine the most prevalent genes in sick and healthy individuals
- To develop methods for studying the functions of bacteria genes associated with specific diseases and to unravel mechanisms of host-microbe interaction

Recognized by the consortium is the need to integrate their findings with those of the global society. To achieve this, the consortium participates in the activities of the International Human Microbiome Consortium (IHMC), transfers technology to industry, and shares project information with the general public. This project has identified 3.3 million different genes among a cohort of people, which is 150-fold higher than in the human genome. Of note, 99% were bacterial genes, which translated into at least 1000 bacterial species in the human gut. Further analysis indicated each individual carries on average 540,000 microbial genes that correspond to 160 species.

14.4 Host Interactions with the Microbiome

Under normal physiologic conditions, the microbiome interacts with the host at three different levels to offset the occurrence of disease. These levels are immune tolerance, barrier defenses, and eubiosis. The microbiome and host have evolved over millions of years to coexist in peaceful relationships that often do not cause disease. These relationships include mutualism, parasitism, and commensalism. Some microbes establish a beneficial and/or nonpathogenic relationship with the host that enables them to carve permanent microenvironmental niches without triggering the immune system. Pathogenic microbes, however, are immunologically removed. A dynamic interplay between the host and microbiome facilitates and maintains this symbiotic ecosystem. An imbalance that involves changes in the relative abundance/richness of many commensal microbes (dysbiosis) is linked to several diseases, including cancer. The microbiota of healthy individuals demonstrates considerable taxonomic variation, albeit with little at the metagenomic level. Infection, inflammation, innate immunity, diet, drugs, and several other factors can alter this taxonomic composition and numbers or amounts. Such perturbations have been associated with cancer in animal models and human correlative studies.

14.5 The Human Microbiome and Cancer

Epidemiologic evidence implicates the human microbiome in cancer development. Several cross-sectional and some case-control studies, albeit mostly of small sample sizes, provide evidence for the association of the microbiome with cancer. While these have mostly been discovery studies, plans to execute prospective studies inclusive of all microbes (fungi, protists, viruses, archaea, bacteria) using different molecular targets and approaches (genome, transcriptome, proteome, metabolome) should augment our understanding of the microbiome in cancer. Such well-executed studies that will confirm the involvement of the microbiome in cancer should usher in another major breakthrough in the fight to conquer cancer at multiple levels (i.e., from prevention to therapy).

14.5.1 Gastric Cancer

Strong epidemiological evidence implicates *H. pylori* infection with >twofold increased risk of gastric carcinoma. *H. pylori* infection causes gastric mucosal inflammation leading to achlorhydria, epithelial atrophy, and eventual dysplasia that progresses to cancer. Additionally, the majority (>90%) of low-grade gastric mucosal-associated lymphoid tissue (MALT) lymphomas are caused by *H. pylori* infection. Because these lymphomas are associated with B-cell chromosomal translocations, it has been mechanistically postulated to be mediated either by the effects of *H. pylori* CagA protein or aberrant inflammation-associated increased B-cell proliferation. Of interest, *H. pylori* eradication leads to regression of these lymphomas. Curiously, however, the few gastric lymphomas not caused by *H. pylori* infections also regress with antibiotic treatment, which suggest a role for other bacteria. Bacterial community dynamics as etiologic factor of gastric cancer has been suggested. Eun et al. used pyrosequencing to provide evidence of gastric microbiome in cancer [1]. In patients with gastric mucosal lesions of increasing severity from gastritis, intestinal mucosal metaplasia, to non-cardia gastric cancer, the diversity of gastric microbiome (specifically the number of different taxa or α-diversity) increased with disease severity [2].

14.5.2 Esophageal Cancer

The achlorhydria associated with *H. pylori* gastritis and gastric atrophy reduces the risk of esophageal adenocarcinoma. However, implicating the salivary microbiome in esophageal cancer development is the finding of the association of tooth loss with a number of cancers including esophageal cancer [3]. Studies of esophageal squamous cell carcinoma (ESCC) microbiome suggest changes in both α- and β-diversities confer increased risk of developing esophageal cancer. Upper GIT fluid (gastric, esophageal, and oral) samples from people with and without esophageal squamous dysplasia (EsSD) were subjected to chip array (HOMIM) analysis of the microbiota. The increase in the number of individual microbial genera (α-diversity) predicted the odds of developing EsSD (the odds were 0–74 per standard deviation increase in α-diversity). Additionally, altered bacterial composition (β-diversity) was associated with EsSD [4]. In another study of gastric corpus tissue microbiota from patients with EsSD and ESCC compared to age/sex-matched healthy controls, no significant difference was detected in α-diversity between groups. However, interindividual bacterial composition or β-diversity models revealed significant differences between matched cases and controls [5].

14.5.3 Lung Cancer

Changes in the oral microbiome, as evidenced in periodontal diseases, are associated with lung cancer risk [3]. Moreover, lung infection increases the risk of lung cancer. A meta-analytical study of tuberculous and non-tuberculous lung infections revealed an infection-associated elevated risk for lung cancer. The pooled RR of tuberculous and non-tuberculous infections and development of lung cancer were 1.76 and 1.43, respectively [6]. A pilot investigation of the microbiome and lung cancer examined 16SrRNA sequences in oral washes and sputum from female patients and matched controls [7]. While community diversity in oral fluids washes did not differ between the groups, it was lower in sputum from lung cancer patients.

However, lung cancer patients had relatively decreased levels of Spirochete (oral washes and sputum), Bacteroidetes (oral washes), and Synergistetes (sputum) associated with increases in *Firmicutes* (oral washes).

14.5.4 Hepatobiliary Cancer

Infectious causes of hepatobiliary cancers have been demonstrated. *H. pylori* infections may contribute to HCC and cholangiocarcinoma. Indeed, a significant increase in biliary tract cancer (OR = 5.47) was associated with *H. pylori* infection in a Finish prospective analysis of serum anti-*H. pylori* antibodies [8]. While association was observed for HCC (OR = 1.20), it failed to reach significance. Several other studies implicate the risk of biliary tract and gallbladder cancers with *Helicobacter* spp. and *Salmonella typhi*, respectively. A meta-analysis of 10 studies of *Helicobacter* spp. and biliary tract cancer found a pooled OR of 3.20 [9]. The pooled risk ratio/RR was 4.28 for gallbladder cancer in people infected with *S. typhi.*

14.5.5 Pancreatic Cancer

The risk of pancreatic cancer is elevated in patients with periodontal disease and tooth loss [3], and this may be associated with alterations in oral microbiome. Changes in oral microbial communities are directly or indirectly implicated with pancreatic cancer. A seroepidemiological study used immunoblot array targeting antibodies from 25 oral bacteria strains [10]. This was a well-designed study with matched cases (n = 405) to controls (n = 416) for sex, age, date, and time of blood draw fasting status and whether or not women were on hormonal therapy. High antibody levels of nonpathogenic commensal oral bacteria were protective against pancreatic cancer with an OR of 0.55. However, a subset of cases (6%) with antibody titer >200 ng/ml, a periodontal microbe, and *Porphyromonas gingivalis* had elevated risk of 2.14 times for pancreatic cancer compared to people with lower levels. A pilot study compared a possible direct link between oral microbiome and pancreatic cancer using the HOMIM array [11]. Of the 410 bacteria taxa, 16 were significantly associated with pancreatic cancer, of which 6 were confirmed by PCR. An attempt to validate this study in an independent sample sets uncovered *Streptococcus mitis* and *Neisseria elongata* as risk agents of pancreatic cancer.

14.5.6 Colorectal Cancer

Being the embodiment of most microbes in the human body, several studies have explored the role of gut microbiome in cancer. Expectedly, consistent findings have not yet being achieved, which may partly be due to lack of knowledge on factors that control microbial community diversity and how changes in α- and β-diversities cause cancer. Studies of precursor lesions found no significant differences in fecal community diversity between patients with colorectal adenomas and healthy controls. Microbial compositional differences have however been uncovered in some studies. Fusobacterium and Porphyromonas/daceae increased risk for adenomas, while both organisms and *Ruminococcus* increased colorectal cancer risk.

14.5.7 Breast Cancer

The gut microbiome is implicated in breast cancer. In a case-control study of postmenopausal women, both changes in microbial composition and low community diversity were associated with breast cancer. Mechanistically, this risk was attributed to enterohepatic estrogen circulation by gut microbiome and possibly to inflammatory mediators or microbial metabolites [12].

14.5.8 Hematologic Malignancy

As sites of immune reactions, lymphoid tissues are exposed to a vast array of microbial components. It has been hypothesized that the microbiome may at least influence lymphoid neoplastic transformation. A pilot study compared fecal microbiome between twins with adolescent/young adult Hodgkin lymphomas to their unaffected co-twins [13]. Community diversity was significantly lower in the cases than controls, offering support to the possible risk of association of clean environment with this affliction, although other confounding variables such as treatment or "cause vs. effect" cannot be ruled out. Additionally, non-gastrointestinal MALT lymphomas have been associated with *Chlamydophila psittaci* (sequences were amplified from lesions) [14]. Seropositivity to causative agents of Lyme disease, *Borrelia burgdorferi*, has been associated with cutaneous B-cell non-Hodgkin lymphoma in one of two studies [15, 16].

14.6 Microbiome and Human Diseases

Partly because of their numerous useful functions, perturbations in the human microbiome are associated with various diseases. Several diseases, including type 2 diabetes, Crohn's disease, and chronic allergies, demonstrate microbial differences between cases and controls. Microbial involvement in human diseases fall under two main categories: (i) pathogenicity of single microbes and (ii) microbial imbalances, i.e., changes in the relative abundances in a community or dysbiosis.

Single microbes including *H. pylori*, HPV, and EBV are associated with specific cancer with defined mechanisms (Table 14.1). These mechanisms include alteration of signaling pathways as well as nonspecific inflammation-associated dysplasia. Recently, much attention has been attracted to the global changes in the microbiome and human diseases. By mass, about 99% of the human microbiome resides in the gastrointestinal tract. These microbes are involved in local and long-distance interactions with the host.

Under physiologic conditions, the microbiome interacts with the host at three levels to offset disease occurrence: immune tolerance, barrier defenses, and eubiosis. Barrier defenses between body fluid microbiome and the internal milieu of the host occur at multiple levels. These include both host and microbial functions. The host defenses include epithelial and mucus layers and their modifications (e.g., stratum corneum), production of antibacterial peptides (e.g., defensins and IgA) by cells such as keratinocytes, Paneth and goblet cells, pH alterations (e.g., low gastric pH),

Table 14.1 Infectious agents that cause cancer

Infectious agents	Associated cancers
Viruses	
HPV	Cervical cancer, head and neck cancer
	Also vulva, vaginal, penile, and anal cancers
HBV	Liver cancer
EBV	Nasopharyngeal cancer, lymphomas (Burkitt lymphoma, Hodgkin lymphoma)
HIV	Kaposi's sarcoma, cervical cancer, non-Hodgkin lymphoma
HHV8	Kaposi's sarcoma
HTLV1	Adult T-cell leukemia/lymphoma (ATL)
MCV	Merkel cell carcinoma of the skin
Bacteria	
Helicobacter pylori	Gastric cancer, gastric lymphoma
Chlamydia trachomatis	Cervical cancer
Parasites	
Schistosoma haematobium	Urothelial bladder cancer
Opisthorchis viverrini, Clonorchis sinensis	Cholangiocarcinoma

HPV human papillomavirus; *HBV* hepatitis B virus; *EBV* Epstein-Barr virus; *HIV* human immunodeficiency virus; *HHV8* human herpes virus 8; *HTLV1* human T-lymphotropic virus 1; *MCV* molluscum contagiosum virus as well as functions of cells such as dendritic cells, γδT cells, and MALTs. Luminal microbes similarly function to prevent overgrowth of pathogenic organisms. Mechanistically, these involve production of substances such as bacteriocins and mucins, as well as metabolic deprivation and stimulation of epithelial turnover. Barrier failure due to inflammation, trauma, injury, or altered expression of component biomolecules can contribute to microbiome-mediated carcinogenesis. However, this interrelationship may be complex, because while inflammation from infection could cause barrier failure, cancer from noninfectious etiology could also lead to barrier failure. Examples of the relationship between barrier failure, inflammation, and microbiome are

- Mutations in genes involved in inflammasome and human diseases
- Antibiotic suppression of gut microbiome and overgrowth of pathogenic *Clostridium difficile* that causes disease (severe colitis)
- Mutations in barrier proteins (e.g., laminin) associated with ulcerative colitis.
- *H. pylori* infection perturbs barrier functions through inflammation, altered gastric pH, and hence microbiome.
- Spontaneous development of colorectal cancer in muc2$^{-/-}$ mice that lack predominant gastrointestinal mucin.

While not completely clarified, there are putative mechanistic explanations for microbial dysbiosis, which include the following.

- The importance of immune and inflammatory responses in causing dysbiosis has been demonstrated in Nod2$^{-/-}$, IL-10$^{-/-}$, Asc$^{-/-}$, and Nlrp6$^{-/-}$ mice [17–20].
- Inflammation-mediated bacterial stress-response gene expression could enhance bacterial fitness, survival, and adaptability. Patwa et al. provided evidence using IL-10$^{-/-}$ mouse model with intestinal inflammation [21]. *Escherichia coli* from these mice demonstrated increased heat shock protein (IbpA, IbpB) expression, which protected them from oxidative stress.
- Inflammation-mediated production of specific metabolites may selectively enhance specific microbial growth. For example, nitrate production (due to inflammation) could favor overgrowth of facultative anaerobes (*Enterobacteriaceae*) in a community dominated by obligate anaerobes because of inefficient electron transport chain activity to metabolize nitrate [22].
- "Keystone pathogens" or "alpha-bugs" could exert dominant effects on bacterial community composition leading to dysbiosis.

14.7 Microbiome Dysbiosis and Carcinogenesis

The role of dysbiosis in cancer has been extensively studied in colorectal cancer (CRC). Other cancers such as esophageal, pancreatic, gallbladder, liver, and colorectal cancer have also been interrogated as cancer caused by dysbiosis (Table 14.2). Several correlative studies associate intestinal luminal fluid bacterial

Table 14.2 Changes in microbiome in cancer compared to controls

Cancer	Body fluid	Microbes
Head and neck	Saliva	Increased levels of *Capnocytophaga gingivalis, C. ochracea, Eubacterium sabureum, Leptotrichia buccalis, Streptococcus mitis*
Barrett's esophagus, esophageal	Saliva	Increased levels of *Campylobacter concisus, C. rectus, Treponema denticola, S. anginosus, S. mitis*
		Decreased levels of *Helicobacter pylori*
Pancreatic	Saliva	Increases levels of *S. mitis* and *Neisseria elongata*
Gallbladder	Bile	Increased levels of *Salmonella typhi, S. paratyphi*
Colorectal	Stool	Increased levels of *S. bovis, Streptococcus* spp., *Escherichia coli, Fusobacterium nucleatum, Clostridium, Bacteroides*
		Decreased levels of *Lactobacillus, Roseburia, Faecalibacterium, Microbacterium, Anoxybacillus, Akkermansia muciniphila*

dysbiosis as etiologic factor of CRC [23–25]. Of the numerous pathogens, *Fusobacterium* spp., which are more enriched in gut microbiome of Crohn's disease patients than healthy individuals, have been identified as causative agent of CRC. Specifically, clinical isolates of *F. nucleatum* promoted CRC development in $APC^{min/+}$ mice [26]. Mechanistically, *F. nucleatum* protein, FadA, interacts with E-cadherin (CDH1) to activate Wnt/β-catenin signaling that plays important role in colorectal carcinogenesis [27]. Further analysis indicated FadA levels were significantly elevated in colorectal cancer tissue samples.

The sufficiency of dysbiosis in cancer promotion has been demonstrated using $Il10^{-/-}$, $Nlrp6^{-/-}$, $Asc^{-/-}$, and $Nod2^{-/-}$ mice models [17, 18]. All these transgenic mice developed dysbiosis-associated cancers. NLRP6 is part of the inflammasome involved in inducing acute inflammation. $Nlr6^{-/-}$ mice develop dysbiosis-associated colitis that contribute to the development of colorectal cancer as a consequence of decreased inflammasome activation and IL-18 production. Consistently, $Asc^{-/-}$ and $Il18^{-/-}$ mice also have increased tendency to develop colorectal cancer. Of interest, the colitis and colorectal cancer developed by these mice could be transmitted to wild-type mice via c0-housing. IL-6 receptor is a component of the mechanism that mediated colorectal cancer development in these mice. First, *Il6r* ablation is associated with reduced colorectal cancer development. Second, in $Nod2^{-/-}$ and $Nlrp6^{-/-}$ mice, treatment with neutralizing IL-6 receptor antibodies reduced colorectal cancer development.

The associated elevated risk of cancer in obese people may partly be accounted for by dysbiosis. Human and mouse model studies suggest increased gut microbial dysbiosis in obese people, often enriched for *Firmicutes* in association with diminished *Bacteroidetes*. Additional observations in obesity are altered metabolism in association with reduced microbial richness. Possible linkage of obesity-associated dysbiosis and abnormal metabolism to carcinogenesis is provided by the following: (i) dietary fat promoted colitis in IL-$10^{-/-}$ mice as a consequence of its induction of increased taurocholic acid production that enhances *Bilophila wadsworthia* levels in the gut, and (ii) obesity-associated increases in *Clostridia* causes increase production of the secondary bile acid, deoxycholic acid (DCA), that promotes hepatocarcinogenesis. DCA, produced by bacterial 7 α-dehydroxylation, has also promoted colon and esophageal cancer development.

14.8 Gnotobiotic Mice

There are established evidences of microbiome alterations in cancer. However, whether these observations implicate microbial compositional changes as etiologic agents or consequence of the carcinogenic process requires clarification. To help resolve this dilemma, investigators have resorted to controlled studies using gnotobiotic mice.

Gnotobiotic (gnotos, Greek for "known") mice are either germ-free animals or those with defined microbial species. These animals are generated via aseptic cesarean section delivery in an isolated chamber and raised in a separate isolator on sterile water and food supplemented with vitamins. Germ-free animals have distinctive features indicative of bioenergetic (malnutrition) and immune (poor immune system) aberrations. They appear leaner than conventional microbe-associated siblings, although they eat more food and have low levels of insulin and glycogen, are hypoglycemic, and resistant to obesity.

Germ-free mice with specific gene knockouts can be used to uncover the interaction of the specific genes with microbes in disease evolution. Germ-free mice inoculated with known microbes (gnotobiotic mice) can also be established to study the effects of these organisms on health. These microbes could be a community of a single microbe (mono-associated mice), a few different microbes (poly-associated mice), or microbes from known human diseases (humanized mice). The designed experiments enable the effects of microbial composition on disease to be uncovered. Moreover, functional associations could be made for specific microbes and their genes or gene products. Such manipulations have enabled the study of the role of microbiota in immunoregulation in cancer. For example, germ-free background *TGFβ1*$^{-/-}$ mice prevented the development of colorectal inflammation and cancer observed in normal littermates [28]. IL-10$^{-/-}$ mice developed colitis, which could be abrogated when raised as germ-free mice [29]. These findings are suggestive of germ-free mice having reduced pro-tumorigenic Th17 cytokine profile (IL-17, IL-22, and IL-23) in the gut [30, 31].

Evidence of microbial interaction with human genetics in disease modulation has also been made possible using mouse models. Single nucleotide polymorphism in Declin-1 gene is associated with severe ulcerative colitis. Corroborative evidence has been provided, whereby declin-1$^{-/-}$ mice were very sensitive to dextran sulfate-induced colitis mediated by changes in gut fungi [32].

14.9 Microbiome and Innate Immunity in Cancer

The microbiome, through activation of pattern recognition receptors (PRRs) that include toll-like receptors (TLRs) and nod-like receptors (NLRs) of the innate immune system, can modulate chemotherapy and immunotherapy responses to cancer. Ample evidence, however, implicates PRR interaction with bacterial components (PAMP or MAMP) in tumorigenesis.

Genetic and pharmacologic manipulations of TLRs, as well as TLR-myeloid differentiation primary response 88 (MYD88) and TLR-IL-17/23 procarcinogenic mice, have been used to demonstrate the innate immune-microbiome interaction in cancer. TLR2, which interacts with bacterial peptidoglycan and lipotechoic acid, promoted gastric cancer growth [33]. *TLR4*$^{-/-}$ mice had reduced tumor formation, while mice constitutively expressing activated epithelial TLR4 had increased tumor load. The tumors modulated by TLR4 signaling are skin, colon, liver, and pancreatic cancers [34–38]. TLRs activate the NF-κB and STAT3 pathways to promote cancer cell survival. Indeed, a point mutation in MYD88 is associated with some lymphomas with activated NF-κB and STAT3 signaling [39]. Activation of TLRs on fibroblast caused secretion of mitogens including hepatocyte growth factor (HGF), amphiregulin and epiregulin, which promoted HCC and colorectal cancer cell proliferation [34, 40, 41]. Additionally, activation of TLRs on myeloid cells by MAMP-induced expression of IL-17 and IL-23 promoted carcinogenesis. These effects were reversed by genetic inactivation of *Tlr2*, *Tlr4*, *Tlr9*, and *Myd88*, as well as microbiome removal by antibiotic treatment. Similarly, blocking IL-17 and IL-23 signaling via pharmacologic or genetic means reduced tumor formation [42].

Substantial evidence also implicates activated NLRs by the microbiome in cancer. Demonstrated are the effects of NOD1, NOD2, and NLRP6, while NLRP3, NLRP12, and NLRC4 although implicated require further mechanistic clarification. Irritable bowel disease is characterized by variants of NOD1, which has a role in intestinal defense against microbes [43]. Consistently, NOD1 deficiency led to intestinal barrier failure and inflammation [44]. Loss of NOD2 is associated with Crohn's disease [45], and inactivating polymorphisms in NOD2 enhanced colorectal carcinogenesis [46]. Indeed, loss of NOD2 caused intestinal dysbiosis and increased susceptibility to colorectal cancer [17, 47, 48]. *NOD2*$^{-/-}$ mice demonstrate increase susceptibility to bacterial infections and inefficient commensal bacterial killing by colonic crypts [47, 49]. The cancer predisposition by *NOD2*$^{-/-}$ mice could be transferred to wild-type mice through cohousing, suggesting that dysbiosis underlay the cancer propensity [17].

14.10 Carcinogenic Mechanisms of the Microbiome

The mechanisms of microbial carcinogenesis have been affirmed for single microbial causes of cancer. Metagenomic studies, however, reveal complex relationships between the microbiome and cancer, suggestive of combined or aggregate effects.

Dysbiosis, inflammation, and disturbed barrier functions are predisposing events in microbial carcinogenesis. Changes in the microbiome can cause alterations in several biologic processes to initiate cancer development. Mechanistically, cellular transformation could result from DNA damage (genotoxicity), cytokine and chemokine signaling, bacterial metabolism, and virulent microbial factors.

14.10.1 Genotoxicity

The microbiome can mediate DNA damage leading to genomic instability and cancer predisposition in several ways. Microbial-mediated inflammation-associated increased ROS production can cause oxidative stress and genotoxicity. Some microbes, such as *Enterococcus faecalis*, can produce large quantities of extracellular superoxide to cause DNA damage [50, 51] that could progress to CRC in *Il10*$^{-/-}$ mice. The tumorigenic effect was abrogated when the *Il10*$^{-/-}$ mice were infected with mutant *E. faecalis* (Δmem B strain) [52, 53]. Other bacteria including *δ-Proteobacteria* and *Fusobacteria* produce genotoxic hydrogen sulfite, and *Fusobacteria* have been associated with colorectal cancer [26].

Bacterial-specific toxins can also induce DNA damage responses. Toxins, including cytolethal distending toxin (CDT), colibactin, *B. fragilis* toxin, and cytotoxic necrotizing factor 1, are involved in cellular responses such as DNA damage response in cancer [20, 54–57]. However, the established genotoxins are colibactin and CDT because they cause direct DNA damage responses and genomic instability [56, 57]. Colibactin and CDT could induce G2/M phase cycle arrest associated with cell swelling through activation of ATM-CHK2 signaling and phosphorylation of histone H2AX.

Colibactin contains a genotoxicity island composed of 54 kb polyketide synthase (*pks*). *Enterobacteriaceae* family, including *E. coli*, mostly produces colibactin. *E. coli* colibactin is linked to colorectal cancer. In colorectal cancer patients, pks-containing *E. coli* was more prevalent in mucosa of patients than controls. Moreover, *E. coli NC101 pks* was associated with *CRC* development in gnotobiotic *Il10*$^{-/-}$ mice [20, 58]. Other *pks*-containing bacteria are *Klebsiella pneumonia* and *Proteus mirabilis*. Both organisms could induce colitis in *Tbet*$^{-/-}$*; Rag2*$^{-/-}$ mice [59]. Pks induces dsDNA breaks, DNA damage response, cycle arrest, and genomic instability [20, 57]. Consequently, cells infected with *E. coli pks*-defective isogenic mutants harbored less genomic damage than those with pks + strains [60].

Gram-negative bacteria such as *E. coli, Helicobacter*, and *S. typhi* produce CDT, which is associated with gastric, gallbladder, and colorectal cancers. CDT has three components: CdtA, CdtB, and CdtC. CdtB is the active component with DNase activity that directly causes DNA damage. CdtA and CdtC enable bacterial attachment to host cell to facilitate delivery of CdtB into the cytoplasm, from where it enters the nucleus to mediate its activities. The active sites of CdtB are highly homologous to those of mammalian DNase I. CdtB mutant strains of *Helicobacter cinaedi* and *C. jejuni* could not induce dysplasia in *Il10*$^{-/-}$ mice and also failed to induce intestinal hyperplasia in mice lacking p50 (Nfkb1) subunit and one allele of p65 (Rela) subunit of NF-κB [61, 62].

14.10.2 Microbial Metabolism

Bacteria metabolize a much more diverse substrates than humans. With over 115 and 21 families of glycoside hydrolases and polysaccharide lyases, respectively, the genome of gut microbiome is much more enriched with carbohydrate-metabolizing enzyme genes than humans. Symbiotic gut microbes thus digest glycans into disaccharides and monosaccharides for absorption by host. Additionally, bacteria contain enzymes for the biosynthesis of vitamins and isoprenoids, as well as metabolism of xenobiotics, nutrients, and bile acids. The interaction between diet and microbial metabolism could result in carcinogenic products. Moreover, risky lifestyles including unhealthy eating, alcohol consumption, tobacco smoking, and obesity are associated with dysbiosis-related carcinogenesis.

Consumption of high-fiber (plant composition) diets may be associated with the production of cancer-protective metabolites. Microbial fermentation of carbohydrates/fiber, for instance, produces short-chain fatty acids such as butyrate that was protective against colon and liver cancer [63–66]. Butyrate is abundant in the colon and is the preferred substrate used to generate about 70% of colonocyte energy. The anticarcinogenic effect of butyrate is also supported by the low abundance of butyrate producing bacteria in colorectal cancer compared to healthy controls. Butyrate, however, has contradictory effects on normal and transformed colonocytes that is referred to as the "butyrate paradox." It decreases colorectal cancer growth through increased apoptosis and reduced proliferation, while it promotes normal colonocyte growth. The effects of butyrate on colorectal cancer cells are due to the Warburg effect of aerobic glycolysis. The Warburg effect, which correlates with increased GLUT expression, leads to increased intake and metabolism of glucose. Butyrate, which is less metabolized, therefore accumulates in the cancer cells and enters the nucleus to inhibit histone deacetylase. This epigenetic regulation impinges on cell cycle and apoptotic genes to decrease colorectal cancer growth.

Phytochemicals including polyphenols derived from plants protect against cancer. Gut microbiome modulates the local and systemic levels of phytochemicals, which has important implications in local/gut and distant tissue cancers. The microbiome also modulates the activity of a class of phytoestrogens called lignans to protect against cancer. In contrast to carbohydrates, bacterial metabolism of proteins could produce potentially toxic intermediates such as amines, natrosamines, sulfides, and phenols, which promote carcinogenesis.

Gut bacteria are involved in the metabolism of bile acids. The secondary bile, deoxycholic acid (DCA) is only produced using bacterial 7-α-dehyroxylase enzyme. DCA is a carcinogen because it causes production of DNA-damaging ROS. Levels of DCA are increased in animals fed on high-fat diets. DCA supplementation of animals on high-fat diet led to the development of HCC, which could be prevented by destroying DCA-producing bacteria with antibiotics [67]. DCA is also implicated in esophageal and colon cancers.

Bacterial control of alcohol metabolism plays important role in alcohol-related cancers including cancers of the oropharynx, esophagus, colorectum, liver, and breast. Bacterial metabolism of alcohol produces acetaldehyde, which mediates the genotoxic and cancer-promoting effects of alcohol. Of interest, germ-free rats harbored significantly lower levels of acetaldehyde than controls [68]. Xenobiotic and hormone metabolism by bacteria have also been implicated in drug-related complications and hormone-related carcinogenesis, respectively.

14.10.3 Virulent Microbiome Factors

Microbial virulent factors are important mediators of their pathogenicity. Some of these virulent factors also appear to alter cellular carcinogenic signaling pathways. For example, transgenic mice expressing *H. pylori* cytotoxin-associated gene A (CagA) developed gastric cancer that was absent in mice expressing phosphorylation-resistant CagA. Carcinogenesis in these mice was associated with activation of SHP2 (PTPN11) tyrosine phosphatase [69]. Moreover, the cellular adherent protein, FadA, interacted with CDH1 to activate Wnt/β-catenin signaling and development of colorectal cancer [27].

14.11 Cancer Prevention Through Prebiotics and Probiotics

The pathogenic effects of gut dysbiosis could be offset by restoring beneficial microbial composition. The use of prebiotics and probiotics enable the establishment and maintenance of normal healthy gut microbiome. Prebiotics are indigestible ingredients in food that stimulate growth and activity of healthy gut microbes. Most commonly used prebiotics are polyphenols. Inulin in dietary fiber is an example of prebiotic that promotes growth of *Bifidobacteria*. Food compounds such as daidzein in soy can be metabolized to equol by sulfate-reducing gut bacteria. Increased levels of equol and equol-producing bacteria correlate with reduced risk of breast and prostate cancer. Another polyphenol present in nuts and berries is ellagic acid. This prebiotic is metabolized to urolithins, which can decrease inflammation mediated by COX-2 activity.

Probiotics are live microbes in the diet or food supplement that exert beneficial health effects. Common probiotics include lactobacilli in yogurt, as well as *Bifidobacteria* and *Streptococcus* in cheese and some drinks. Genetically engineered bacteria in food supplements have also been produced and used as probiotics. Examples include *Lactobacillus casei* and *Lactococcus lactis* engineered strains that produce elafin. Elafin controlled inflammation in mouse models of colitis and decreased cytokine production and cell permeability when added to inflamed human colitis epithelial cells. *Lactobacillus gasseri* engineered to overproduce superoxide dismutase could improve colitis in *Il10*$^{-/-}$ mice. *Lactobacillus acidophilus* strain with deleted phosphoglycerol transferase gene is unable to produce lipoteichoic acid. Importantly, administration of this probiotic strain to Apc$^{\Delta/\text{floxed}}$ mice caused regression of established colonic polyps.

14.12 Summary

- The human microbiome is the conglomerate of all microbes that have established permanent relationship with the host.
- The human microbiome and MetaHIT projects are deciphering the role of the microbiome in health and disease.
- Epidemiological studies establish a role for alterations in the microbiome and cancer.
- While the causes of cancers by microbes such as *H. pylori*, HPV, and EBV are well known, the role of microbial dysbiosis in cancer requires further investigation.
- Proposed mechanisms of microbial carcinogenesis include genotoxicity, altered microbial metabolism, and microbial virulence factors.
- Useful gut microbes maintained by prebiotics and probiotics may exert anticarcinogenic effects through reduced inflammation.

References

1. Eun CS, Kim BK, Han DS, et al. Differences in gastric mucosal microbiota profiling in patients with chronic gastritis, intestinal metaplasia, and gastric cancer using pyrosequencing methods. Helicobacter. 2014;19:407–16.
2. Brawner KM, Morrow CD, Smith PD. Gastric microbiome and gastric cancer. Cancer J. 2014;20:211–6.
3. Meyer MS, Joshipura K, Giovannucci E, Michaud DS. A review of the relationship between tooth loss, periodontal disease, and cancer. Cancer Causes Control. 2008;19:895–907.
4. Yu G, Gail MH, Shi J, et al. Association between upper digestive tract microbiota and cancer-predisposing states in the esophagus and stomach. Cancer Epidemiol Biomark Prev. 2014;23:735–41.
5. Nasrollahzadeh D, Malekzadeh R, Ploner A, et al. Variations of gastric corpus microbiota are associated with early esophageal squamous cell carcinoma and squamous dysplasia. Sci Rep. 2015;5:8820.
6. Brenner DR, McLaughlin JR, Hung RJ. Previous lung diseases and lung cancer risk: a systematic review and meta-analysis. PLoS One. 2011;6:e17479.
7. Hosgood HD 3rd, Sapkota AR, Rothman N, et al. The potential role of lung microbiota in lung cancer attributed to household coal burning exposures. Environ Mol Mutagen. 2014;55:643–51.
8. Murphy G, Michel A, Taylor PR, et al. Association of seropositivity to helicobacter species and biliary tract cancer in the ATBC study. Hepatology. 2014;60:1963–71.
9. Zhou D, Wang JD, Weng MZ, et al. Infections of helicobacter spp. in the biliary system are associated with biliary tract cancer: a meta-analysis. Eur J Gastroenterol Hepatol. 2013;25:447–54.
10. Michaud DS, Izard J, Wilhelm-Benartzi CS, et al. Plasma antibodies to oral bacteria and risk of pancreatic cancer in a large European prospective cohort study. Gut. 2013;62:1764–70.
11. Farrell JJ, Zhang L, Zhou H, et al. Variations of oral microbiota are associated with pancreatic diseases including pancreatic cancer. Gut. 2012;61:582–8.
12. Goedert JJ, Jones G, Hua X, et al. Investigation of the association between the fecal microbiota and breast cancer in postmenopausal women: a population-based case-control pilot study. J Natl Cancer Inst. 2015;107(8):pii: djv147.

13. Cozen W, Yu G, Gail MH, et al. Fecal microbiota diversity in survivors of adolescent/young adult Hodgkin lymphoma: a study of twins. Br J Cancer. 2013;108:1163–7.
14. Aigelsreiter A, Gerlza T, Deutsch AJ, et al. Chlamydia psittaci infection in nongastrointestinal extranodal MALT lymphomas and their precursor lesions. Am J Clin Pathol. 2011;135:70–5.
15. Schollkopf C, Melbye M, Munksgaard L, et al. Borrelia infection and risk of non-Hodgkin lymphoma. Blood. 2008;111:5524–9.
16. Chang CM, Landgren O, Koshiol J, et al. Borrelia and subsequent risk of solid tumors and hematologic malignancies in Sweden. Int J Cancer. 2012;131:2208–9.
17. Couturier-Maillard A, Secher T, Rehman A, et al. NOD2-mediated dysbiosis predisposes mice to transmissible colitis and colorectal cancer. J Clin Invest. 2013;123:700–11.
18. Hu B, Elinav E, Huber S, et al. Microbiota-induced activation of epithelial IL-6 signaling links inflammasome-driven inflammation with transmissible cancer. Proc Natl Acad Sci U S A. 2013;110:9862–7.
19. Elinav E, Strowig T, Henao-Mejia J, Flavell RA. Regulation of the antimicrobial response by NLR proteins. Immunity. 2011;34:665–79.
20. Arthur JC, Perez-Chanona E, Muhlbauer M, et al. Intestinal inflammation targets cancer-inducing activity of the microbiota. Science. 2012;338:120–3.
21. Patwa LG, Fan TJ, Tchaptchet S, et al. Chronic intestinal inflammation induces stress-response genes in commensal Escherichia coli. Gastroenterology. 2011;141:1842–1851 e1841-1810.
22. Winter SE, Winter MG, Xavier MN, et al. Host-derived nitrate boosts growth of E. coli in the inflamed gut. Science. 2013;339:708–11.
23. Chen W, Liu F, Ling Z, et al. Human intestinal lumen and mucosa-associated microbiota in patients with colorectal cancer. PLoS One. 2012;7:e39743.
24. Sanapareddy N, Legge RM, Jovov B, et al. Increased rectal microbial richness is associated with the presence of colorectal adenomas in humans. ISME J. 2012;6:1858–68.
25. Sobhani I, Tap J, Roudot-Thoraval F, et al. Microbial dysbiosis in colorectal cancer (CRC) patients. PLoS One. 2011;6:e16393.
26. Kostic AD, Chun E, Robertson L, et al. Fusobacterium nucleatum potentiates intestinal tumorigenesis and modulates the tumor-immune microenvironment. Cell Host Microbe. 2013;14:207–15.
27. Rubinstein MR, Wang X, Liu W, et al. Fusobacterium nucleatum promotes colorectal carcinogenesis by modulating E-cadherin/beta-catenin signaling via its FadA adhesin. Cell Host Microbe. 2013;14:195–206.
28. Engle SJ, Ormsby I, Pawlowski S, et al. Elimination of colon cancer in germ-free transforming growth factor beta 1-deficient mice. Cancer Res. 2002;62:6362–6.
29. Sellon RK, Tonkonogy S, Schultz M, et al. Resident enteric bacteria are necessary for development of spontaneous colitis and immune system activation in interleukin-10-deficient mice. Infect Immun. 1998;66:5224–31.
30. Ivanov II, Frutos Rde L, Manel N, et al. Specific microbiota direct the differentiation of IL-17-producing T-helper cells in the mucosa of the small intestine. Cell Host Microbe. 2008;4:337–49.
31. Atarashi K, Nishimura J, Shima T, et al. ATP drives lamina propria T(H)17 cell differentiation. Nature. 2008;455:808–12.
32. Iliev ID, Funari VA, Taylor KD, et al. Interactions between commensal fungi and the C-type lectin receptor Dectin-1 influence colitis. Science. 2012;336:1314–7.
33. Tye H, Kennedy CL, Najdovska M, et al. STAT3-driven upregulation of TLR2 promotes gastric tumorigenesis independent of tumor inflammation. Cancer Cell. 2012;22:466–78.
34. Dapito DH, Mencin A, Gwak GY, et al. Promotion of hepatocellular carcinoma by the intestinal microbiota and TLR4. Cancer Cell. 2012;21:504–16.
35. Ochi A, Nguyen AH, Bedrosian AS, et al. MyD88 inhibition amplifies dendritic cell capacity to promote pancreatic carcinogenesis via Th2 cells. J Exp Med. 2012;209:1671–87.
36. Mittal D, Saccheri F, Venereau E, et al. TLR4-mediated skin carcinogenesis is dependent on immune and radioresistant cells. EMBO J. 2010;29:2242–52.

37. Fukata M, Chen A, Vamadevan AS, et al. Toll-like receptor-4 promotes the development of colitis-associated colorectal tumors. Gastroenterology. 2007;133:1869–81.
38. Fukata M, Shang L, Santaolalla R, et al. Constitutive activation of epithelial TLR4 augments inflammatory responses to mucosal injury and drives colitis-associated tumorigenesis. Inflamm Bowel Dis. 2011;17:1464–73.
39. Ngo VN, Young RM, Schmitz R, et al. Oncogenically active MYD88 mutations in human lymphoma. Nature. 2011;470:115–9.
40. Fukata M, Abreu MT. TLR4 signalling in the intestine in health and disease. Biochem Soc Trans. 2007;35:1473–8.
41. Neufert C, Becker C, Tureci O, et al. Tumor fibroblast-derived epiregulin promotes growth of colitis-associated neoplasms through ERK. J Clin Invest. 2013;123:1428–43.
42. Grivennikov SI, Wang K, Mucida D, et al. Adenoma-linked barrier defects and microbial products drive IL-23/IL-17-mediated tumour growth. Nature. 2012;491:254–8.
43. McGovern DP, Hysi P, Ahmad T, et al. Association between a complex insertion/deletion polymorphism in NOD1 (CARD4) and susceptibility to inflammatory bowel disease. Hum Mol Genet. 2005;14:1245–50.
44. Chen GY, Shaw MH, Redondo G, Nunez G. The innate immune receptor Nod1 protects the intestine from inflammation-induced tumorigenesis. Cancer Res. 2008;68:10060–7.
45. Khor B, Gardet A, Xavier RJ. Genetics and pathogenesis of inflammatory bowel disease. Nature. 2011;474:307–17.
46. Cho JH. Inflammatory bowel disease: genetic and epidemiologic considerations. World J Gastroenterol. 2008;14:338–47.
47. Kobayashi KS, Chamaillard M, Ogura Y, et al. Nod2-dependent regulation of innate and adaptive immunity in the intestinal tract. Science. 2005;307:731–4.
48. Rehman A, Sina C, Gavrilova O, et al. Nod2 is essential for temporal development of intestinal microbial communities. Gut. 2011;60:1354–62.
49. Petnicki-Ocwieja T, Hrncir T, Liu YJ, et al. Nod2 is required for the regulation of commensal microbiota in the intestine. Proc Natl Acad Sci U S A. 2009;106:15813–8.
50. Huycke MM, Gaskins HR. Commensal bacteria, redox stress, and colorectal cancer: mechanisms and models. Exp Biol Med (Maywood). 2004;229:586–97.
51. Wang X, Huycke MM. Extracellular superoxide production by Enterococcus faecalis promotes chromosomal instability in mammalian cells. Gastroenterology. 2007;132:551–61.
52. Wang X, Yang Y, Moore DR, et al. 4-hydroxy-2-nonenal mediates genotoxicity and bystander effects caused by Enterococcus faecalis-infected macrophages. Gastroenterology. 2012;142:543–551 e547.
53. Balish E, Warner T. Enterococcus faecalis induces inflammatory bowel disease in interleukin-10 knockout mice. Am J Pathol. 2002;160:2253–7.
54. Wu S, Rhee KJ, Albesiano E, et al. A human colonic commensal promotes colon tumorigenesis via activation of T helper type 17 T cell responses. Nat Med. 2009;15:1016–22.
55. Travaglione S, Fabbri A, Fiorentini C. The rho-activating CNF1 toxin from pathogenic E. coli: a risk factor for human cancer development? Infect Agent Cancer. 2008;3:4.
56. Nesic D, Hsu Y, Stebbins CE. Assembly and function of a bacterial genotoxin. Nature. 2004;429:429–33.
57. Cuevas-Ramos G, Petit CR, Marcq I, et al. Escherichia coli induces DNA damage in vivo and triggers genomic instability in mammalian cells. Proc Natl Acad Sci U S A. 2010;107:11537–42.
58. Buc E, Dubois D, Sauvanet P, et al. High prevalence of mucosa-associated E. coli producing cyclomodulin and genotoxin in colon cancer. PLoS One. 2013;8:e56964.
59. Garrett WS, Gallini CA, Yatsunenko T, et al. Enterobacteriaceae act in concert with the gut microbiota to induce spontaneous and maternally transmitted colitis. Cell Host Microbe. 2010;8:292–300.
60. Nougayrede JP, Homburg S, Taieb F, et al. Escherichia coli induces DNA double-strand breaks in eukaryotic cells. Science. 2006;313:848–51.

61. Fox JG, Rogers AB, Whary MT, et al. Gastroenteritis in NF-kappaB-deficient mice is produced with wild-type Campylobacter jejuni but not with C. jejuni lacking cytolethal distending toxin despite persistent colonization with both strains. Infect Immun. 2004;72:1116–25.
62. Shen Z, Ajmo JM, Rogers CQ, et al. Role of SIRT1 in regulation of LPS- or two ethanol metabolites-induced TNF-alpha production in cultured macrophage cell lines. Am J Physiol Gastrointest Liver Physiol. 2009;296:G1047–53.
63. Bindels LB, Porporato P, Dewulf EM, et al. Gut microbiota-derived propionate reduces cancer cell proliferation in the liver. Br J Cancer. 2012;107:1337–44.
64. Donohoe DR, Garge N, Zhang X, et al. The microbiome and butyrate regulate energy metabolism and autophagy in the mammalian colon. Cell Metab. 2011;13:517–26.
65. Hu S, Dong TS, Dalal SR, et al. The microbe-derived short chain fatty acid butyrate targets miRNA-dependent p21 gene expression in human colon cancer. PLoS One. 2011;6:e16221.
66. Maslowski KM, Vieira AT, Ng A, et al. Regulation of inflammatory responses by gut microbiota and chemoattractant receptor GPR43. Nature. 2009;461:1282–6.
67. Yoshimoto S, Loo TM, Atarashi K, et al. Obesity-induced gut microbial metabolite promotes liver cancer through senescence secretome. Nature. 2013;499:97–101.
68. Seitz HK, Stickel F. Molecular mechanisms of alcohol-mediated carcinogenesis. Nat Rev Cancer. 2007;7:599–612.
69. Ohnishi N, Yuasa H, Tanaka S, et al. Transgenic expression of helicobacter pylori CagA induces gastrointestinal and hematopoietic neoplasms in mouse. Proc Natl Acad Sci U S A. 2008;105:1003–8.

Index

G. D. Dakubo, *Cancer Biomarkers in Body Fluids*,
https://doi.org/10.1007/978-3-030-24725-6

MIX
Papier aus verantwortungsvollen Quellen
Paper from responsible sources
FSC® C105338

FSC
www.fsc.org

If you have any concerns about our products,
you can contact us on
ProductSafety@springernature.com

In case Publisher is established outside the EU,
the EU authorized representative is:
Springer Nature Customer Service Center GmbH
Europaplatz 3, 69115 Heidelberg, Germany

Printed by Libri Plureos GmbH
in Hamburg, Germany